*For Gwen & Payton
Enjoy*

LunchBox Envy™

An adventure in healthy eating for kids and families

Locally Delicious™, Inc.

Ann Anderson, Pat Bitton, Lauren Cohn-Sarabia, Martha Haynes,
Kate Jamison-Alward, Ann King, Carol Moné, Suzanne Simpson

Created by:
Locally Delicious, Inc.
P.O. Box 309
Arcata CA 95518
info@locally-delicious.org
orders@locally-delicious.org
www.locally-delicious.org

Published by:
North Coast Co-operative
811 I Street
Arcata CA 95521
707-826-8670
www.northcoastco-op.com

Copyright 2013, Locally Delicious, Inc. A 501(c)(3) non-profit corporation
All profits from this book are used to educate and further the cause of healthy food for all.

The views stated in this book are those of Locally Delicious, Inc. and do not necessarily represent the views of the publisher or supporting organizations.

Authors: Ann Anderson, Lauren Cohn-Sarabia, Martha Haynes, Kate Jamison-Alward, Carol Moné, and Suzanne Simpson

Copy Editors and Proofreaders: Pat Bitton, Ann King and Jessie M. Cretser-Hartenstein

Art Director: Suzanne Simpson

Photographer: Lauren Cohn-Sarabia

Project Coordinators: Ann Anderson and Kate Jamison-Alward

Artwork and Book Design:
  Illustration Team: John Nordberg, Kelsey Tomfohr and Morgan Tomfohr
  Graphics Design Team: Treyce Meredith and Mahayla Camp
    Arcata Arts Institute under the direction of Anne Bown-Crawford
    Arcata High School, Arcata, CA 95521
    www.artsinstitute.net

Consultants: Lonny Grafman, Corey Lee Lewis, Ph.D., Linda Prescott and Megan Russin

Art and Graphic Consultants: Susan Abbott, Joanne Berke, Anne Bown-Crawford and Treyce Meredith

Photo credits: Lauren Cohn-Sarabia (all except as noted); Alexandre EcoDairy Farm (pages 26 and 55); Ann Anderson (pages 14, 20, 99 (peas), 104 (kale), 123 (beans), 131 (apples), 133 (strawberry), 134, 135, 140, 146 (kale), 151 (lemons), 161 (lemons), 165 (basil), 166 (peas)); Kate Jamison-Alward (page 105); Martha Haynes (page 147); Cory Myers (page 16); Patrick Sarabia (page 201); Chris Wisner (pages 54, 76 (apples), 119 (squash), 126 (raw beans), 131 (plums and nectarines), 144 (beans), 150 (raspberries), 163 (beans)). Chris Wisner photographs are Copyright Chris Wisner.

ISBN 978-0-9829426-1-1

Some of the recipes in this book were contributed by community members. Every attempt has been made to verify originality; however, recipes are often passed between people many times and their origins are sometimes lost. We apologize to any recipe author whose work has come to us in this manner as our intent is to protect the author's rights.

LunchBox Envy is dedicated to a healthy future for all children.

Acknowledgements

Susan Abbott, Abbott and Company, Inc.
Robert Arena, Bug Press
Janel Apple, Janel Claire Design
JoAnne Berke, M.F.A., Humboldt State University
Melanie Bettenhausen, Outreach Director, North Coast Co-op
Donovan Clark, Arcata Arts Institute, Arcata High School
Anne Bown-Crawford, Director, Arcata Arts Institute, Arcata High School
Steven Dugger, Chef
Tibora Bea Girczyc-Blum, Reduce, Reuse, Recycle and Rot Innovator
Lonny Grafman, Lecturer, Humboldt State University, President, Appropedia Foundation, Locally Delicious, Inc., Board Member
The Chris and Violet Hardee Family, Kayleb, 14, and Dylynn, 10
Anne Holcomb, Executive Director, Food For People
The Shana and Kevin Jamison Family, Andie, 9, and Parker, 8
Betsy Lambert and KIEM-TV
Corey Lee Lewis Ph.D., Professor, Humboldt State University, Locally Delicious, Inc., Board Member, and family, Hunter, 12, and Bodie, 7
David Lippmann, General Manager, North Coast Co-op
Lewis Litzky, Locally Delicious Inc., Board Member
Kathy Marshall
Johanna Mauro, Arcata Arts Institute, Arcata High School
Lisa McNaney, Local & Delicious
Lou Moerner, Northern California Indian Development Council and Humboldt Community for Activity and Nutrition
Cory Myers
The Danielle Newman Family, Althea, 13, and Ursula, 9
Marianne Pennecamp, Community Development Advocate
Linda Prescott, Humboldt County Office of Education, Child Nutrition Consultant, State of California
The Ginny Prince Family, Jordyn, 12, and Gemma, 9
Annie Reid, Instructor, Humboldt State University
The Marnin Robbins and T Griffin Family, Levi, 10, and Sophia, 5
Megan Russin, Nutrition Educator, Humboldt County Office of Education
Mariah Sarabia
The Scott and Tina Stenborg-Davies Family, Westleigh, 16, and Serena, 6
Connie Stewart, Director, California Center for Rural Policy
Eddie Tanner, Deep Seeded Farm
Amy Waldrip, Newsletter Coordinator, North Coast Co-op
Donna Wheeler, Dep. Dir., Humboldt Co. Dept. of Health & Human Services; Social Services
E. Christian Wisner, E. Christian Wisner Photography
Michelle Wyler, Regional Manager, Community Alliance with Family Farmers, Humboldt

Thanks to all our models and to the many people who contributed to funding.

Special acknowledgement and heartfelt thanks to: The Topeka Community Foundation for their on-going support; The Rick Foundation; and Peter Wendell.

Special thanks to our spouses: Robert Haynes, Lewis Litzky, Harvey Raider and Patrick Sarabia and to our intern, Kate Jamison-Alward, who provided project coordination for thousands of details, helped us navigate the world of social media and did much of the typesetting for the book.

Foreword

As a single parent raising children in the 21st century, I've found that many things in our home are different than they were when I was a kid. My Grandma Dot, who is now 92 and still cooking, ran a traditional homesteader's kitchen for most of her life: one filled with vegetables from the garden, locally raised meat, whole milk and cheese, and meals made with nothing more than whole ingredients, family recipes, and real cooking. When I was a child my mother also gardened, cooked from scratch with favorite family recipes, and put real care into our meals. We rarely ate out, never ate frozen or pre-cooked meals, and always had homemade lunches for school, each and every day.

I remember Grandma telling me about growing up in rural Wyoming, about her one-room schoolhouse with grades 1-8 all in one classroom, about walking several miles to school, and about her lunches. Most often they consisted of homemade bread slathered with freshly churned organic butter (that was the only kind back then), and perhaps an apple or a raw potato, some carrots, and fresh well-water. For most of my school life, my lunches consisted of a peanut butter and jelly sandwich, fruit, a juice or milk drink, sometimes soup, often a snack like crackers, or homemade fruit leather. It was not uncommon also to get a sweet note of encouragement from Mom, written on a napkin and hidden discreetly in my lunch.

Over time, however, my mom went back to college, and as I got older, she gardened less. Chips and store-bought fruit snacks replaced homemade ones. The number and variety of products on grocery store shelves increased; bleached-flour breads rapidly replaced whole wheat varieties; corn-based products, from chips to drinks, flooded our lives; and highly processed foods became the norm. By the time I began making my boys' lunches, it was not uncommon for parents to send day-old fast-food meals to school with their kids. I, however, was making the same sandwiches and packing the same snacks and drinks as my mom had done, and carrying on my Grandma Dot's tradition of caring for the family through food . . . or so I thought. Boy, was I wrong.

My kitchen, just like my local grocery store, was a Frankenstein's laboratory of fake foods, chemicals and non-nutritious food products, when compared with my mother's or grandmother's kitchens. My sandwiches were made of bleached white bread with no nutritional value and meats and cheeses

Foreword

that were loaded with carcinogens and other unhealthy toxins. My snacks were made primarily from industrially grown corn, in the form of corn syrup, and dyes of every color. And my school lunches were quickly filling my boys' young and growing bodies with those toxins and carcinogens while missing important basic nutrients.

But I was lucky. And my boys were lucky. We got caught up in a stampede of savvy, determined women, a group we lovingly call the "Heirloom Tomatoes" or just the "Tomatoes." These eight women, wise in years and experience, have written and published one book about local food. The book you're about to read, *LunchBox Envy*, is their second book. It focuses on ways to make better, healthier food choices for children to take to school in their lunch boxes. Those Tomatoes have taught us a new way, which is really an old way, to eat, a way that doesn't depend on chemicals and laboratories, but instead trusts in the natural nutrients in plants and animals, a way of eating that looks to farmers for food instead of to corporations.

And now you are lucky, too. And your kids are lucky. Because you hold in your hands the Tomatoes' most helpful advice and most useful suggestions for taking back control of your kitchen, and for showing your love for your children through the food you put into their bodies.

In short, this book is the tool that many parents like me need, parents who care about the health of our children and our planet, and who want to nourish both through the lunches we make each and every day. Now, thanks to *LunchBox Envy,* we can do just that.

Corey Lee Lewis, Ph.D., Professor, Humboldt State University

Contents

Foreword	v
Introduction	vii
Chapter 1 Planning and Packing	1
Chapter 2 Where to Get Food	13
Chapter 3 What is Healthy Food?	25
Chapter 4 Getting Started Cooking	39
Chapter 5 Recipes	51
Introduction	52
Cooking the Basics	54
The Main Dishes	67
Sandwiches and Wraps	68
Grains and Noodles	88
Egg Dishes	100
Salads	108
Soups	116
Vegetables	125
Fruit	131
Drinks	140
Treats and Snacks	141
Dips and Spreads	158
Chapter 6 Do It Yourself Projects	169
Worm Bin Composter	170
Solar Dehydrator	174
Solar Food Warmer	178
Growing Your Own Food	182
Resources	185
Glossary	186
Read More	189
Food Labels	190
Portions	192
Spice Mixes	193
Index	194
About the Artists	199
About the Authors	200

Introduction

The U.S. is experiencing a childhood obesity epidemic directly related to poor nutrition and lack of sufficient exercise. Statistics show that one in three children born today will have diabetes by the time they are 21. Two out of three adults are currently overweight or obese. It's important to us, as parents, grandparents and concerned citizens, to contribute to a solution.

Many children eat lunches provided by schools, and many of these lunch programs are contributing to the problem, not to the solution. There is a growing movement to improve school lunches, but healthy lunch programs are not yet in place across the country. Information on nutrition and healthy food in this book can help people talk with schools about providing healthier options.

We have chosen to work toward a solution to the childhood obesity problem by focusing on lunches that kids take to school. The resulting book, *LunchBox Envy*, is a how-to guide and cookbook combined. It provides tools for balancing nutrition, planning meals, finding and affording healthy food, cooking efficiently, and building a more sustainable food system. Simple do-it-yourself projects are included to empower children with the knowledge that they can control part of their own food production and processing.

The book addresses families at all income levels with school-aged children. Its focus is how to make a healthy lunch, but its lessons apply to all meals and snacks.

Cooking at home opens a world of possibilities for more affordable, healthier and better tasting food. But many families have not had an education in cooking. *LunchBox Envy* provides basic tools in the "Getting Started Cooking" chapter. The recipes are easy to make, healthy and geared to the tastes of children.

Producing this book was much harder than we anticipated. The more we researched problems around eating healthy food on a budget, the bigger the problem seemed to be, but we found many ways that work to share with readers. This has been a transformational journey for all of us. Our goal is to enable families across the country to take that journey, too. We truly believe that families can change the course of their lives by:

- adapting their eating habits
- understanding what healthy food is and how to build healthy meals
- learning how to plan, shop; and cook as a family, even in "food deserts."

The Heirloom Tomatoes
Authors of *LunchBox Envy*

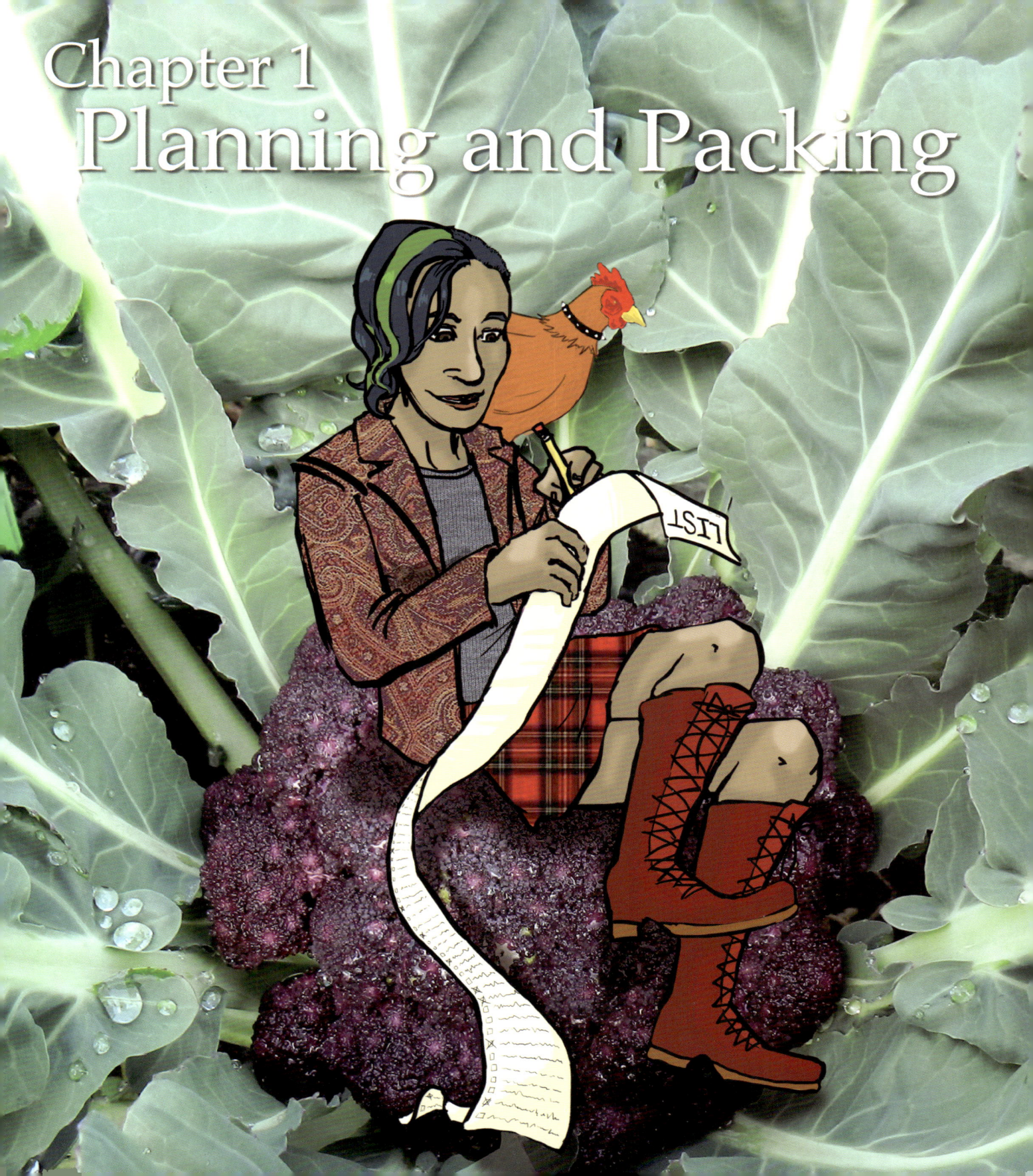

Chapter 1
Planning and Packing

The Morning Rush

It's 7:15 A.M. and the school bus arrives at 7:30. The kids gather up their backpacks and jackets and then—OOPS! The lunch box. But it's not ready. Panic! What to throw together in five minutes?

Sound familiar?

A calmer morning can be enjoyed with a little planning, and making school lunches with kids can be a family activity.

When children help plan their own lunches, they feel they have control and want to eat the lunch they made. At the same time children learn about a healthy diet, families learn how to save money by planning to use up leftovers and by buying from a list rather than impulse or last-minute shopping.

Planning allows time to consider a wider variety of options. The result? Lunches that will be the envy of the other kids, who might then ask their parents to start making enviable lunches too.

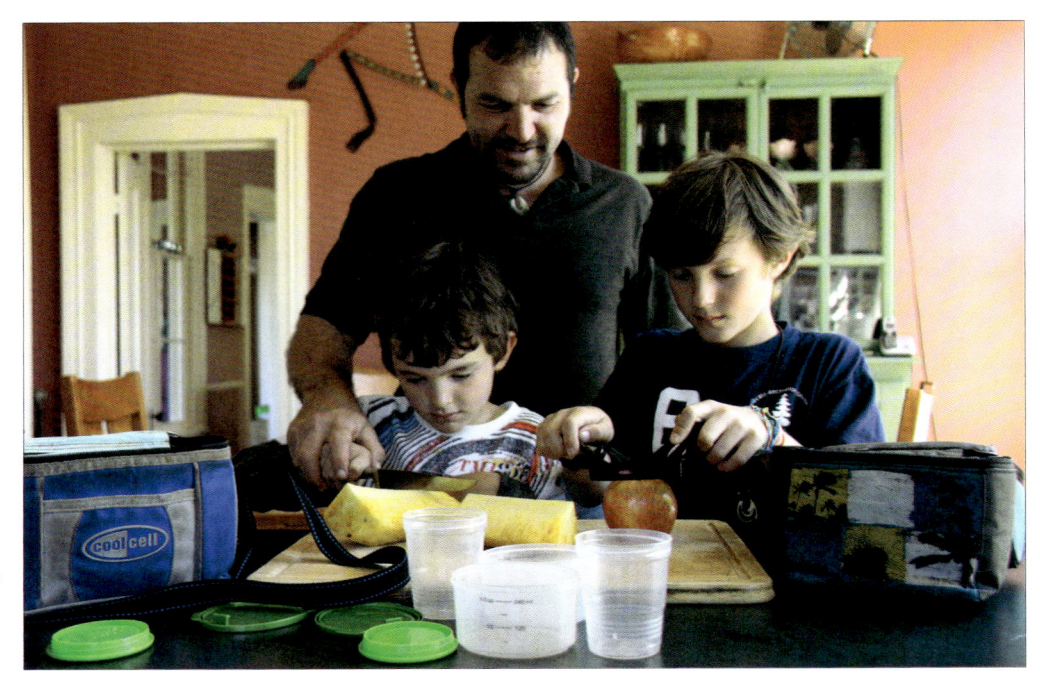

This "How-To" chapter explains the planning process and provides ideas for lunch containers.

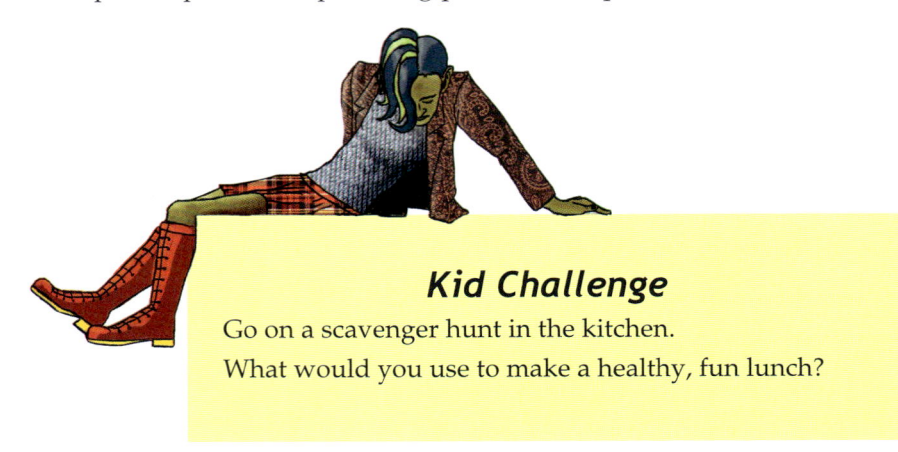

Kid Challenge
Go on a scavenger hunt in the kitchen.
What would you use to make a healthy, fun lunch?

2 Planning and Packing

The Planning Process

Follow the six steps to plan, prepare, cook and pack the lunch. After school, talk about that day's lunch. What was good? What wasn't eaten? Talk about what to change to make it better.

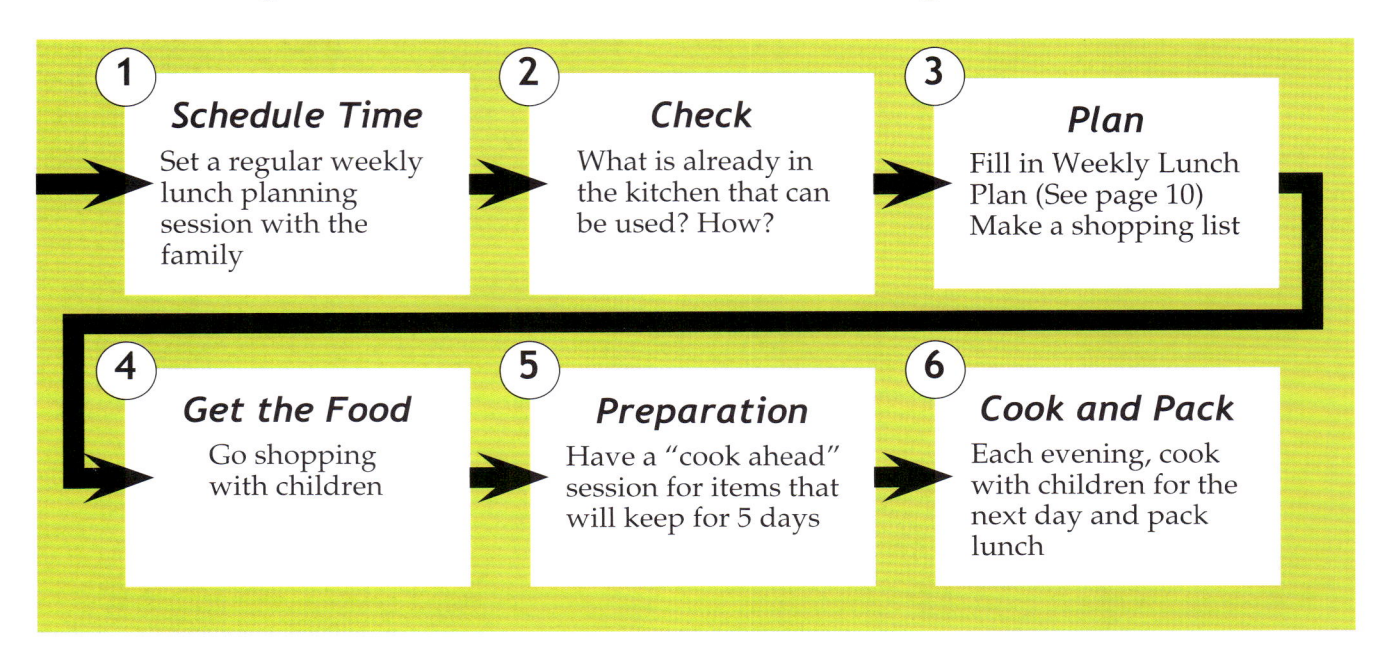

1. Schedule Time — Set a regular weekly lunch planning session with the family

2. Check — What is already in the kitchen that can be used? How?

3. Plan — Fill in Weekly Lunch Plan (See page 10) Make a shopping list

4. Get the Food — Go shopping with children

5. Preparation — Have a "cook ahead" session for items that will keep for 5 days

6. Cook and Pack — Each evening, cook with children for the next day and pack lunch

Follow the adventures of student investigative journalists as they explore the industrial food system in "The Yuck Factor."

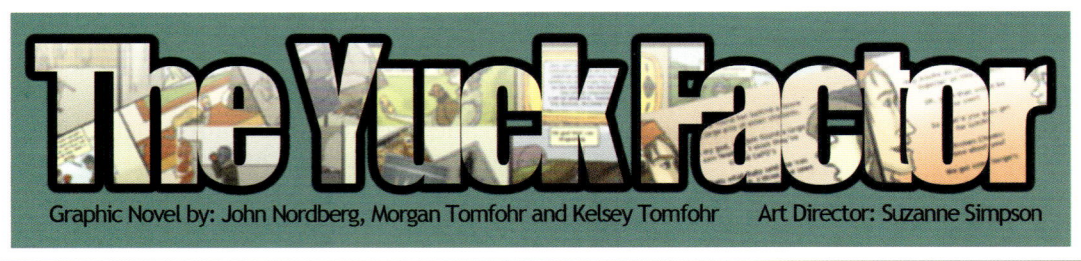

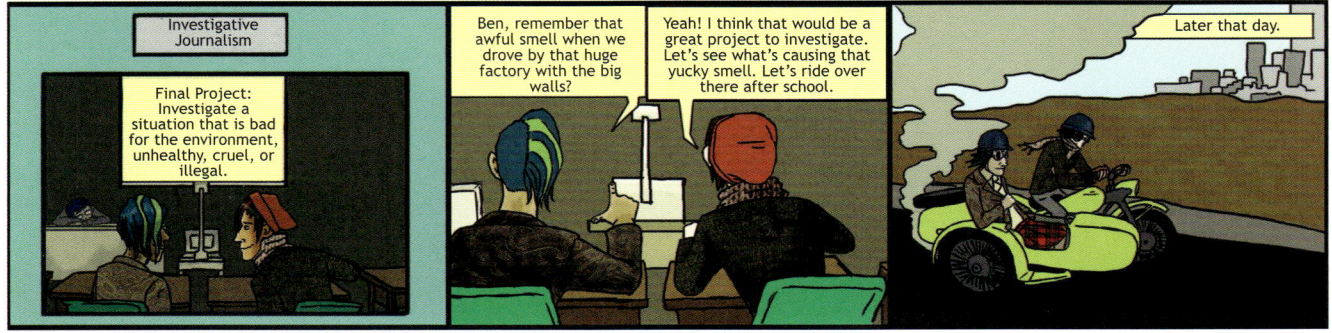

The Yuck Factor

Graphic Novel by: John Nordberg, Morgan Tomfohr and Kelsey Tomfohr   Art Director: Suzanne Simpson

Investigative Journalism

Final Project: Investigate a situation that is bad for the environment, unhealthy, cruel, or illegal.

Ben, remember that awful smell when we drove by that huge factory with the big walls?

Yeah! I think that would be a great project to investigate. Let's see what's causing that yucky smell. Let's ride over there after school.

Later that day.

Planning and Packing 3

What Makes a Lunch Everyone Envies?

An enviable lunch is one that's full of the great-tasting foods kids need in order to grow, to be healthy and to have lots of energy. These foods are fruits, grains, dairy*, vegetables and proteins. The United States Department of Agriculture has created the "MyPlate" resource as a simple way to show us these foods and the relative amount of each type we need. The MyPlate website (www.ChooseMyPlate.gov) is a valuable source for information about food and nutrition. More information on nutrition is also available in the glossary of this book (see page 186).

What's on MyPlate?

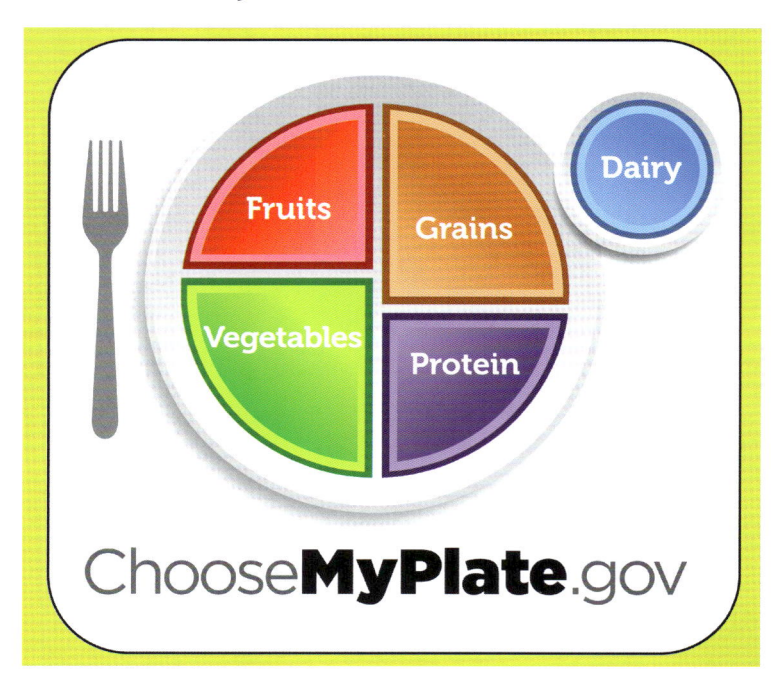

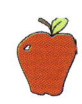

Fruit: Is full of energy and contributes vitamins and minerals for better eyesight, skin, hair and muscles. Helps the body heal.

Grains: Provide major source of energy. Whole grains are better than refined ones.

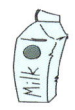

Dairy: Builds strong bones and teeth because it contains calcium.*

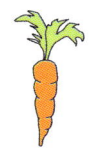

Vegetables: Provide vitamins, minerals, fiber, and hundreds of micro-nutrients to keep the body working. Starchy vegetables provide energy.

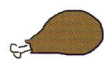

Protein: Builds muscles, nerves and brain.

* Many people don't eat dairy. There are plenty of other great non-dairy sources of calcium. You'll find some non-dairy alternatives on the next page.

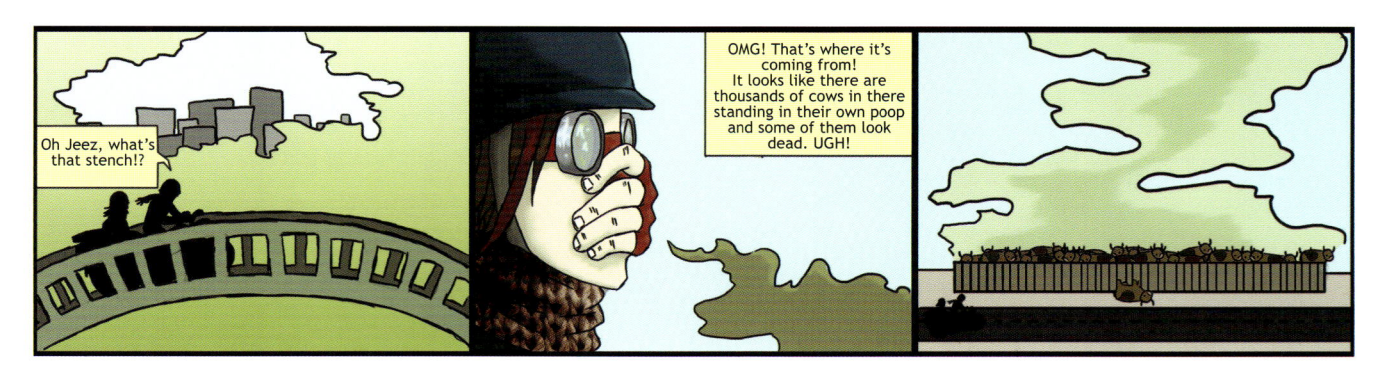

Oh Jeez, what's that stench!?

OMG! That's where it's coming from! It looks like there are thousands of cows in there standing in their own poop and some of them look dead. UGH!

4 Planning and Packing

Examples of MyPlate Foods

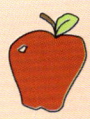

Fruit

Citrus: Lemons, limes, oranges, grapefruit, tangerines

Berries: Strawberries, blueberries, raspberries, blackberries

Melons: Cantaloupe, honeydew, watermelon

Tropical: Bananas, mangoes, papaya, pineapple

Stone Fruit: Apricots, cherries, nectarines, peaches, plums

Other: Apples, grapes, pears; and raisins, prunes and other dried fruit

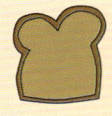

Grains

Whole Grains: Brown rice, bulgur, oatmeal, popcorn, rolled oats, quinoa, whole grain barley, whole grain cornmeal, whole rye. Whole wheat bread, crackers, pasta, sandwich buns and rolls, whole grain tortillas, cereal flakes, wild rice and muesli

Refined Grains: Cornbread, corn and flour tortillas, couscous, crackers, grits, noodles, pitas, pretzels, white bread, white sandwich buns and rolls, white rice, pastas, and most ready-to-eat breakfast cereals

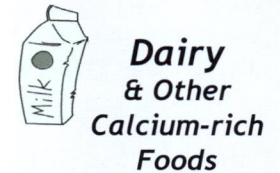

Dairy & Other Calcium-rich Foods

Milk Products: Cheese, yogurt, cottage cheese, milk and milk-based desserts such as ice cream, frozen yogurt

Soy: Tofu and calcium-fortified soy milk

Other Calcium Sources: Dark green vegetables, oranges, beans, peas, peanuts, almonds, sardines, salmon

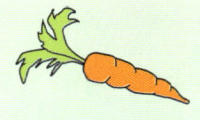

Vegetables

Dark Greens: Bok choy, broccoli, dark green leafy lettuce, kale, spinach, watercress

Starchy: Corn, black-eyed peas (cowpeas), green peas, lima beans, potatoes

Red & Orange: Acorn, butternut and Hubbard squash, carrots, pumpkin, red peppers, sweet potatoes

Beans and Peas: Black, kidney, navy, white, pinto, garbanzo, and soy beans, lentils, split peas

Other: Artichokes, asparagus, avocado, bean sprouts, beets, Brussels sprouts, cabbage, cauliflower, celery, cucumbers, eggplant, green beans, green peppers, lettuce, okra, onions, parsnips, turnips, wax beans, zucchini

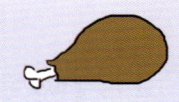

Protein

Meats: Beef, pork, lamb, game meat (bison, rabbit, venison)

Poultry: Chicken, duck, goose, turkey

Eggs: Chicken, duck, goose, quail

Beans and Peas: Black, kidney, navy, white, lima, black-eyed peas (cowpeas), lentils, garbanzo beans, adzuki, mung, fava

Processed Soy and Milk Products: Tofu, tempeh, yogurt, cheese, cottage cheese

What to Put into the Lunchbox

Use the chart on page 10 to plan lunches for the week. We've provided two weeks of suggested plans to get you started. Use the recipes in Chapter 5, other cookbooks and your family's imagination to decide what goes in the lunchbox.

The recipes in this book are organized into Main Dish, Vegetables, Fruit, Drinks, Treats and Snacks and Dips and Spreads sections.

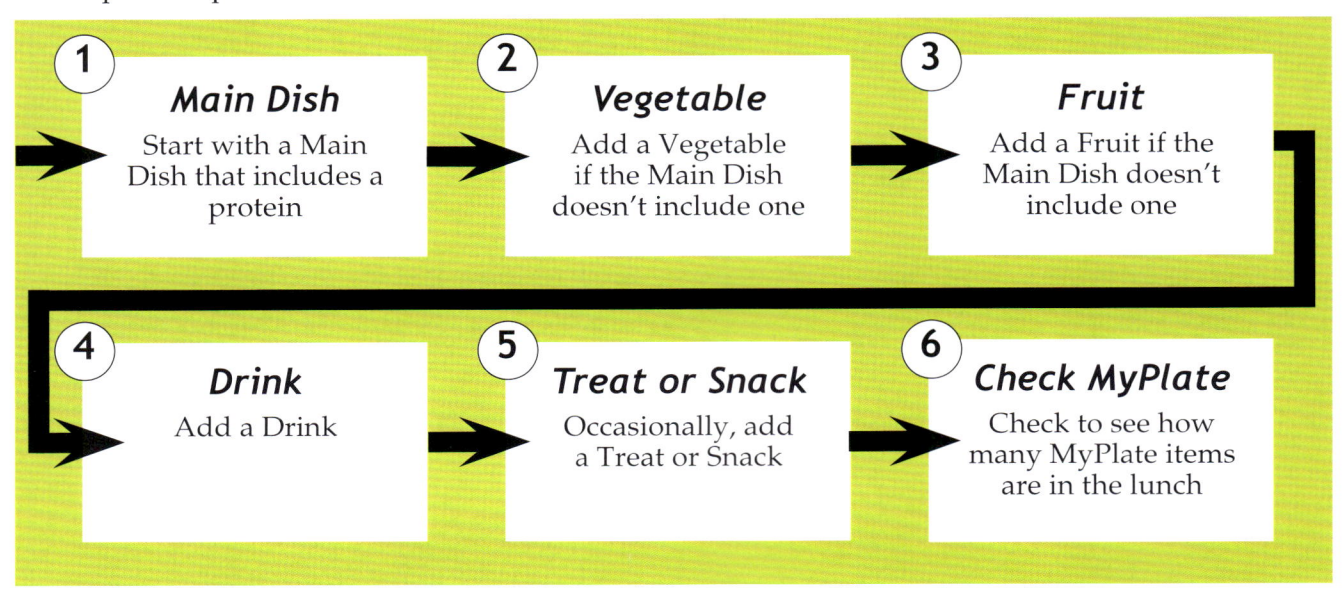

1. Main Dish — Start with a Main Dish that includes a protein

2. Vegetable — Add a Vegetable if the Main Dish doesn't include one

3. Fruit — Add a Fruit if the Main Dish doesn't include one

4. Drink — Add a Drink

5. Treat or Snack — Occasionally, add a Treat or Snack

6. Check MyPlate — Check to see how many MyPlate items are in the lunch

The Weekly Lunch Plan Charts have an extra column to use to check your selections against the MyPlate recommendations. The recipes in this book include icons for the MyPlate foods. Some of your lunch selections will include more than one of the MyPlate foods—a tuna sandwich, for example, can include protein (tuna), grains (bread) and vegetable(s) (lettuce or celery).

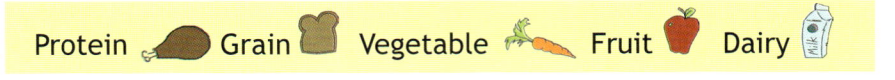

Protein Grain Vegetable Fruit Dairy

The Weekly Lunch Plan Chart on page 10 may be copied, or downloaded and printed from the Locally Delicious website: www.locally-delicious.org/LunchBoxEnvy/lunchchart

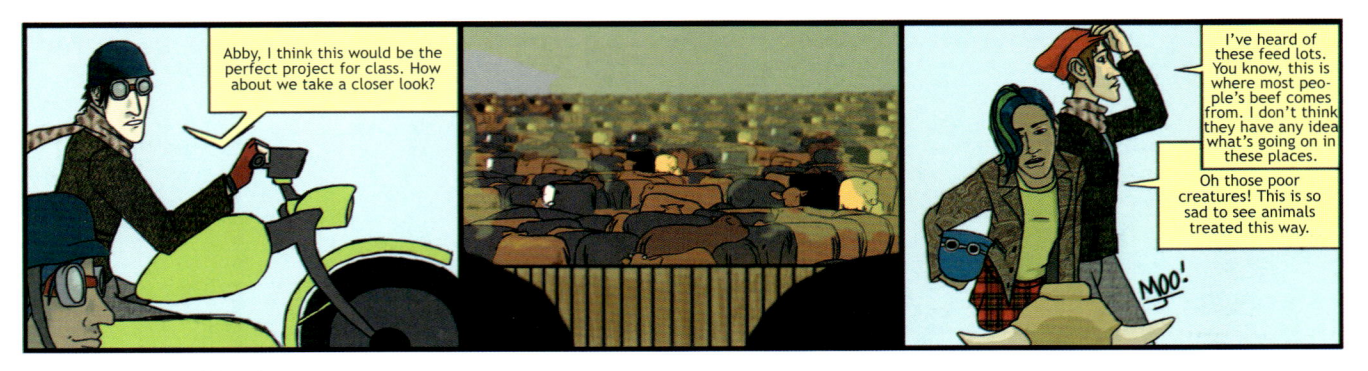

6 Planning and Packing

How Much to Put into the Lunchbox

The amount of food to put into the lunchbox depends on the size and activity level of your child. These guidelines are a starting point and the MyPlate.gov website provides details.

- Notice what was eaten out of each lunch, to learn how much your child needs. If the apple is half eaten, just send a half next time. But ask a few questions first: Did they eat the food or trade it or throw it away? Did they have enough time to eat the whole lunch?
- When lunches contain healthy food choices, children will eat what they need. Their bodies know what to do. Trust them. Hint: Kids like fruit and vegetables better if they are cut into smaller pieces. Ask them what they like.
- On the MyPlate diagram, the biggest sections are for grains and vegetables. Fruit and meat sections are smaller. Pack more grains than meat and more vegetables than fruit, and be cautious about putting in too many treats. Kids often eat those first and may not have room for the healthy food.
- Portions in restaurants have become too large, leading people to assume that these are the right portion sizes for all meals. You'll find healthier portion sizes described on page 192, but a rough guide is that a serving of fruit, vegetable or grain is about the size of a baseball. A serving of protein is about the size of the child's palm.

Did you know that 20 percent of what you eat is used to power your brain? So whether your favorite subject is math or soccer, you need energy from grains, fruit and some vegetables.

Need to Make a Lunch in a Hurry?
- Leftovers are already cooked and are good options for a fast-to-make lunch.
- Many items can be "No-Prep." See the ideas at the beginning of each section in the recipe chapter.

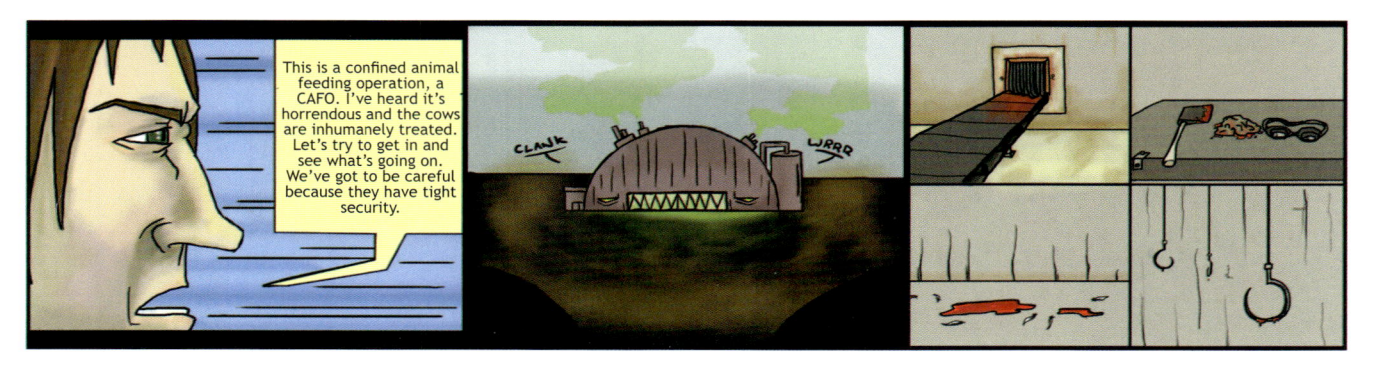

This is a confined animal feeding operation, a CAFO. I've heard it's horrendous and the cows are inhumanely treated. Let's try to get in and see what's going on. We've got to be careful because they have tight security.

CLANK WRRR

Planning and Packing

Weekly Lunch Plan Example

Make your food selections and check to see how many MyPlate foods they include. It's important to eat something from each of the MyPlate food groups every day but they don't have to be in every meal. Note that many of the lunch items can be made on the weekend and used during the week.

What to Pack	Main Dish (Protein)	Vegetable	Fruit	Drink	Treat/Snack Some days	Does it include?	
Monday	homemade stackable sandwiches (page 70), cut on Sunday night		applesauce (page 136)	milk	2 cookies	Protein	✓
						Grain	✓
						Veggie	✓
						Fruit	✓
						Dairy	✓
Tuesday	macaroni & cheese (page 90) left over from weekend	carrot & cucumber sticks, ranch dressing (page 162)		apple juice	nuts	Protein	✓
						Grain	✓
						Veggie	✓
						Fruit	✓
						Dairy	✓
Wednesday	peanut butter & jam pinwheels (page 72)			fruit smoothie	kale chips (page 146)	Protein	✓
						Grain	✓
						Veggie	✓
						Fruit	✓
						Dairy	
Thursday	chicken noodle soup (page 124)		sliced fruit in yogurt	water	corn muffin (page 152)	Protein	✓
						Grain	✓
						Veggie	✓
						Fruit	✓
						Dairy	✓
Friday	burrito (page 78)		fruit leather (page 134)	milk		Protein	✓
						Grain	✓
						Veggie	✓
						Fruit	✓
						Dairy	✓

The No-Waste Lunchbox

A "No-Waste Lunchbox" means the box and all the containers are washable and reusable.

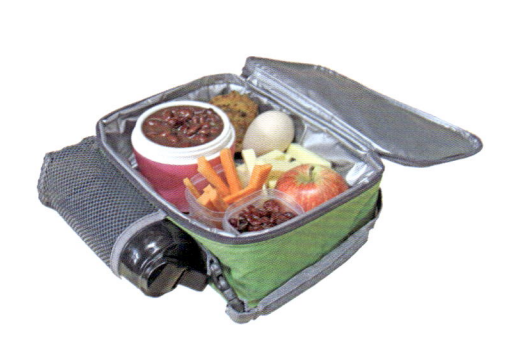

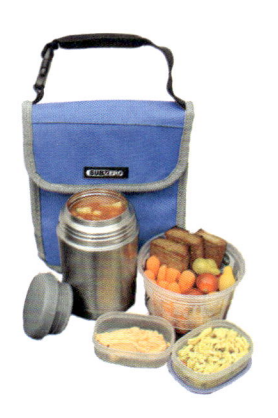

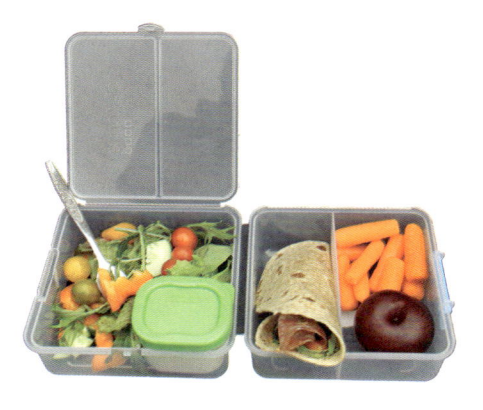

Lunchbox, Container and Utensil Ideas

- Insulated or non-insulated lunchboxes
- Cloth or vinyl totes
- Bento boxes
- Homemade cloth or vinyl lunch bags*
- Stainless steel–lined containers for hot food
- Insulated (vacuum or thermos) plastic or steel containers for cold food
- Recycled yogurt, salsa or other plastic containers used for food
- Cloth napkins
- Metal forks and spoons

For Safety

- Keep foods that contain meat, eggs and mayonnaise cold in insulated containers.
- Plastic containers should be recycle types 1, 2, 4, 5, or 6— NOT types 3 or 7, which could contain Bisphenol A (BPA) (See Glossary, page 186). Find the recycling type on the bottom of the container.
- When re-heating food, do not microwave plastic wrap, plastic or metal containers.

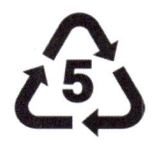

*See Locally Delicious website for do-it-yourself containers.
www.locally-delicious.org/LunchBoxEnvy/DIYContainers

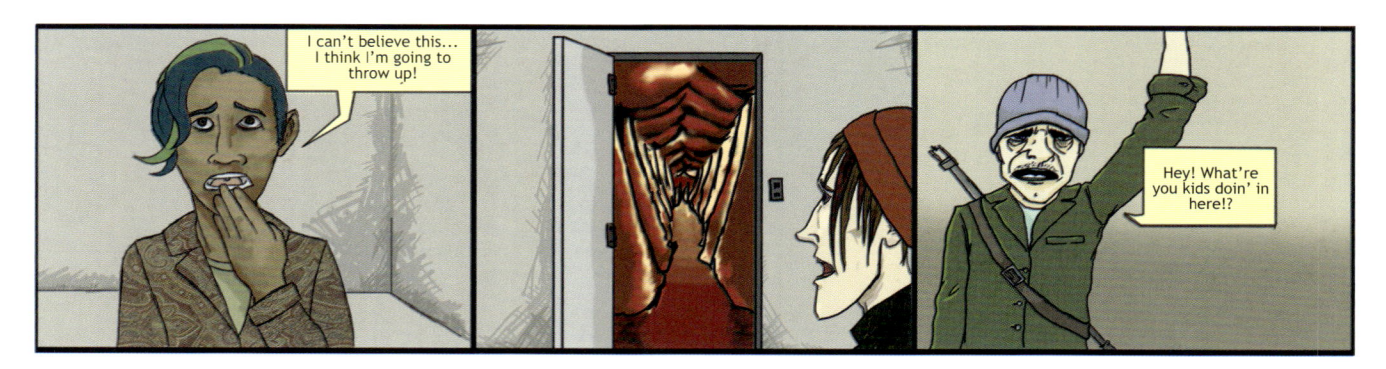

Planning and Packing 11

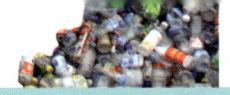

Where Does the Waste Go?

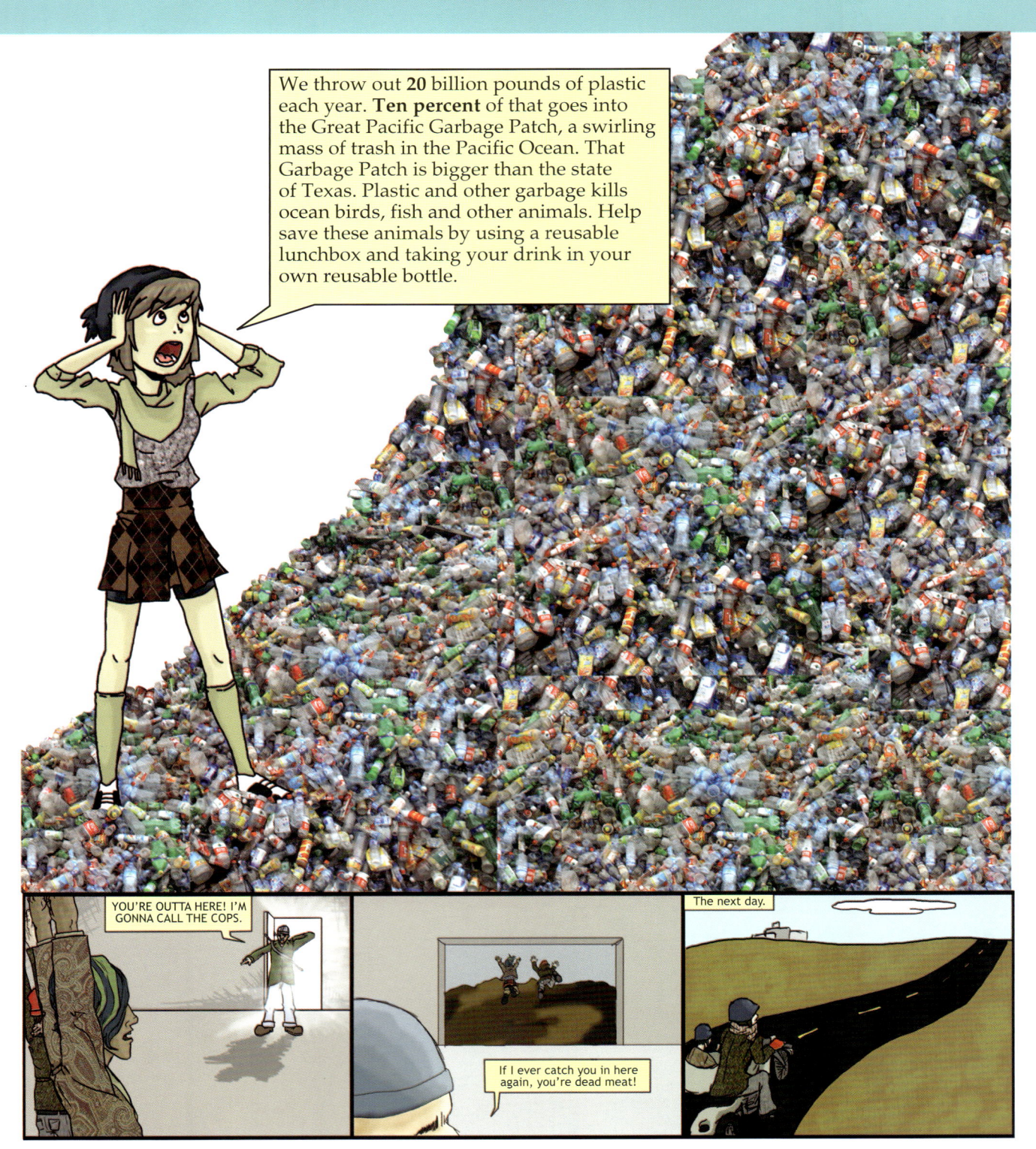

> We throw out **20** billion pounds of plastic each year. **Ten percent** of that goes into the Great Pacific Garbage Patch, a swirling mass of trash in the Pacific Ocean. That Garbage Patch is bigger than the state of Texas. Plastic and other garbage kills ocean birds, fish and other animals. Help save these animals by using a reusable lunchbox and taking your drink in your own reusable bottle.

> YOU'RE OUTTA HERE! I'M GONNA CALL THE COPS.

> If I ever catch you in here again, you're dead meat!

The next day.

Planning and Packing

Chapter 2
Where to Get Food

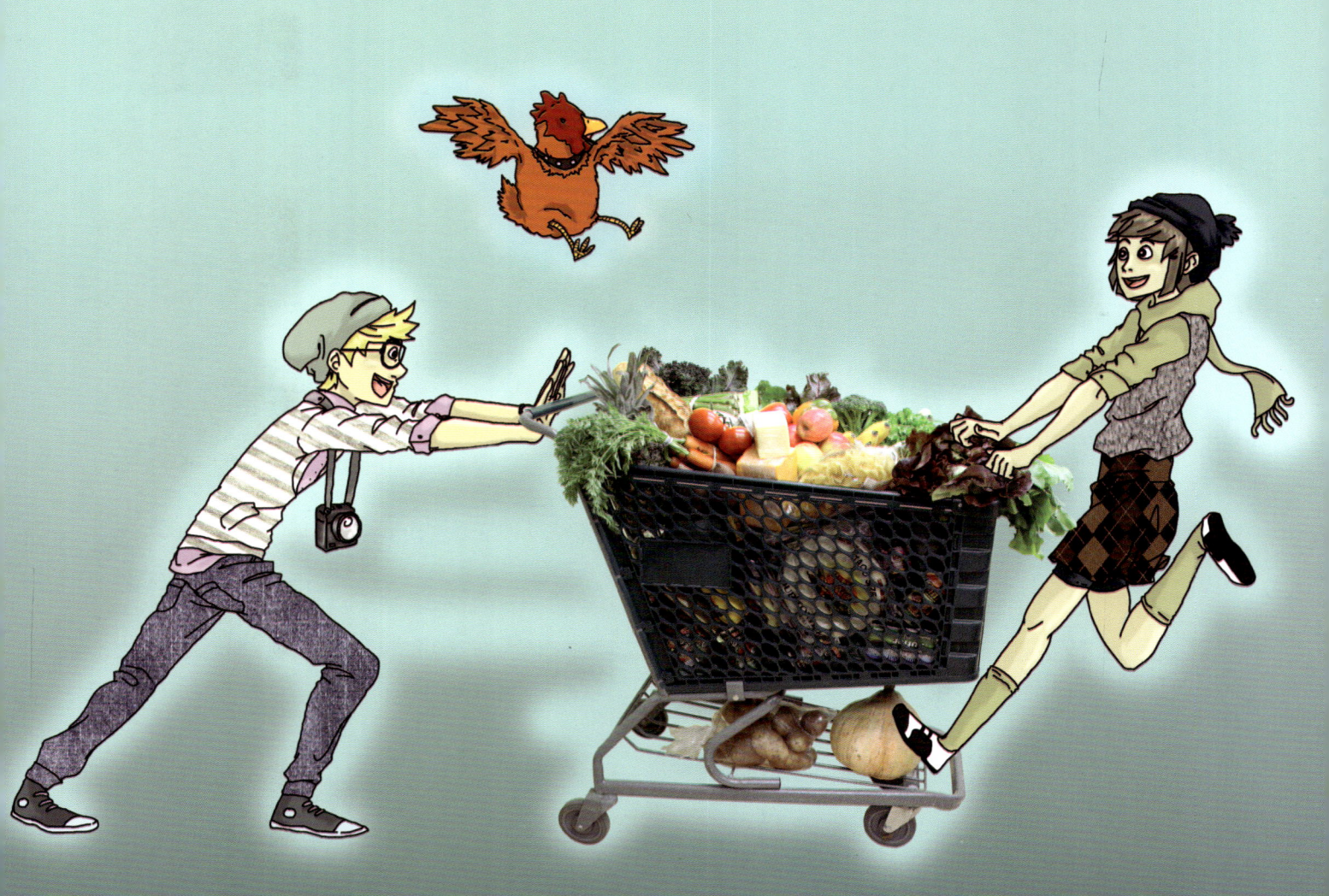

Healthy Food Sources

There are many ways to get healthy food:
- Supermarkets, regional grocery stores
- Natural food stores
- Food cooperatives and buying clubs
- Big-box stores
- Corner markets
- Directly from farmers
  - Farmers' Markets
  - Community Supported Agriculture Farms (CSAs)
  - Farm Stands
- Food banks
- Home and community gardens

This chapter discusses how to find the highest quality of food available for the lowest cost from each of these sources.

Not all of these options are available to everyone. We hope this chapter helps you to do the best you can with the food sources you have. If we all make the best choices we can, the entire food system will improve over time.

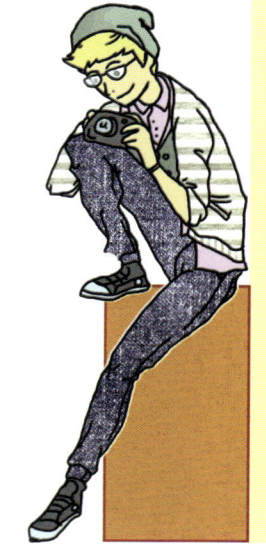

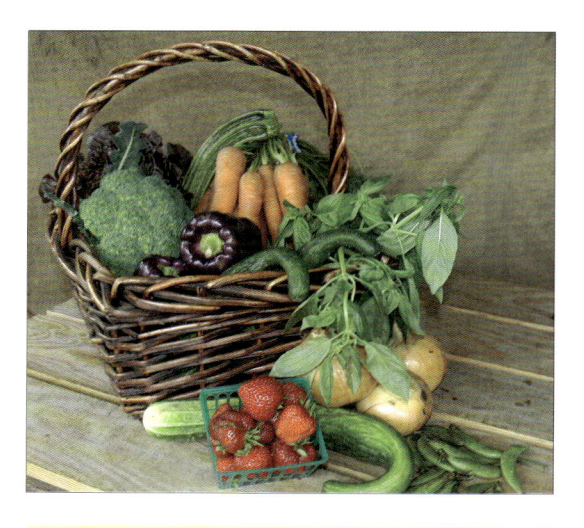

I like whole grains.

A Few General Tips for Saving Money on Your Food

- Make a shopping list and stick to it.
- Check what is in your refrigerator before you go shopping. Use that food, whether it's leftovers or still-fresh food that has not yet been used.
- Don't shop when you're hungry.

Did you know that 15-20 percent of the food we bring home is wasted? We throw out leftovers and let food go bad before we even use it.

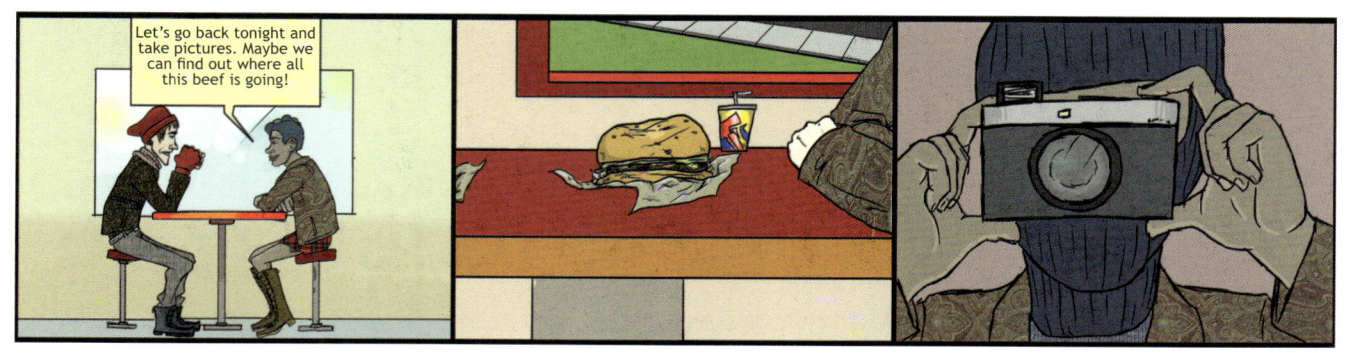

Let's go back tonight and take pictures. Maybe we can find out where all this beef is going!

14   Where to Get Food

Grocery Stores

Grocery stores come in many varieties: supermarkets, regional grocery stores, co-ops and natural food stores. Wherever you shop, there are some common elements.

For Healthier Options

- Shop the outside walls. In most markets, this is where the freshest food is found—fruits, vegetables, meat, poultry, fish, dairy products, fresh-baked goods and bulk foods.
- Reduce shopping in the center of the store, which usually has packaged, highly processed food.

To Save Money

- Buy fruits and vegetables in season.
- Buy generic or store brands; they usually cost less and are often identical to "national" brands.
- Stock up on necessary items when they are on sale, then freeze, dehydrate or can fresh food when possible.
- Check the shelf label for the unit price—the price per ounce or pound. Larger packages are usually less expensive per unit, but not always!
- Buy only needed quantities of meat and other perishable foods.
- Buy block cheese and slice it yourself.
- Roast your own lunch meats. Example: cook a turkey breast or a whole chicken; use the meat in lunches.
- Look at food on the top and bottom shelves. Items at eye level on shelves are often the most expensive.
- Buy from bulk bins. Items are usually less expensive.

What is a Co-op Grocery Store?

- A food cooperative (co-op) is a grocery store owned and directed by its members. Their focus is to make organic and whole foods more affordable. Most co-ops are open to everyone, not just members. A recent listing showed about 400 co-ops or buying clubs throughout the U.S. Local food is usually easier to find in a co-op.
- In a co-op, organic food is:
  - More easily found than in a supermarket
  - Often less expensive than in a supermarket.

Buying Clubs

A buying club is a form of co-op that's usually made up of a small group of families or households in search of a better or more economical method of purchasing food or other items. To locate one or find out how to start one, go to www.coopdirectory.org

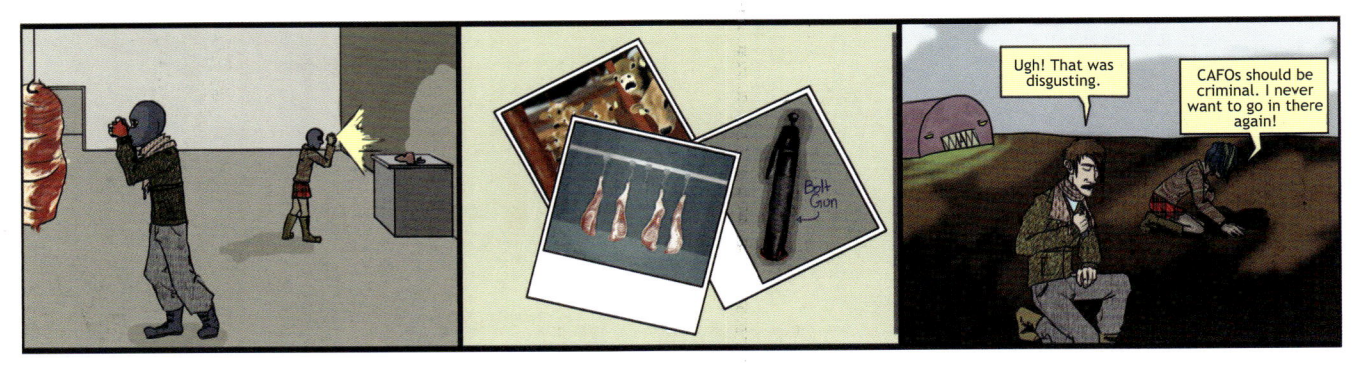

Why Buy in Bulk?

Supermarkets, regional grocery stores, co-ops and natural food stores usually have food sold from bulk bins.

- Bulk foods are less expensive. You could pay 50 percent less for peanut butter and up to 70 percent less for popcorn if you buy in bulk.
- Bulk items are often fresher than packaged items.
- Dry bulk foods (beans, grains, rice, flour, or dried fruit) store well.
- Organic bulk items are generally available for the same or lower price than packaged conventional items.
- Bulk buying eliminates packaging, which reduces waste.

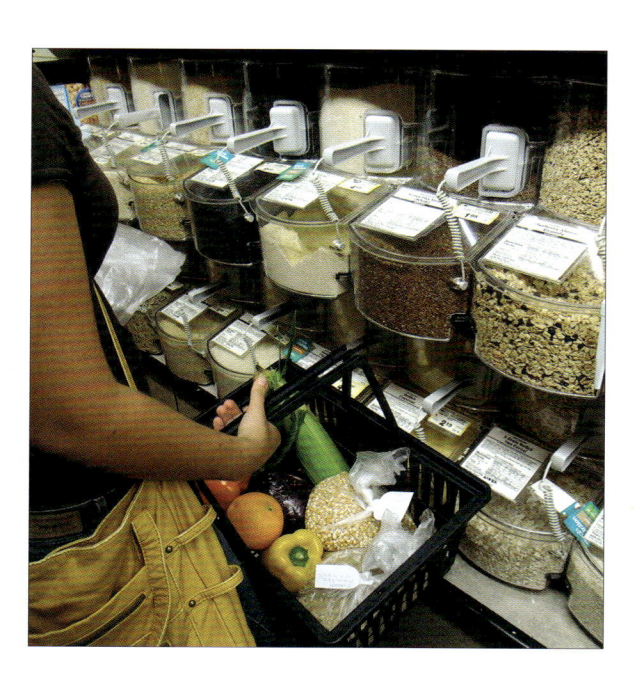

Cost Comparison*
Granola

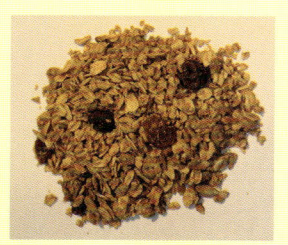

Bulk
27¢ per ounce

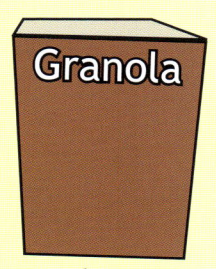

Packaged
44¢ per ounce

Or Homemade (page 149)
18¢ per ounce

*Prices vary. Estimate based on nationwide chain grocery store generic brands, 2012

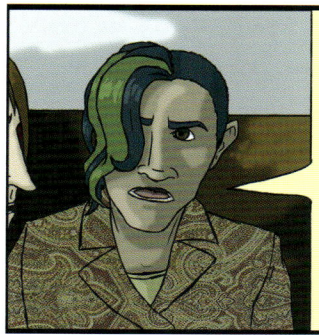

I did some research on CAFOs, and besides being cruelly treated, animals are forced to eat food that makes them sick, then they're given antibiotics which are needed because of the crowded and unsanitary conditions they live in.
I found out that because of the heavy use of antibiotics in livestock, antibiotics are becoming less effective in humans. Let's do something about this.

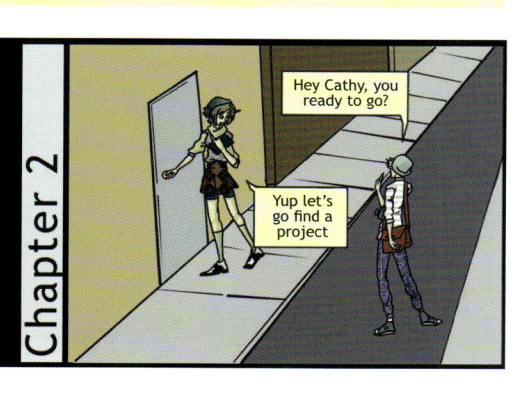

Chapter 2

Hey Cathy, you ready to go?

Yup let's go find a project

16 Where to Get Food

Grocery Store Scavenger Hunt

Let the kids learn about what they're eating while you shop together. Use the Scavenger Hunt ideas below or make up your own. Arrange the clues in the order you move through the store. Additional games are available on the Locally Delicious website: www.locally-delicious.org/LunchBoxEnvy/games.

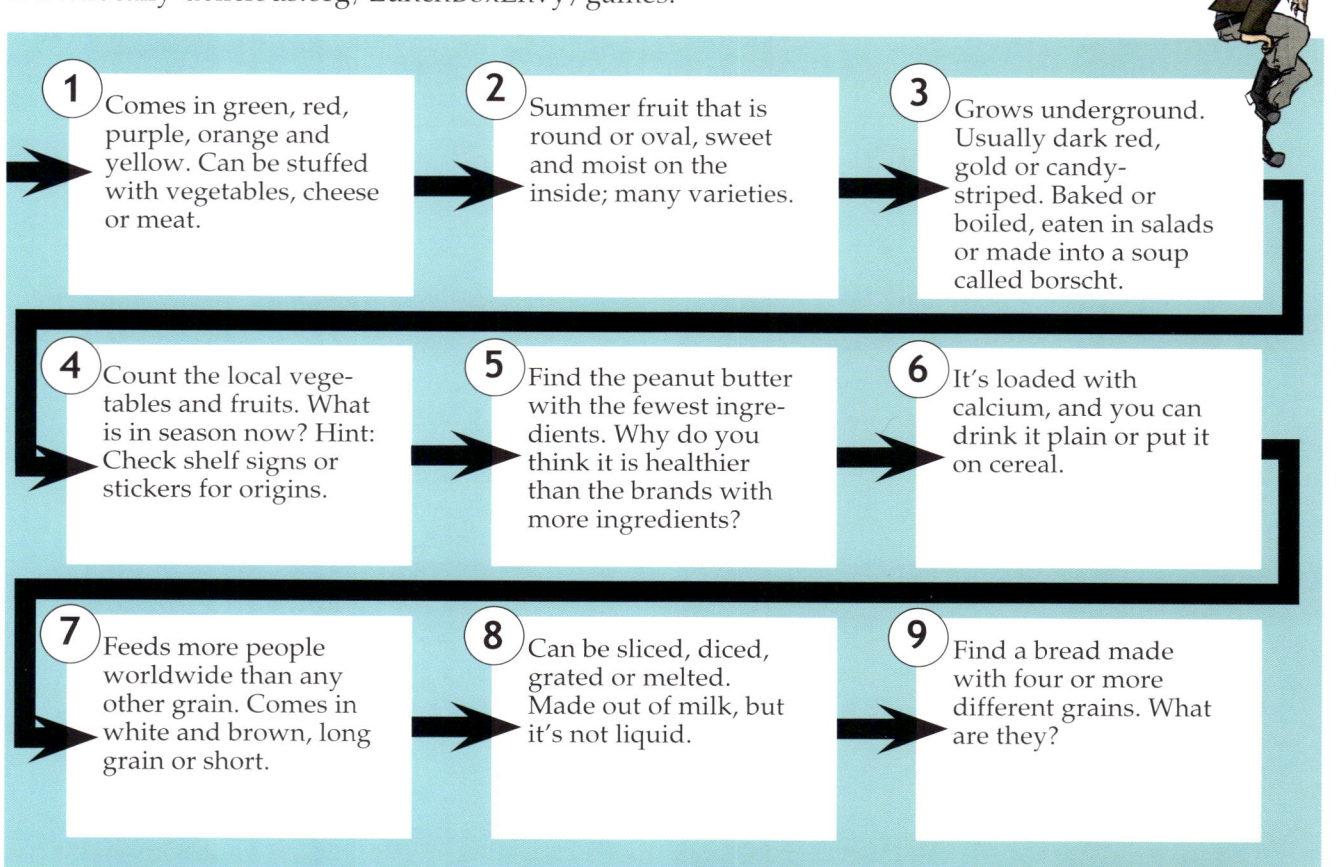

1. Comes in green, red, purple, orange and yellow. Can be stuffed with vegetables, cheese or meat.

2. Summer fruit that is round or oval, sweet and moist on the inside; many varieties.

3. Grows underground. Usually dark red, gold or candy-striped. Baked or boiled, eaten in salads or made into a soup called borscht.

4. Count the local vegetables and fruits. What is in season now? Hint: Check shelf signs or stickers for origins.

5. Find the peanut butter with the fewest ingredients. Why do you think it is healthier than the brands with more ingredients?

6. It's loaded with calcium, and you can drink it plain or put it on cereal.

7. Feeds more people worldwide than any other grain. Comes in white and brown, long grain or short.

8. Can be sliced, diced, grated or melted. Made out of milk, but it's not liquid.

9. Find a bread made with four or more different grains. What are they?

Answers: 1-bell peppers; 2-melons; 3-beets; 5-no preservatives, just real food; 6-milk; 7-rice; 8-cheese; 4 and 9 are specific to your shopping trip

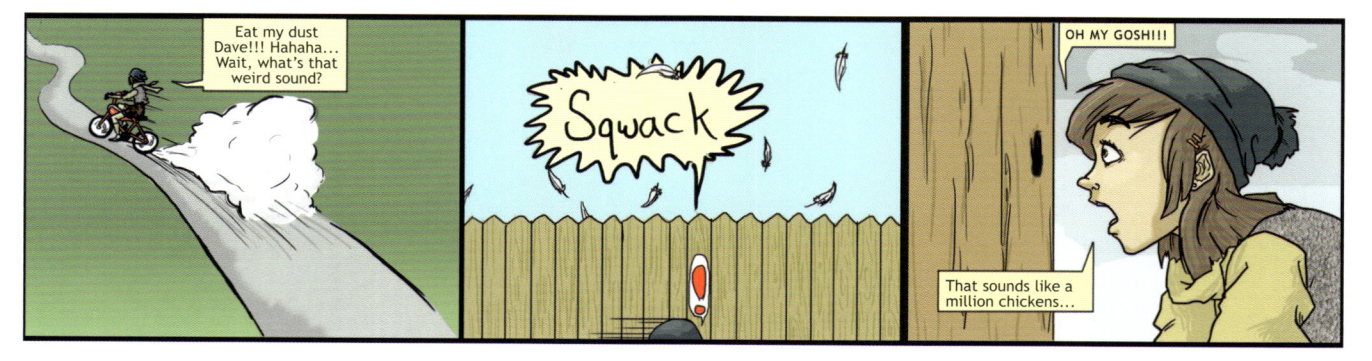

Where to Get Food 17

Tips for Shopping at Big-box Stores

For Healthier Items

- Big-box stores that sell fresh food often have organic choices—if so, take advantage of the savings.

To Save Money

- Price savings can be large, but it's easy to buy too much, as items are often pre-packaged in large quantities.
- Have a strategy for using the food before it goes bad, or preserve it by freezing, refrigerating, cooking or dehydrating for a longer life.
- Shop with a friend and split up packages that are too large for either of you individually.

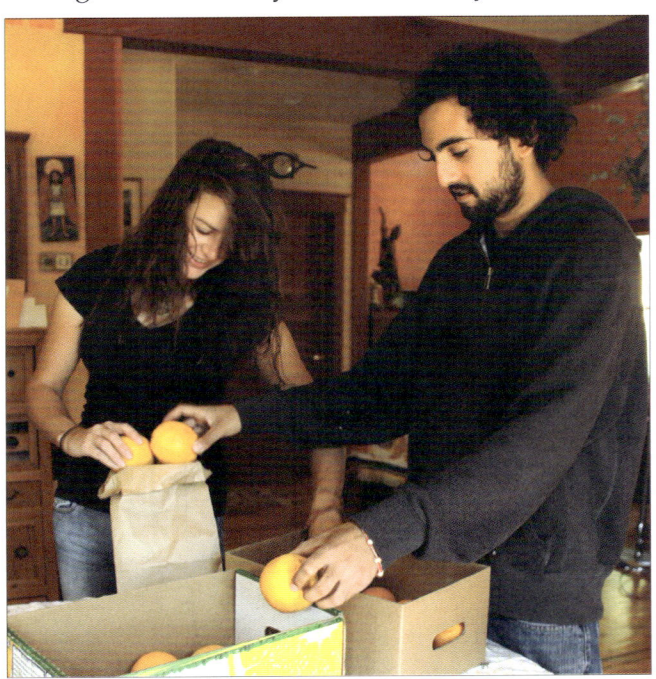

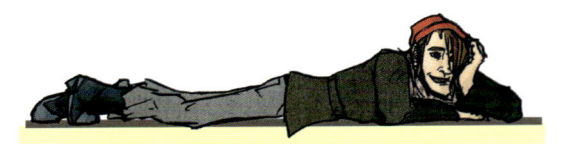

Cooking with Friends

When I lived in Elk Grove, I belonged to a Moms' Club chapter. Once a month, we got together and made meals to freeze for the upcoming month.

Everyone had a signature recipe that all the kids liked, and we found recipes online and in cookbooks. We planned the menus during our kids' weekly play dates and divided up the shopping between us.

On "Cooking Day" (usually a Sunday), we would arrive at the designated host's house in the morning with empty containers and lots of ingredients, and leave with anywhere from 5 to 10 meals each. It was a great day of fun and friendship, and everyone went home with dinner ready to be put into the oven and an array of things for the freezer to have on hand for the next month.

Ginny Prince
Mother of two girls, aged 8 and 12

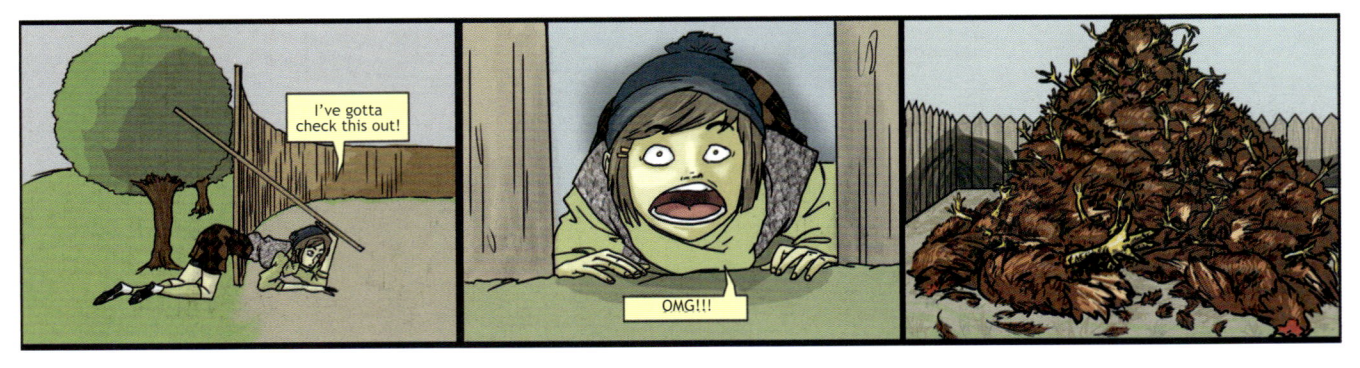

I've gotta check this out!

OMG!!!

Buying at a Farmers' Market

Buying directly from a local farmer ensures that the food is in season. Money goes into the local community—a dollar spent with a local producer has three times the economic benefit to a community as a dollar spent for food grown outside the area.

Farmers' Markets

America has seen a rebirth of local organic farms selling directly to consumers. Currently more than 7,000 farmers' markets operate in the U.S.

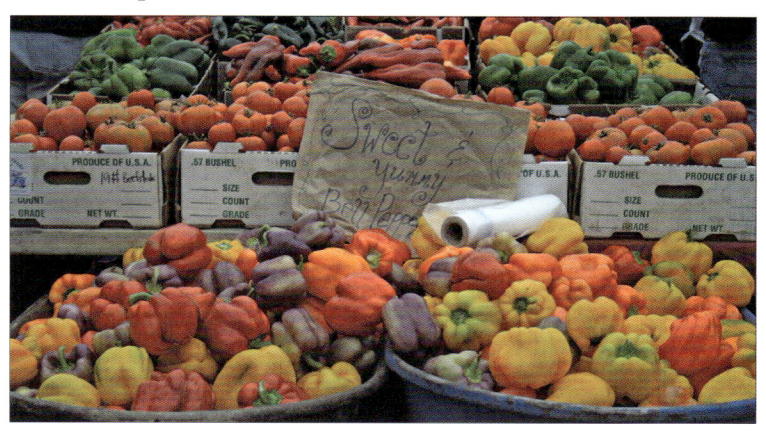

Why Shop at a Farmers' Market

- Kids love them.
- It's fun and a great way to stay connected with your community.
- The produce is seasonal, usually local and organic.
- The food tastes better. Imported produce is bred for travel hardiness, not taste, and is generally harvested before it's ripe. Compare the taste of a local tomato picked at peak ripeness with a typical supermarket variety.
- There are many more varieties of fruit and vegetables. Instead of one kind of tomato in July, there could be 20! Learn about foods you may not have seen before.
- Animal products sold at farmers' markets are not from CAFOs (factory farms).

To Save Money

- Bargain with the farmers. Many farmers reduce prices at the end of the day.
- Ask farmers for quantity discounts, and share with others.
- Ask if damaged produce (example: an apple with blemishes) can be marked down.
- Take advantage of farmers' markets that accept WIC and SNAP (EBT). See page 21.

Some farmers at farmers' markets sell produce that may not be certified organic, but may exceed the legal requirements for certification. Organic certification is an expense that many small farmers can't afford. But if you know the farmer, you'll probably trust him or her to tell you whether the food is organic.

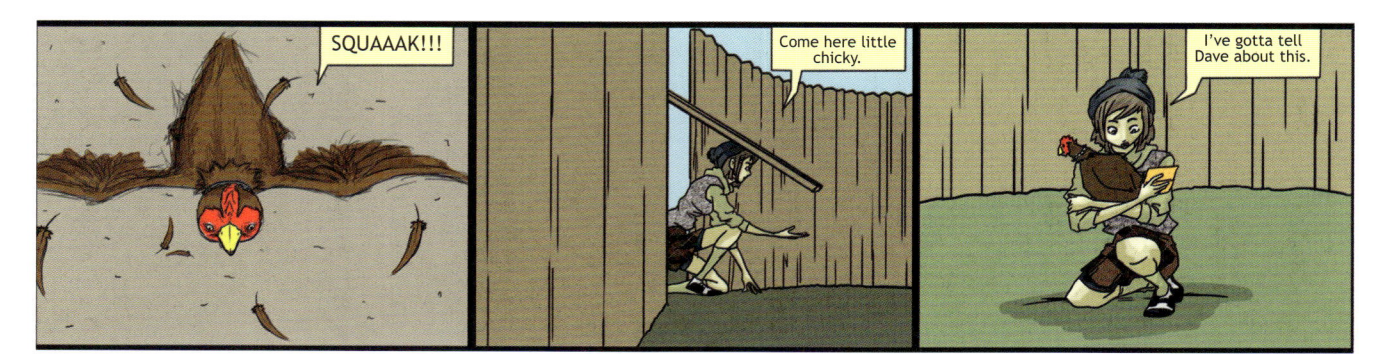

Where to Get Food 19

Buying at the Farm

Community Supported Agriculture (CSA) Farm

CSA members purchase shares in the farm at the start of the season and receive a box or bag of fresh food each week during the season.

- Buying a CSA share lowers the costs for fresh, organic food.
- CSAs provide an educational opportunity. If children learn how their food is grown they are more likely to eat it.
- CSAs make it easy to eat seasonally.
- CSAs provide opportunities to experiment with new foods.
- CSAs support and extend local food production and help the local economy.

Discounts may be available in exchange for work time on the farm.

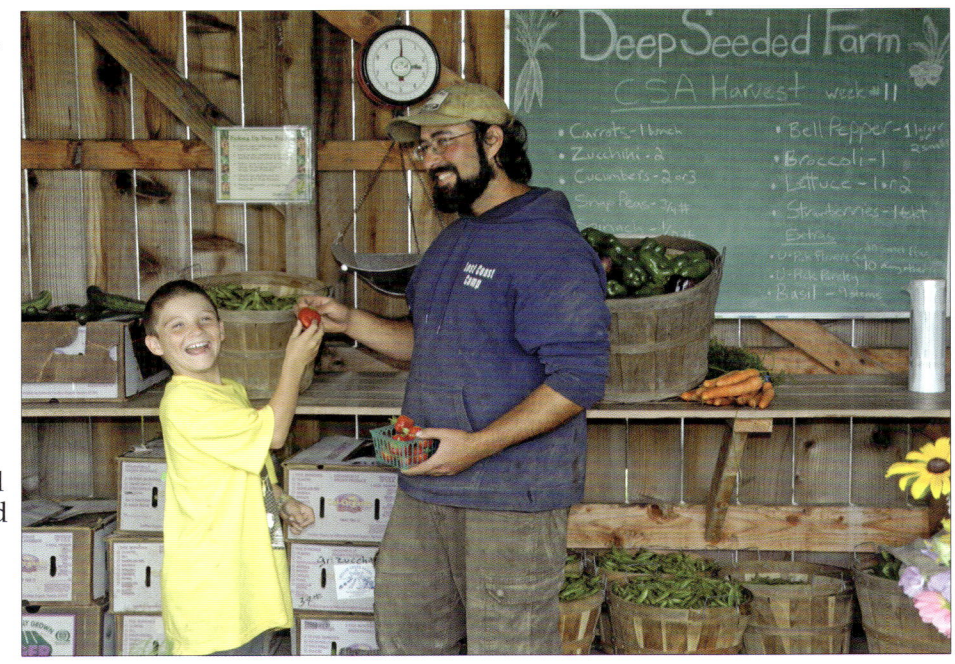

Farm Stands

- Farm stands are generally next to the farm that grows the food and are most commonly found in rural areas.
- Food is fresh and visiting a farm is a great adventure!
- Some farms have the option to let you pick your own food.
- Prices may be lower than in grocery stores.

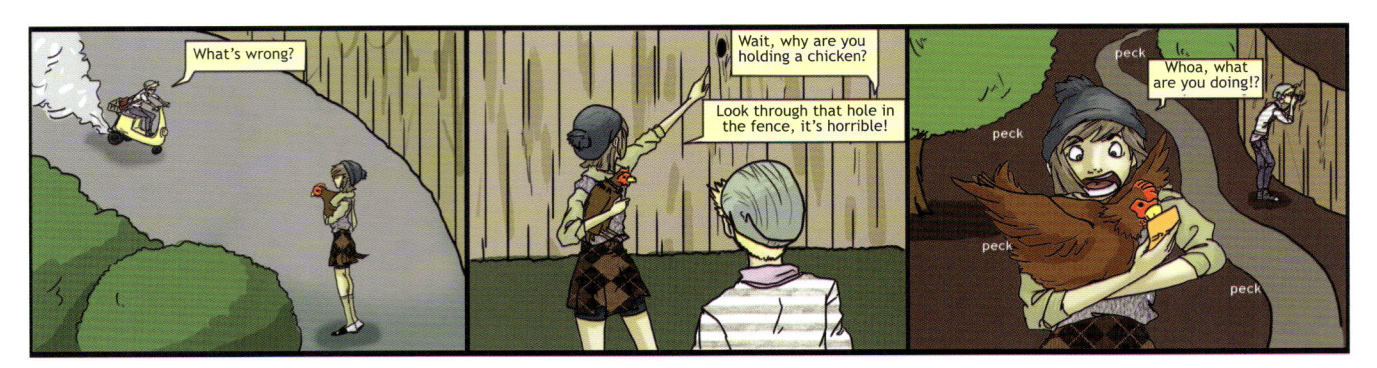

Where to Get Food

What Programs Are There to Help?

About 50 million Americans do not know where their next meal is coming from and are experiencing food insecurity. Programs are available to help, but many people do not use them. Use of these programs is encouraged to help families be healthier.

WIC and SNAP

- New rules make it easier to qualify, and government agencies encourage their use.
- Organic choices are available with WIC coupons and SNAP EBT cards. See sidebar.
- EBT cards and WIC coupons can be used to buy fresh produce at many farmers' markets. If your state does not provide this option, talk with your local representative and let them know you want it.
- WIC and SNAP bring money into local communities.

Food Banks

- Local food banks often have information on how to create healthy meals using the food bank foods.
- If the food bank doesn't have local, fresh items, ask the director if there are farms with whom they can work. There may be opportunities for gleaning or direct purchase of food.
- Ask what special programs are available. Many food banks have become very innovative. As an example, Food for People in Humboldt County partners with Locally Delicious, Inc., St. Joseph Hospital Foundation and community members to hire local farmers to grow food specifically for the food bank. Clients of the food bank get the freshest food and the local farm economy benefits.
- If you don't need a food bank, please support the important activities of these organizations through donations or volunteer work.

WIC

(Special Supplemental Nutrition Program for Women, Infants and Children) provides federal grants to states for supplemental foods, health care referrals, and nutrition education for low-income pregnant, breast feeding, and non-breast feeding postpartum women, and to infants and children up to age five who are found to be at nutritional risk.

SNAP

(Supplemental Nutrition Assistance Program) is the new name for the Food Stamp program. Each state may have a different name. For example, it is called CalFresh in California. Clients receive an Electronic Benefit Transfer (EBT) card that can be used at grocery stores and many farmers' markets.

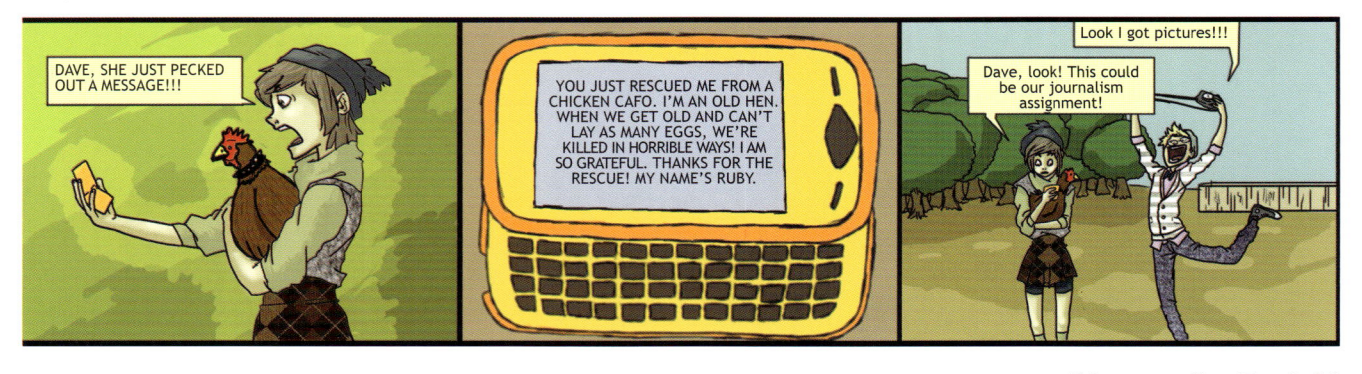

How to Maximize Options in a Food Desert

Some communities don't have grocery stores, but have convenience stores, small corner markets or liquor stores that carry food. These communities are called "food deserts." These sources do not have a wide choice of fresh food and prices are often high.

Healthy Eating in a Food Desert

- Buy the healthiest items available, such as dairy, produce, bread, tortillas, packaged beans, rice and canned vegetables.
- Encourage the store owner to offer more fresh produce.
- Participate in a community garden. acga.localharvest.org
- Grow food in your garden or in containers. Some ideas for getting started are in Chapter 6.
- Join or form a community food project. www.apps.ams.usda.gov/fooddeserts/grantOpportunities.aspx
- Check out what the Market Maker Team is doing in South Central Los Angeles to green the food desert, one corner store at a time. The site has many ideas including videos for kids. www.marketmakeovers.org

If you don't live in a food desert, support community efforts to make healthy food available to everyone.

Making Change in Food Deserts

Food Deserts are places where there is a lack of healthy, fresh, affordable and culturally appropriate food. Sadly, there is an overabundance of highly processed and fast foods. West Oakland, California, has been described as a food desert. For over 30,000 residents there are more than 50 liquor stores and fast food chains, but only one small produce market on the outskirts of the community.

Healthy food should be available to everyone regardless of race, class or neighborhood.

The People's Grocery, a community-based organization, supports a grass-roots movement fighting to improve the health and economy of West Oakland. They work to ensure that the community plays a large part in the revitalization of neighborhoods. Learn more about the organization and see some great videos of their work at www.peoplesgrocery.org

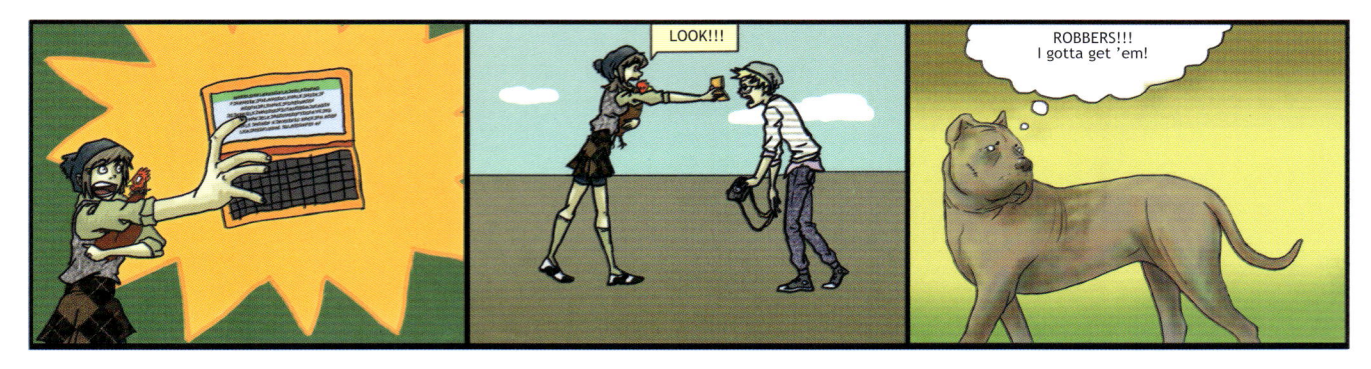

Grow Your Own Food

Raising food in a home garden or a community garden has gained in popularity over the last few years. There are more than 18,000 community gardens in the U.S. today. During World War II, up to 40 percent of all produce was grown at home in what were called Victory Gardens.

- Food from the garden is freshest and tastes the best.
- Because it is fresh, it is higher in nutrients.
- It can save money.
- A large amount of food can be grown in a small space.
- Children are more likely to eat food they have grown themselves.

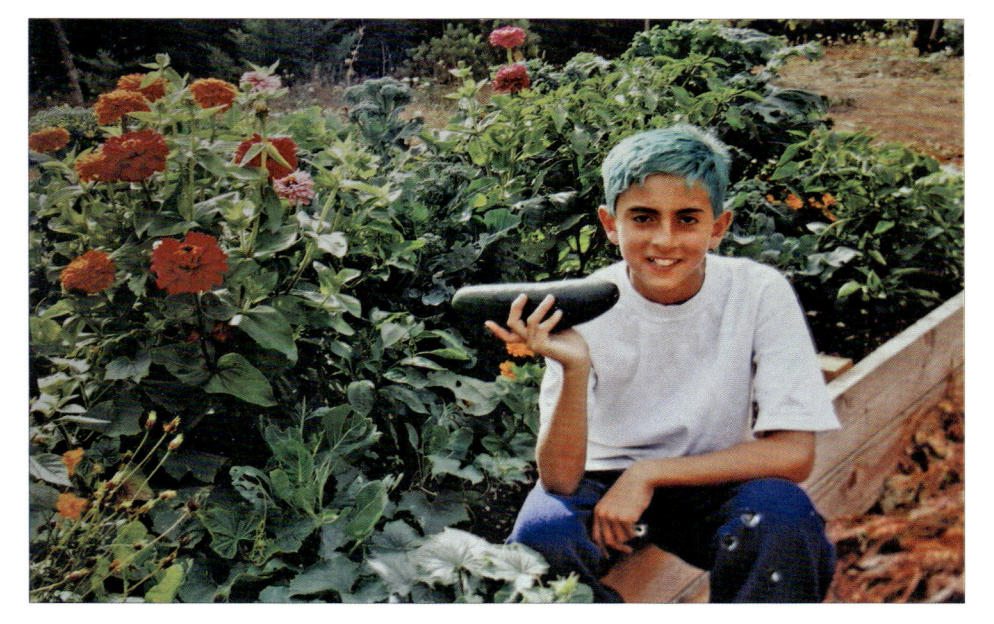

Chapter 6 has ideas for growing your own food, including growing in containers or in a small garden space. Grow food for the recipes that your children like. If you don't have room for a garden at home, take a space in a community garden.

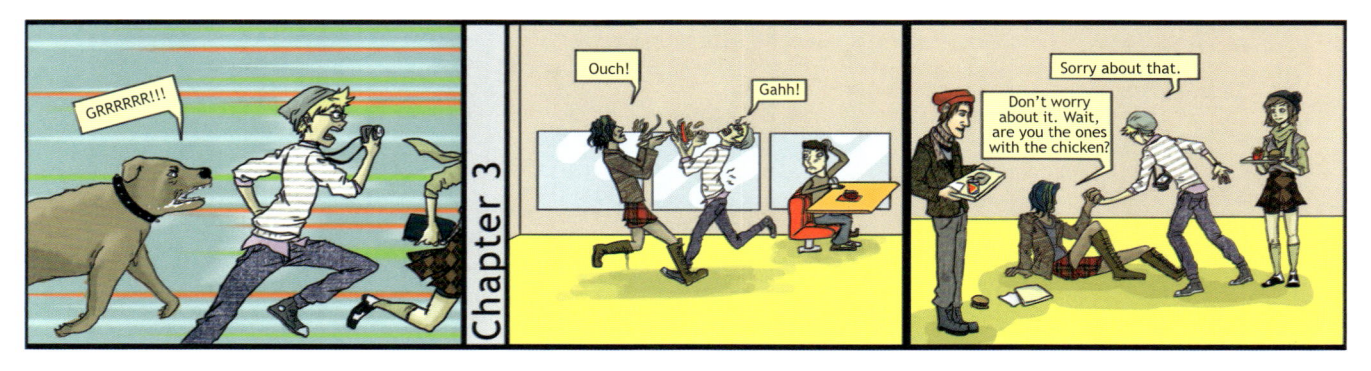

How to Help Improve Our Food System

Everyone deserves healthy food. Be an active consumer and ask the grocer questions. Make a positive change! Change happens when people demand it. Vote with your dollars.

Ask the owners of the corner stores if they can carry more produce.

Ask the grocer:
- "Can you carry more organic fruits, vegetables, dairy and meat?"
- "Is the beef grass-fed?" and "Are the poultry pasture-raised and the eggs from pasture-raised chickens?"
- "Would you label food with country, state or county of origin? Can you show which local farm has grown it? Can you buy from local farmers?"

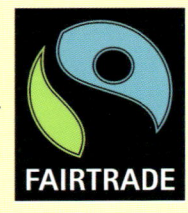

Buying Local

Food security exists when all people, at all times, have physical, social and economic access to sufficient, safe and nutritious food. Food security will increase if the food system becomes more local and each community produces much of its own food, as was the case before the 1940s and again when there were Victory Gardens.

- Having local farms all across the country creates more food security, as crops are well suited to each climate. The diversity of seed makes the food system less likely to be destroyed by a single pest (insect, fungus or bacteria).
- Having many sources of food grown all over the country adds security in case one area is hit by droughts or floods.
- Industrially produced food travels an average of 1,500 miles from farm to table and uses lots of fuel that adds CO_2 to the atmosphere.
- A greater variety of locally grown foods makes for a more interesting diet.
- Local food is automatically in-season and will be fresher and taste better.

Please support your local food system with your dollars by buying locally.

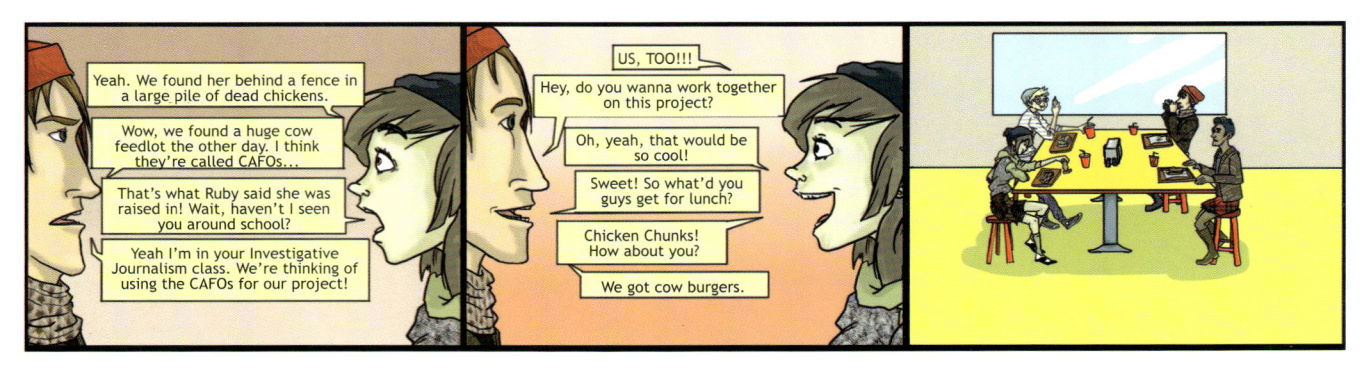

What about food that can't be grown in the U.S.?

Some foods we just can't give up. For these, buy products labeled Fairtrade if you can. It contributes to sustainable development and helps protect farm workers around the world.

For example, some cacao is harvested using slave labor—sometimes by children. If you buy Fairtrade chocolate, you are assured that it is NOT from slave labor.

24 Where to Get Food

Chapter 3
What is Healthy Food?

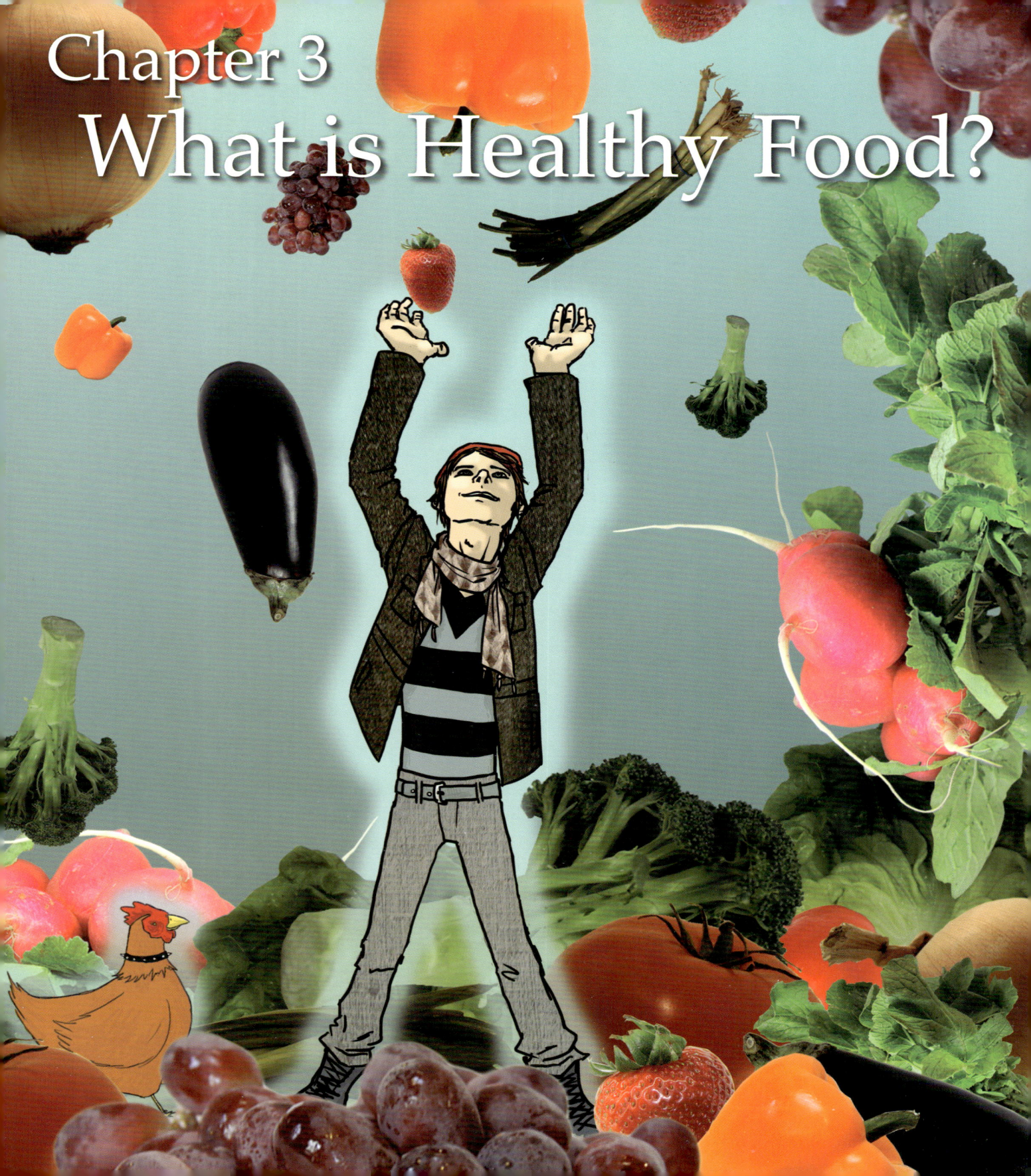

A Little History

Before 1940 most of the food we ate was "whole", meaning that it had little or no processing. Farming was organic—that was just how things were done.

After 1945, our agricultural system became more specialized—farmers increasingly focused on growing just one crop and not integrating plants and animals on the same farm. Farmers began to use more pesticides and synthetic fertilizers. They began to raise animals in confined spaces on diets that weren't natural for them. Hormones were used to stimulate growth and antibiotics were used to keep the animals from getting sick in the confined spaces. More recently, genetic engineering has created plants that combine DNA from other, different plants, animals and bacteria.

At that same time, our food started to come in packages and contained chemicals to make it last longer when traveling or sitting on a store shelf. Fast food became part of our world.

Not all of these changes to the food system have helped us.

This chapter describes food that is healthy for our bodies, our communities and our Earth. You'll find some strategies to save money, but the best way to save money and to have delicious, healthy food is to prepare it at home. Yes, cooking takes more time, but it's worth the effort.

Every healthy choice you make provides everyone in your family with a better diet, and also helps protect the environment.

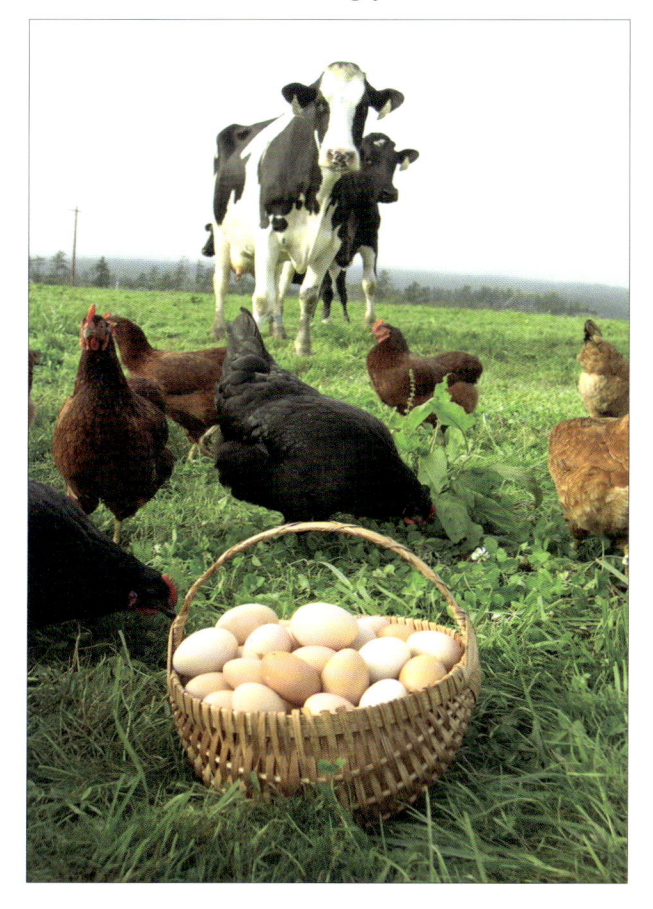

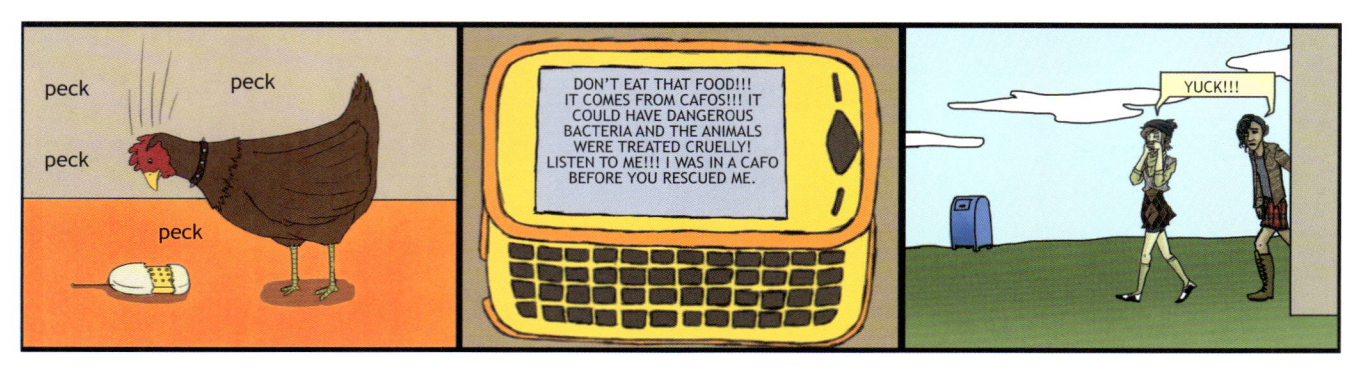

26 What is Healthy Food?

Whole, Unprocessed Food

A healthy diet includes whole, unprocessed food.

What is whole, unprocessed food? It...

- can be identified as what it is: an apple, a carrot or a piece of chicken.
- is simply packaged or unpackaged: fresh fruit, vegetables, meat and dairy products, rice, whole grains, whole-grain flours, beans.
- has no ingredient list—the food IS the ingredient.
- is food your great-grandmother would have recognized.

What's good about whole, unprocessed food? It...

- contains the full range of nutrients your body needs including vitamins and minerals, as well as important nutrients (phytochemicals and micronutrients, see Glossary, page 188) that we're just now learning about.
- is generally less expensive than processed foods.

What's bad about processed food? It can...

- contain added chemicals that do your body no good and could do harm.
- have extra sugar and fat that contribute to obesity.
- have extra salt that contributes to high blood pressure.
- depend on highly subsidized corn and soy products that are often genetically modified (GMOs).
- be made from ingredients that contain pesticide levels that are not good for you or for helpful insects like bees and butterflies.
- be over-packaged, which consumes energy and creates waste.

How Can Whole, Unprocessed Food be Less Expensive?

You buy only the food—not the processing, packaging, shipping and advertising. Only 15 percent of the money you spend for processed food is for the food itself.

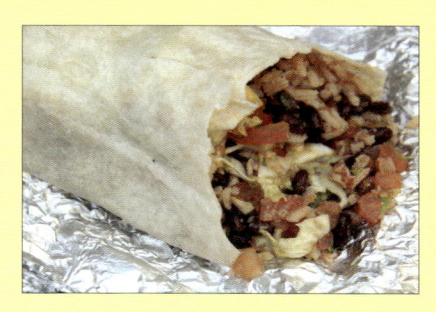

A homemade burrito with beans and cheese (see recipe, page 78) will cost about $1.20. A purchased burrito may cost $3.00 or more and may contain many synthetic ingredients in addition to the tortilla, beans and cheese.

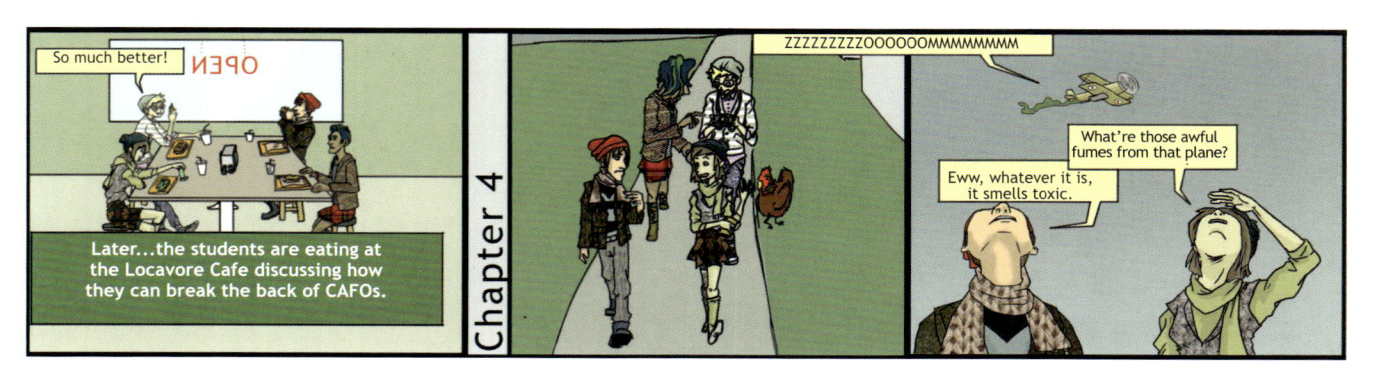

What is Healthy Food?

Processed Foods

Despite a goal of eating only unprocessed food, there are probably some packaged foods we still have to buy. What strategies can we use to avoid the worst ingredients in processed food? Look at the ingredient list on the container and choose the products with:

- names you can pronounce—they're more likely real food, not chemicals.
- ingredients that you might have in your cupboard. For example, you probably have flour but not butylated hydroxyanisole or sodium carboxymethyl cellulose.
- food items that don't have much sugar, fat and salt.
- fewer ingredients.

See "Food Labels," page 190, to help you understand what is in the food.

Why Are All These Extra Ingredients in the Packaged Food?

Preservatives help the products last longer on the shelf. Extenders make the products bulkier. Artificial colors make the food look fresher or more appealing. Articial flavors change the taste. None of these adds to the food value. In fact, some ingredients such as added sugar, salt and fat may make the food more addictive and worse for your health.

Comparison of Two Peanut Butters

Peanut Butter Number 1	Peanut Butter Number 2
Roasted peanuts	Roasted peanuts
	Sugar
	Hydrogenated vegetable oils (cottonseed, soybean and rapeseed)
	Salt

The added ingredients are sugar, fat and salt and can be bad for your health.

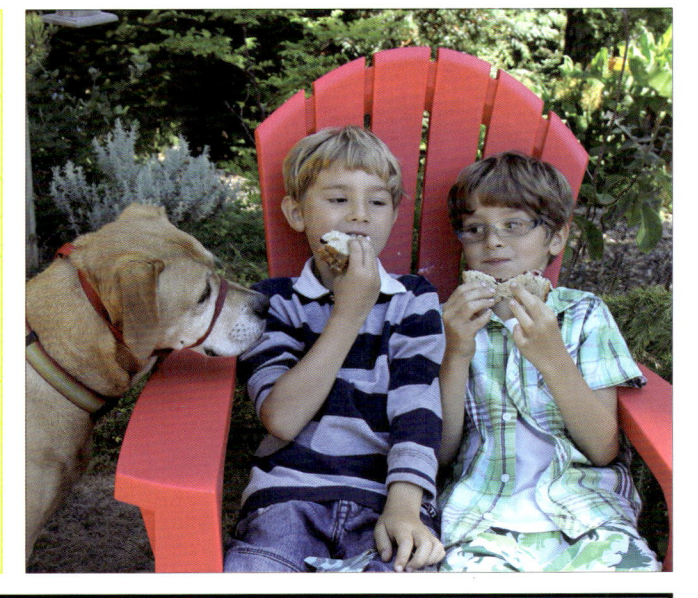

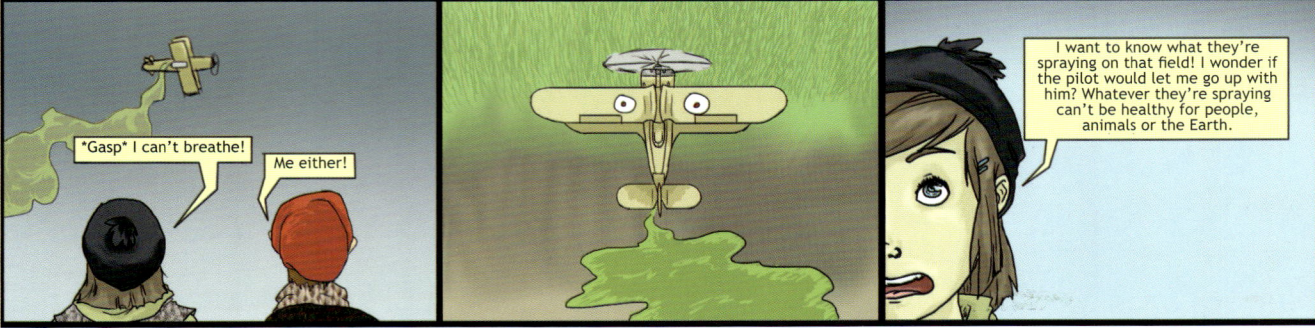

Gasp I can't breathe!

Me either!

I want to know what they're spraying on that field! I wonder if the pilot would let me go up with him? Whatever they're spraying can't be healthy for people, animals or the Earth.

28 What is Healthy Food?

Fresh and In-season Food

Fresh and in-season food tastes better and is better for you. Consider choosing what to buy based on the season—buy peaches in the summer, switch to apples in the fall and citrus in winter. In-season foods will also cost less than out-of-season ones.

How to Tell if It's In-season Food
If it's fresh and from:

- the U.S., Mexico or Canada
- a local farm
- your garden

Labels on the store shelf or stickers on produce give the origin of the food. The food distributor is usually listed, but look for the "made in" or "produced in" or "product of" wording. Ask your grocer to provide that information if it isn't obvious.

Why Is Food From the Southern Hemisphere Fresh in the Winter Here?

When it's winter in the U.S., it is summer in the Southern Hemisphere in countries like New Zealand, Chile, Ecuador and Argentina. That's why we can get summer crops, like peaches, from South America during our winter. These foods travel long distances using lots of fossil fuel and adding CO_2 into the air.

Other Options: Frozen, Canned and Dried
People have been preserving food for thousands of years. Now more people are preserving their own food, as they are growing more of their own food. Commercially preserved food can also be a good option, but when food is fresh and in-season, choose that first.

- Frozen food retains most nutrients when frozen directly after harvest. It keeps its color well and has a fresher taste than canned food.
- Canned food doesn't need refrigeration, and is an alternative. It often has a lot of added salt. Compare products and choose the one with lower salt. If the food is still high in salt, rinse it before using. If organic options are available, buy those whenever possible.
- Dried food stores well and is convenient. Raisins and dried fruit are handy snacks, for instance.

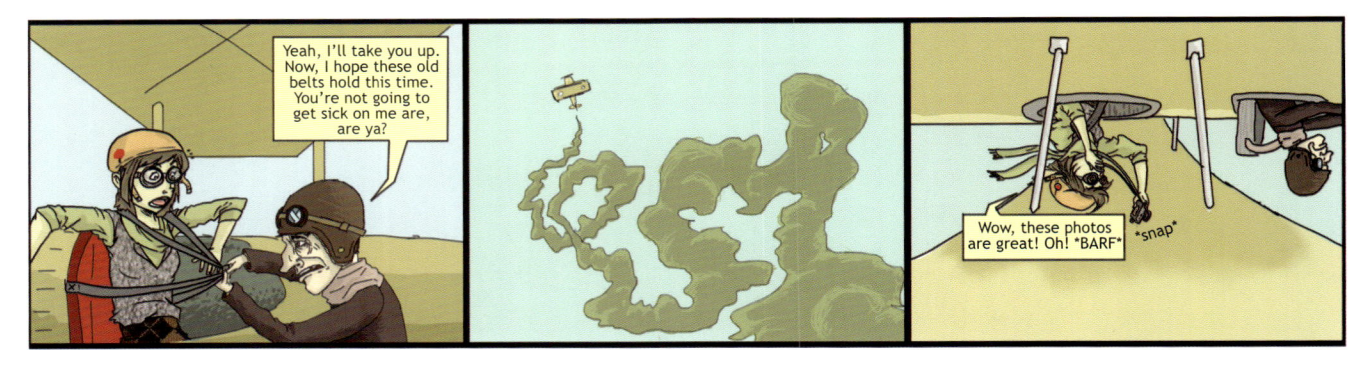

What is Healthy Food?

Protein from Meat and Poultry

Most beef, pork and poultry in the U.S. is raised in factory farms, also called "Concentrated Animal Feeding Operations" (CAFOs). There is, however, an increase in the number of farms raising meat in the traditional way—in open fields on grass or other food natural for the animal. If the meat at the market isn't labeled pasture-raised, grass-fed or organic, it almost certainly comes from a CAFO.

Pasture-raised meat is not available everywhere and is usually more expensive. Over time, customer demand may change this, but for now, many of us have few options. Do the best you can.

Benefits of Pasture-raised Meat
- Animals that have been fed well produce more nutritious meat.
- Animals have a better life and eat food that is natural for them.

Problems with Factory-farmed Meats
- Animals are usually treated cruelly.
- Animals are fed antibiotics to combat their unnatural diets and unsanitary housing. This has created disease bacteria that are now resistant to antibiotics. In people, resistant bacteria can cause illness that antibiotics will not cure. *E. coli* is one example that's often in the news.
- CAFO meat has higher levels of bad fats and lower levels of good fats.
- CAFOs are a serious source of water, air and soil pollution.

Pasture-Raised Meat Can Be Affordable
- Buy only what you need. Most of us eat about twice what our bodies need. Less than half a pound daily of animal protein (or three cups of grains, beans and legumes) will maintain optimal health.
- Instead of buying packaged meat, ask the butcher to make a package with just the amount you want.
- Use meat as an ingredient, not the main course. Include meat in stews or soups along with beans, grains or vegetables.

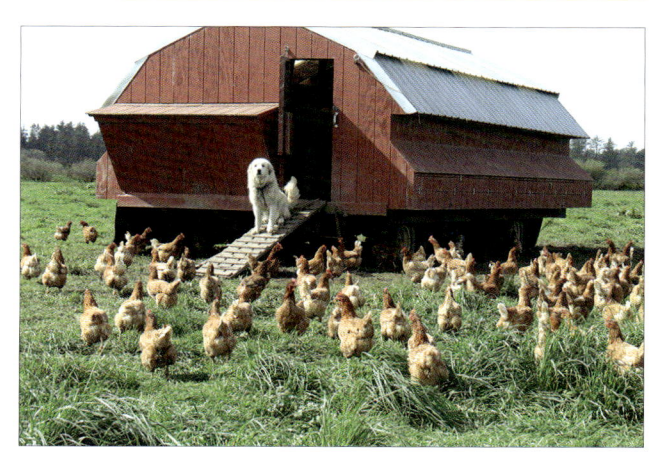

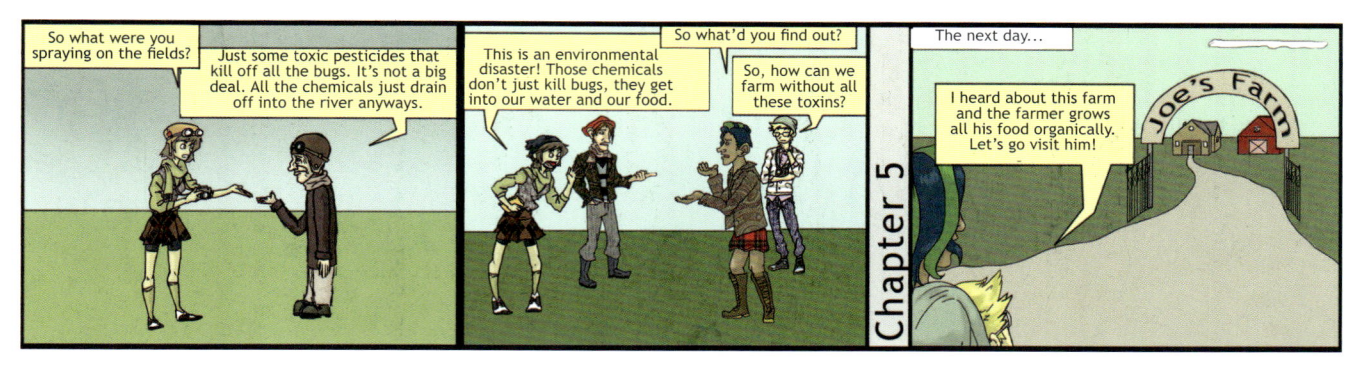

Protein from Plants, Eggs, Dairy and Fish

Many world cultures depend on a mostly plant-based diet. Some add eggs, dairy and fish. These are all good sources of protein.

A Plant-based Diet

- Provides the protein your body needs. When it comes to nutrients, your body doesn't know beef from beans.
- Helps with weight loss, and improves overall vitamin absorption.
- Costs less than a meat-based diet.
- Includes a wide variety of high-protein foods such as nuts, seeds, beans, legumes, some grains and tofu.

Egg and Dairy Products . . .

- can save you money.
- are available from many types of stores.
- offer many creative meatless meal possibilities.

Fish

- Is a healthy source of protein, but needs to be selected carefully.
- When canned, fish such as tuna and salmon are convenient and ready to eat.

My favorite plant-based food is a peanut butter and jam sandwich.

Problems with Fish

Fish is frequently farmed. Some types of farmed fish are healthy for your body and the Earth, but many are not. The issues with farmed fish are:

- Interbreeding with wild fish, thereby destroying native species.
- PCB (see Glossary, page 186) and antibiotic contamination of wild fish from fish farms
- Water pollution

Many wild fish species may be, or are currently, overfished and in danger of becoming extinct.

The Monterey Bay Aquarium's Seafood Watch is a good guide for the "Best Choice," "Good Alternative" and "Fish to Avoid." www.montereybayaqarium.org/cr/seafoodwatch.asps

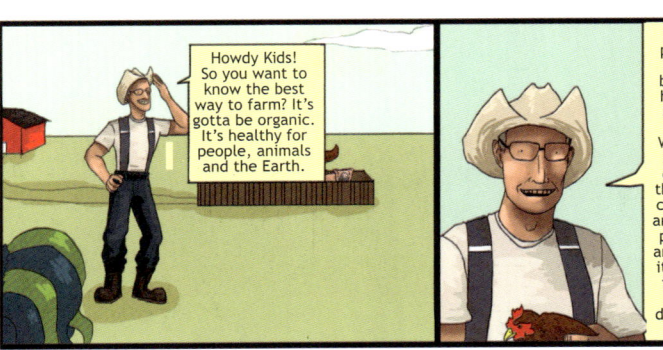

Panel 1: Howdy Kids! So you want to know the best way to farm? It's gotta be organic. It's healthy for people, animals and the Earth.

Panel 2: We don't use harmful pesticides or chemicals that kill good bugs, bees, and butterflies. It's important to have healthy soil, and do ya know where it comes from? Poop!!! We rotate the animals in the pasture. Cows are first and eat the long grasses, and... they poop. Then the chickens come and eat the small grass and bugs and then...yup, they poop. Last, the pigs come in and rototill and...you guessed it, they poop. That's the way it was done in the old days. Modern farming practices destroy land, rivers, streams, and create pollution.

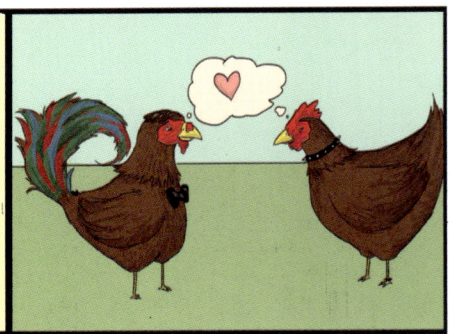

What is Healthy Food? 31

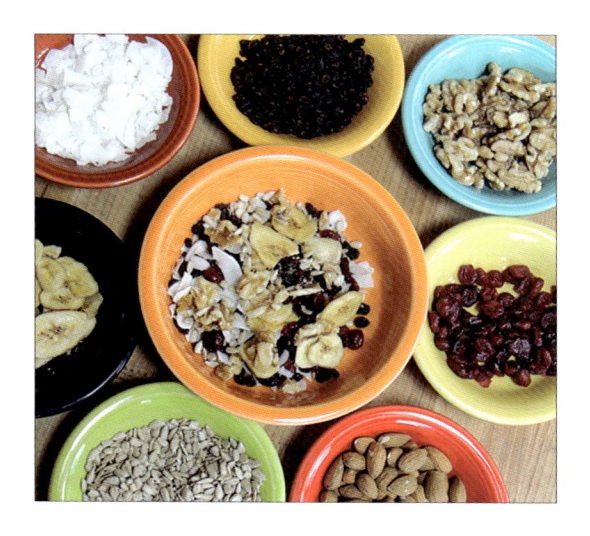

The Evil Trio: Sugar, Fat and Salt

Excess sugar, fat and salt are the main dietary causes of obesity and obesity-related diseases such as type 2 diabetes, heart disease, high blood pressure and cancer. The current generation of children has a shorter life expectancy than their parents. Much of the problem is due to what the children are eating.

Extra salt, fat and sugar sneaks into our diets through processed snack foods and sugared drinks. Too much of these foods is bad. Moderation is the key.

Children don't always recognize the negative consequences of eating extra sugar, fat and salt, so it's important to give them healthy snack and drink options.

For delicious snack and drink options, pack...

- trail mix you've made with items from the bulk bins at the market.
- homemade muffins or cookies that include fruit and vegetables and lower sugar and fat levels.
- a selection of nuts.
- fresh fruit. Buy extra when it's in season and dry it for a convenient snack. Make your own fruit leather (see page 154).
- bags of home-popped popcorn. Make up your own bags of microwave popcorn (see page 144).
- water, sparkling water, vegetable juice, diluted fruit juices, or milk instead of soft drinks, energy drinks and sugary flavored waters. Ideas for low-sugar flavored waters are in the recipe chapter on page 140. A special note on energy drinks: they also contain high levels of stimulants that may be harmful to kids.

Why People Like Sweet, Fat and Salty food.

In ancient times, when food was scarce, the best strategy to survive was to get fat when there was food and hope you didn't starve when there was none. For this reason, it's natural for humans to like sweets and fats, which are rich in calories. Salt was crucial to replenish sweat from hard work. Nowadays we lead less harsh and more predictable lives, but we still need these three —in moderation!

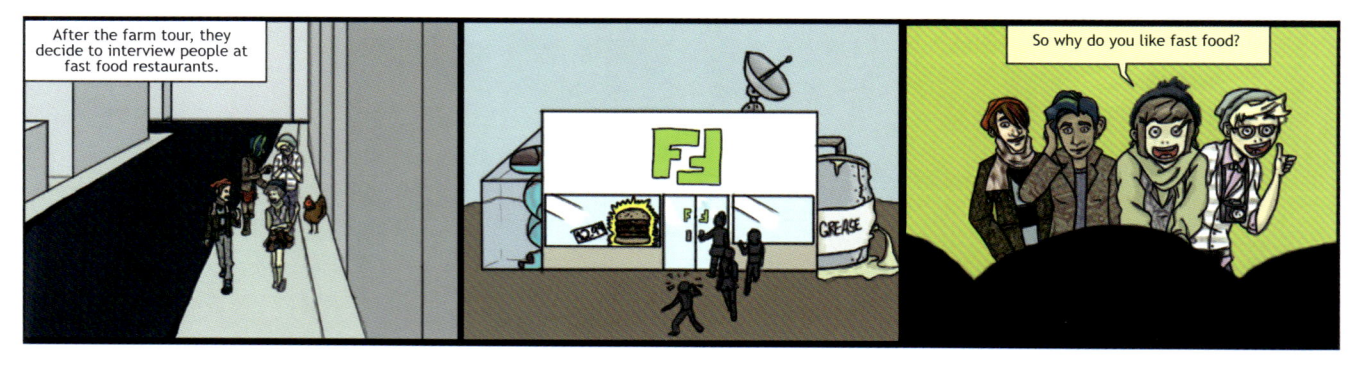

32 What is Healthy Food?

The Evil Trio: Sugar, Fat and Salt

Why is it easy to eat too much sugar, fat and salt?

- Manufacturers heavily advertise foods that contain these items. Look at kids' TV programming and count how many foods fall into this category.
- These products are sold everywhere. Is it easier to find a soda or a fresh carrot?
- These foods are addictive.
- They are cheap because they often use government-subsidized corn and soybean products, including high-fructose corn syrup. Fresh fruits and vegetables have little or no subsidy. Reversing the subsidies would help make healthy food less expensive and unhealthy food more expensive.

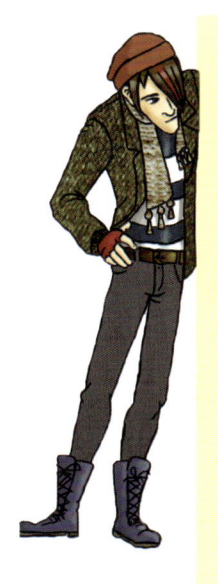

Find the Hidden Sugar

How do you spell "sugar"? Look at package labels and find how much sugar processed food really contains.

Here are some other names for sugar:

Barley malt	Brown sugar
High-fructose corn syrup	Powdered Sugar
Corn syrup	Raw Sugar
Maple syrup	Honey
Cane juice	Molasses
Glucose	Fructose
Maltodextrin	Dextrose
Sucrose	Lactose

Kitchen Test

There are about 17 teaspoons of sugar in a 20-ounce soda. Get a teaspoon and bag of sugar and measure this into a bowl.

Next, pour the sugar into 20 ounces of water and taste it. What do you think?

If you drink three 20-ounce sodas a day, that's 720 calories, or almost half of all the calories you need in a day.

Amount of Sugar you Consume if you Drink 1, 2 or 3 20-ounce Sugary Drinks a Day

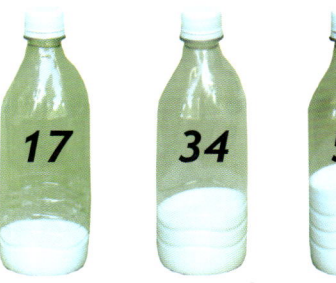

17   34   51

Teaspoons of Sugar

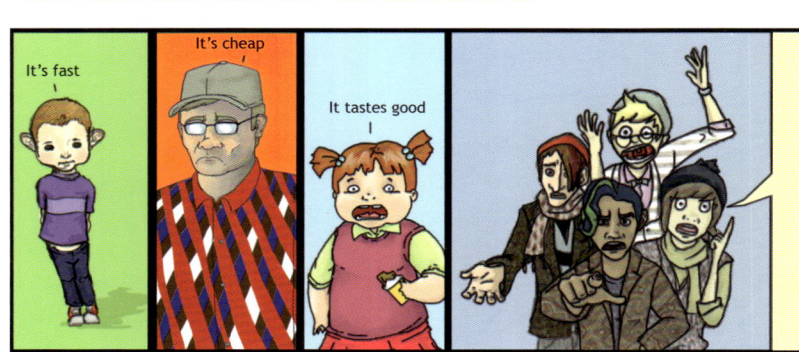

It's fast | It's cheap | It tastes good

What!!!

Fast food can make you sick!
It's bad for you!!
That food is so filled with sugar, fat and salt that it's even addictive. It can cause obesity, which leads to other diseases, like type 2 diabetes, heart disease, cancer, high blood pressure, and a shortened life. Yuck!
You can avoid these problems if you eat healthy snacks like fresh fruit, vegetables, and trail mix.
And by the way, lay off those sugary drinks!

What is Healthy Food?

Rethink Your Drink

Did You Know?

- The average person eats almost 100 pounds of added sugar a year — that's about one quarter of a pound of added sugar a day!
- Soda is the #1 source of added sugar in the American diet.
- Over 30% of all calories from added sugars consumed daily are from sweetened beverages.
- Extra calories from all this sugar may lead to weight gain, putting people at risk for lifelong health problems such as diabetes and heart disease.
- 2 out of 3 Americans are overweight or obese.

Be Sugar Savvy!

Take a look at how much sugar is in these popular drinks:

	Soda	Orange Drink	Sweetened Tea Drink	Tamarindo	Big Pouch	Grass Jelly Drink	Sports Drink	Water
Size	20 oz.	16 oz.	20 oz.	13.5 oz.	11.25 oz.	11 oz.	20 oz.	
Calories	250	260	220	186	152	143	140	0
Teaspoons of Sugar	17	15	13	12	9.5	8.6	9	0

Challenge yourself to make a difference in your health. Commit to drinking:

- Water
- Non-fat or low-fat milk
- Unsweetened iced tea
- 100% fruit juice in limited amounts

rethink YOUR DRINK

Commit to drinking water or unsweetened beverages!

I, _____, will drink water instead of sugary drinks this month.
(print your name)

Keep track of your healthy drink days! Check ✓ a box for every day that you drink water instead of sugary drinks.

WRITE IN THE DATES:	SUN	MON	TUE	WED	THU	FRI	SAT
Week:							
Week:							
Week:							
Week:							

Bay Area Nutrition & Physical Activity Collaborative   www.banpac.org   Reprinted with permission.

Dairy and Grain Products

Real Dairy Products

- Choose real cheese. Processed cheese is less than 51 percent milk and may be mostly vegetable oil.
- Use plain yogurt, or make your own. Commercially flavored yogurt contains excess sugar and many additives, including "natural" flavorings that can be questionable (see sidebar). Add your choice of fresh fruit to plain yogurt.

Whole Grains

- Whole grains are the entire seed and include wheat, corn, brown rice, oats, barley, sorghum, spelt, rye and more (See "Grains of the World, page 96).
- The original outer layer of the grain contains healthy fats and vitamins that get lost in the milling process. "Enriched" grains have some, but not all, of the nutrients added back in an artificial form.
- White flour is so highly processed that it is like sugar—nearly pure carbohydrate that contributes to obesity, diabetes and heart disease.
- Eating whole grains reduces the risk of obesity, diabetes, heart disease, stroke and cancer.

Weird Source of Natural Fruit Flavors

Did you know that some yogurts, ice creams and candies are flavored with castoreum? This natural flavor enhancer comes from an anal gland of beavers. Flavor manufacturers extract it from the glands of beavers that have been killed for their fur.

The word "natural" can mean a lot of things! How about just using real fruit instead of stuff from beavers' butt glands?

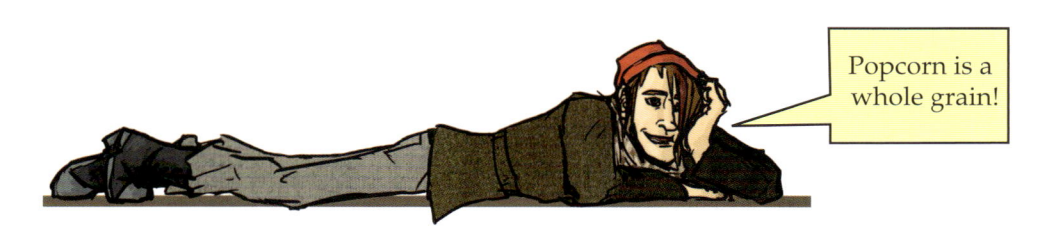

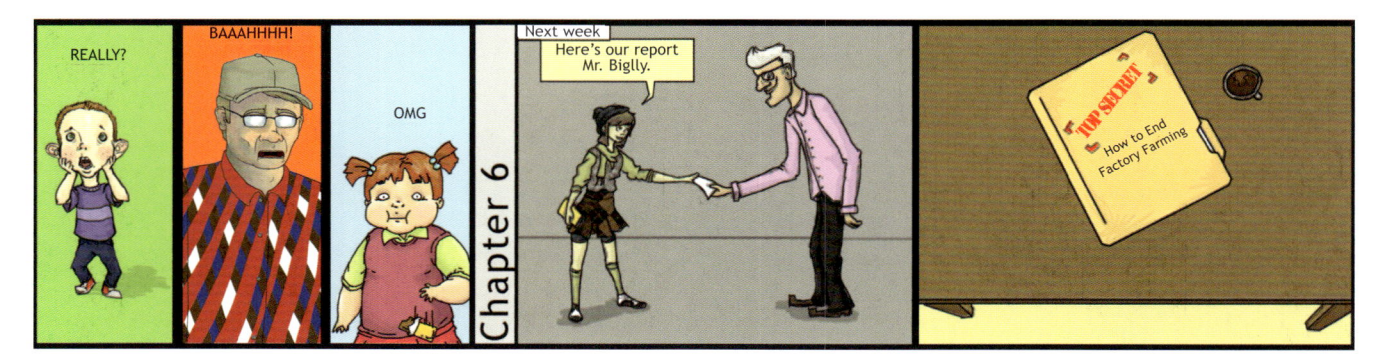

Popcorn is a whole grain!

What is Healthy Food?

Organic

The labels "organic" and "certified organic" have legal definitions, so you know what you are buying. Organic food does not contain pesticides, hormones, antibiotics, artificial ingredients or Genetically Modified Organisms (GMOs). Buying organic is a way to assure yourself that you will not be affected by the negative aspects of these substances.

When available and affordable, consider buying organic because it...

- contains no pesticide residue.
- is safer for farmers and farm laborers because no toxic chemicals are used.
- does not cause water pollution because it does not contribute excessive fertilizer to the water system, thus preventing ocean dead zones.
- does not destroy topsoil, as does much of industrial farming.
- does not create air pollution produced by the use of synthetic fertilizers.

To Save Money

- Shop for organic food at a co-op.
- Grow your own food.
- Use money-saving tips for buying directly from the farmer (see pages 19 and 20).
- Check price of organics at big-box stores. Look for the U.S. Department of Agriculture (USDA) approved organic label.
- Buy organic. If more people demand organic foods, it will again become more available and prices will drop.

What About Buying Products labeled "Natural"?

Unlike organic, "natural" has no legal definition—good, bad or neutral. However, the word "natural" has been hijacked by advertisers to convince consumers that natural is equal to organic. It isn't. Read the ingredients on all food labels to know what you are buying. (See page 190)

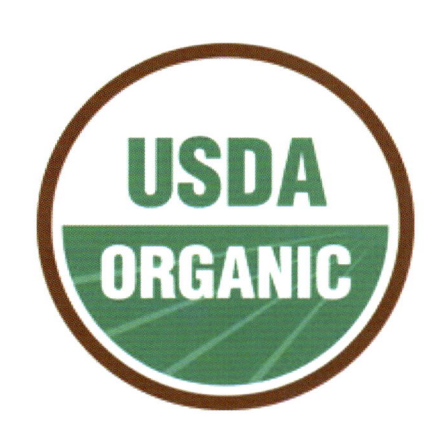

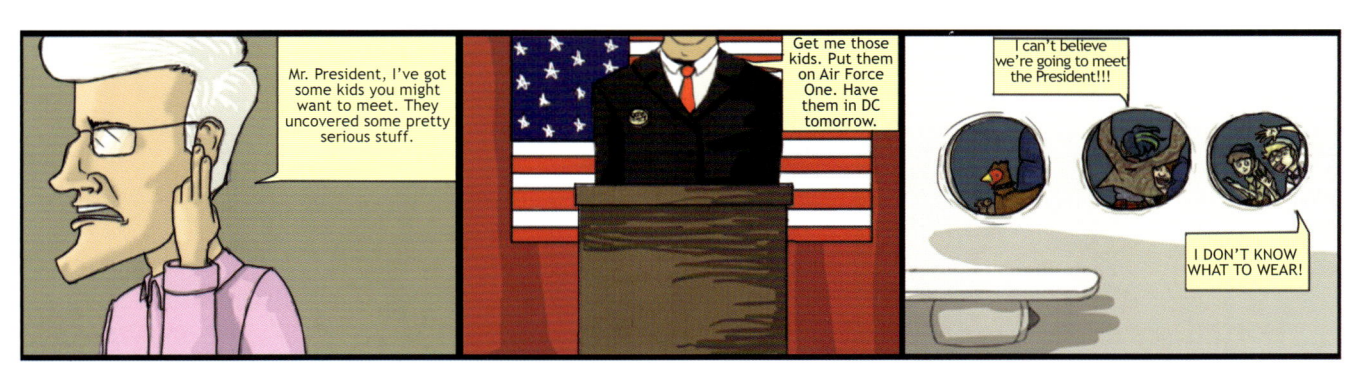

36 What is Healthy Food?

Does It Have to Be Organic?

Organic food is not available everywhere and can be more expensive than industrially grown food. Do your best to buy organic when you can.

Where to Put Your Money If You Can't Buy All Organic

Some foods have more pesticide residues than others. Use the tables on the right to help decide where organic is most important to reduce pesticide exposure. The list shows conventionally grown foods with the highest and lowest pesticide levels. Go to the Environmental Working Group's website (www.ewg.org) to learn more and download a pocket guide to keep in your wallet when you're shopping.

Other Ways to Reduce Pesticide Exposure:

- Trim outer portions of leafy vegetables and peel root vegetables.
- Wash all produce before eating.
- Buy produce grown in the U.S. that's regulated by the USDA.

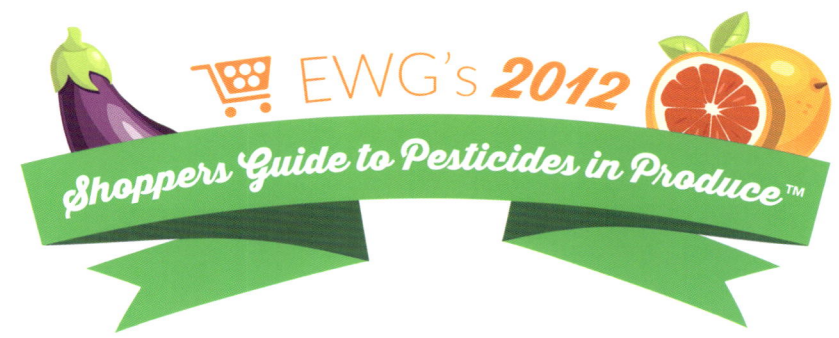

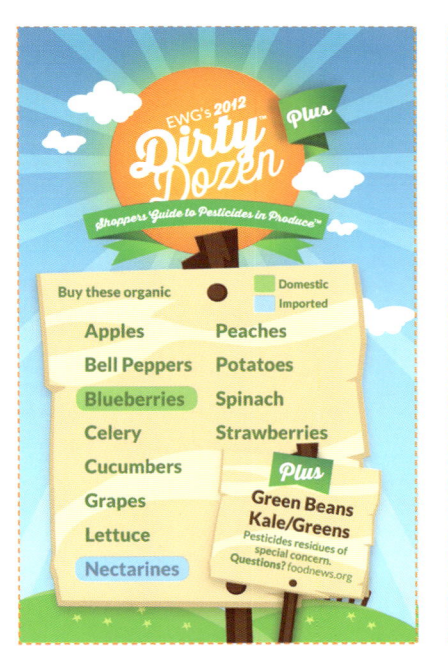

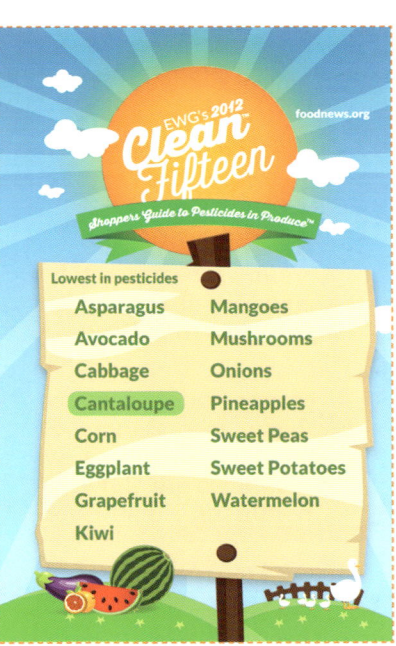

EWG's 2012 Shoppers Guide to Pesticides in Produce™

EWG's 2012 Dirty Dozen Plus — Buy these organic (Domestic / Imported):
- Apples
- Bell Peppers
- Blueberries
- Celery
- Cucumbers
- Grapes
- Lettuce
- Nectarines
- Peaches
- Potatoes
- Spinach
- Strawberries

Plus: Green Beans, Kale/Greens — Pesticides residues of special concern. Questions? foodnews.org

EWG's 2012 Clean Fifteen — Lowest in pesticides:
- Asparagus
- Avocado
- Cabbage
- Cantaloupe
- Corn
- Eggplant
- Grapefruit
- Kiwi
- Mangoes
- Mushrooms
- Onions
- Pineapples
- Sweet Peas
- Sweet Potatoes
- Watermelon

Copyright © Environmental Working Group, www.ewg.org
Reprinted with permission

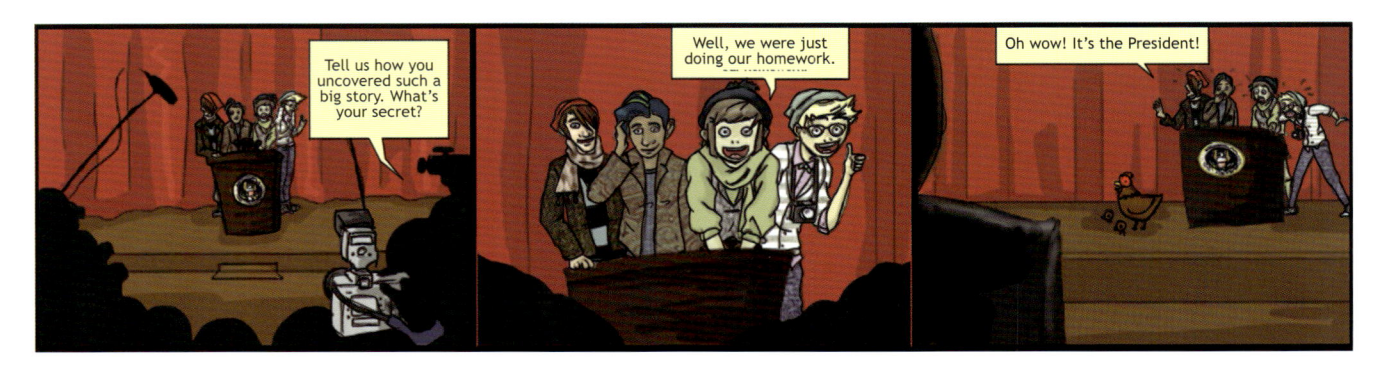

What is Healthy Food?

Genetically Modified (GMO) Food

GMOs are genetically modified organisms. This means the genetic code (DNA) in plants, animals or bacteria have been changed or mixed together. Genetic modifications allow big companies to profit from seed and pesticide sales. GMO seeds are more expensive for farmers and often require the use of specific pesticides manufactured by the company that produced the seeds.

Are GMOs safe? This is what we know:

- GMOs have not been proven to be safe for animals or humans.
- There is conflicting evidence as to whether GMOs can cause health problems, especially in children.
- GMOs increase the use of pesticides.
- Some GMO foods contain bacterial genes that create an insecticide inside the food itself. If the insecticide is in the food, you can't wash it off. You eat it!
- GMOs can cross pollinate with, and contaminate, non-GMO plants.

As products containing GMOs are not usually labeled in the U.S., the only way to guarantee their absence in your food is to buy USDA Organic or grow your own food from organic seeds.

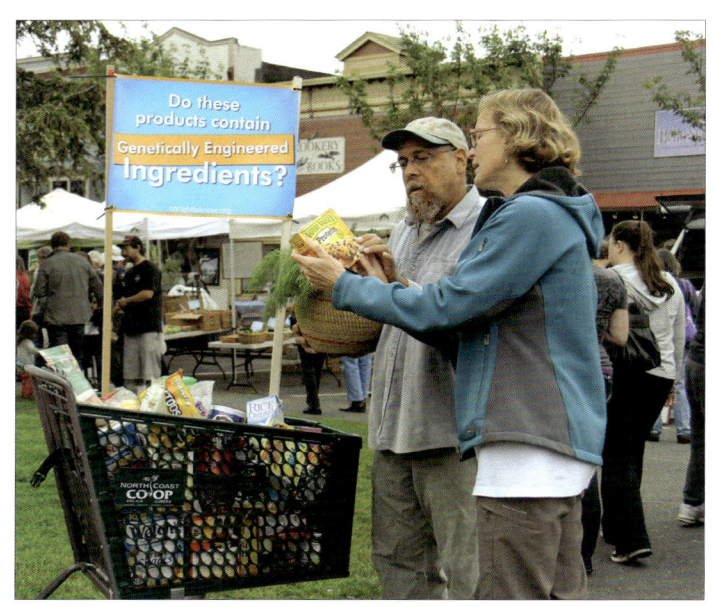

The most common GMO foods are...

- corn, cornstarch and corn syrup, including high-fructose corn syrup
- cottonseed and canola oils
- soy products
- beet sugar

These foods are also the most common ingredients in processed foods, including most snacks and sugary drinks. Most conventional (non-organic) processed foods contain GMOs. Avoiding processed food products will lower your exposure to GMO foods.

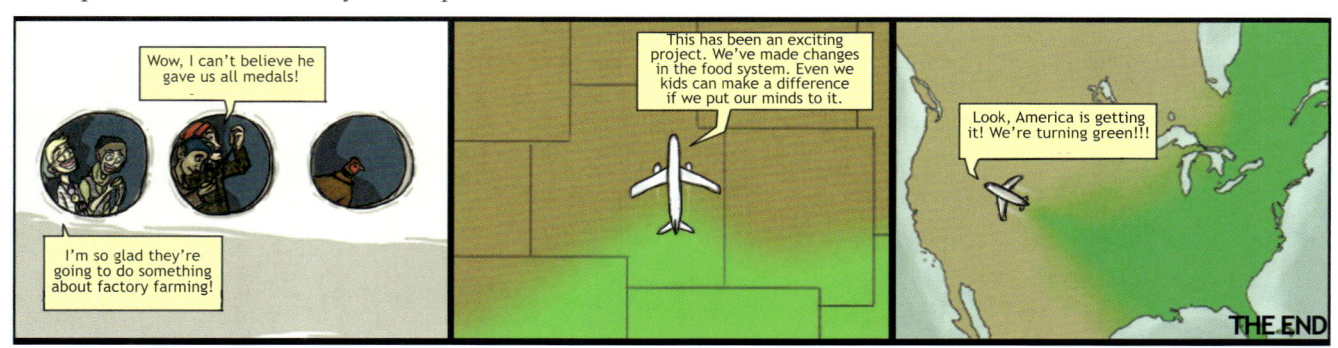

Chapter 4
Getting Started Cooking

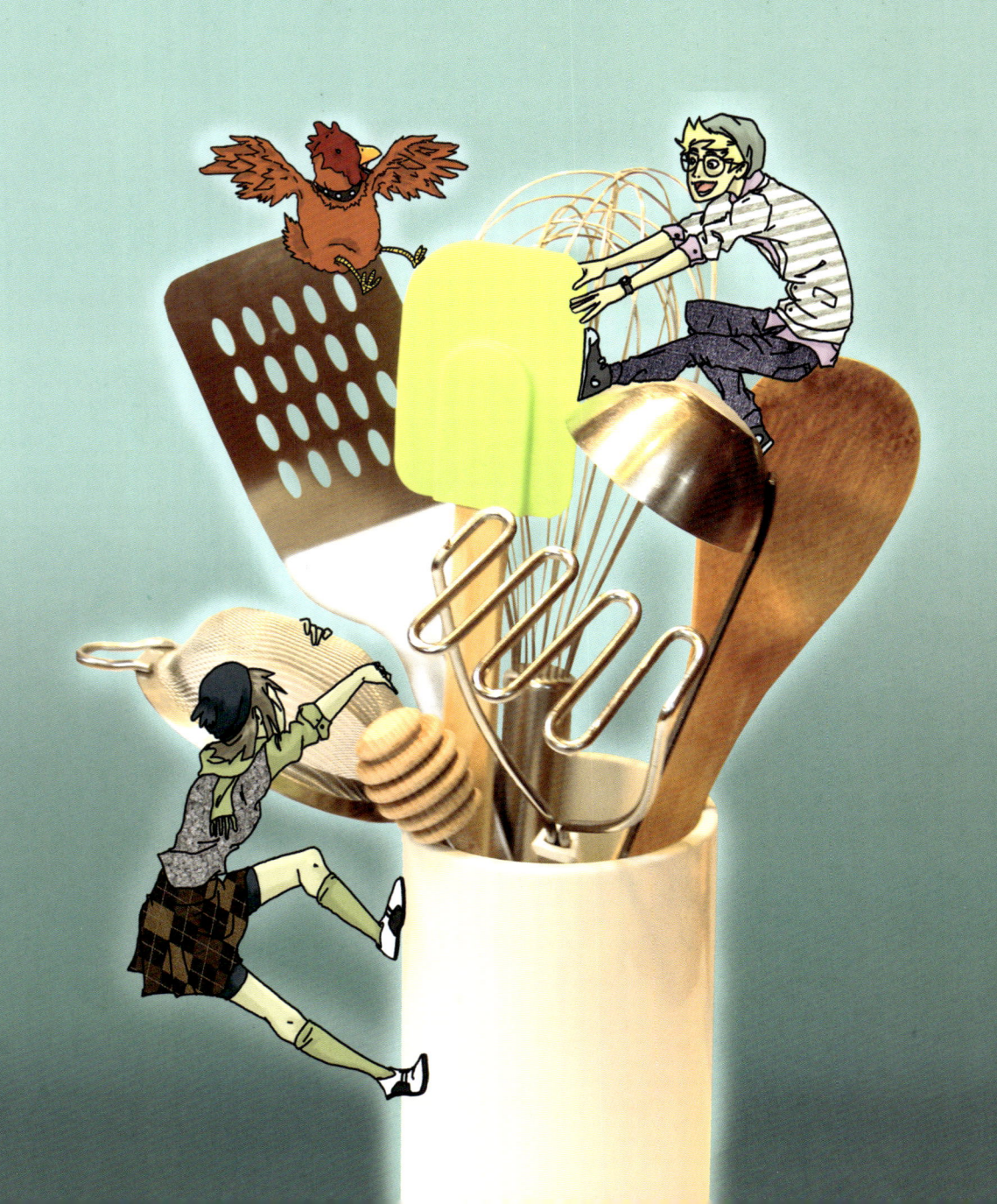

Why Cook?

Cooking is a satisfying experience. Planning your meals and budgeting your time makes it even more so. Although this book's focus is on preparing delicious, nutritious lunches, this chapter will help make cooking any meal easier. Directions for cooking basic foods such as rice, beans and pasta are at the beginning of the recipe chapter. (See pages 54-66.)

Using whole, nutritious foods and cooking from scratch will cost less and be healthier for you and your family.

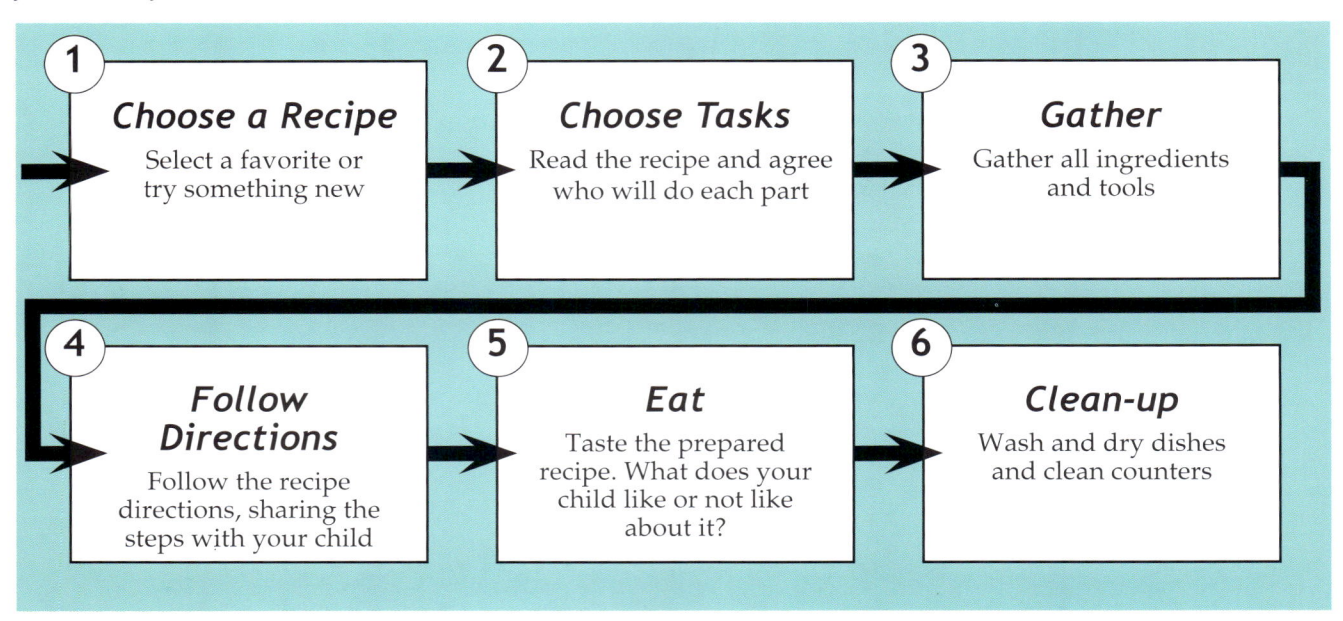

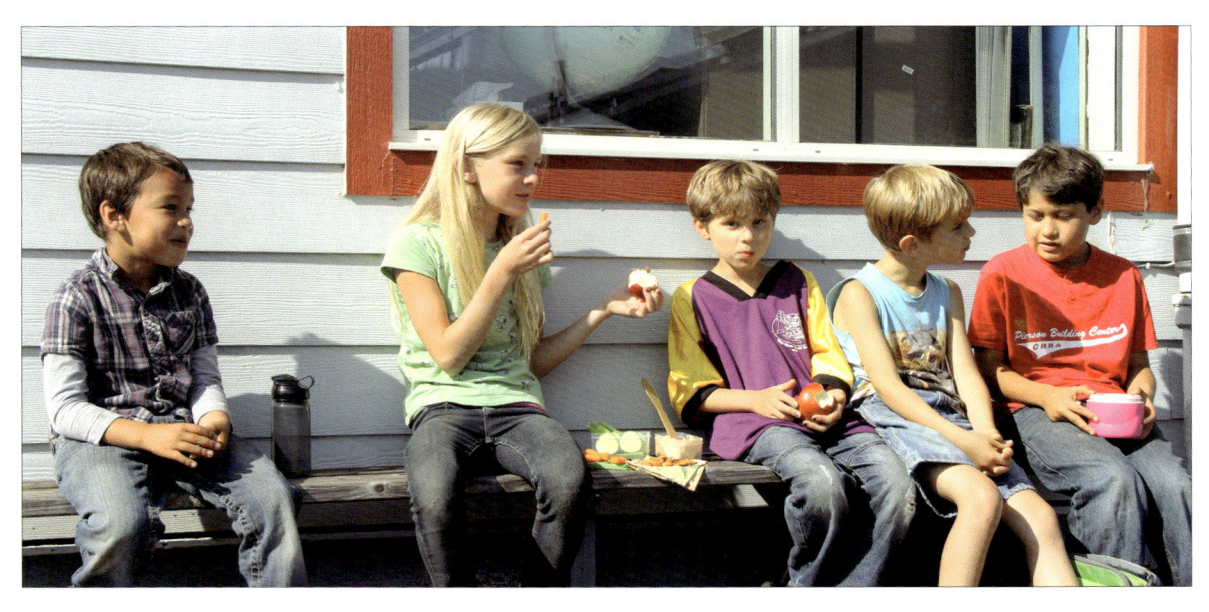

1. Choose a Recipe — Select a favorite or try something new

2. Choose Tasks — Read the recipe and agree who will do each part

3. Gather — Gather all ingredients and tools

4. Follow Directions — Follow the recipe directions, sharing the steps with your child

5. Eat — Taste the prepared recipe. What does your child like or not like about it?

6. Clean-up — Wash and dry dishes and clean counters

40 Getting Started Cooking

How Can Kids Help with Cooking?

When children help to plan and to cook, they are more likely to enjoy the results.

Recipes in Chapter 5 include icons showing the level of difficulty. If the small hand is filled in, the recipe is appropriate for children working by themselves. Recipes showing both a small hand and a big hand filled in require adult assistance until the child can handle a knife, electrical appliances and hot items. Recipes with the chef's hat filled in require an additional level of skill. The levels are explained in detail in the recipe chapter.

There are many ways that even the youngest child can help.

Getting Ready
- Help plan the menu
- Help shop
- Gather ingredients and tools

Prepare Ingredients
- Wash vegetables and fruit
- Peel vegetables and fruit
- Wash and dry lettuce
- Tear lettuce
- Toss a salad
- Measure ingredients (learn about fractions)

Help with Cooking
- Add and mix ingredients
- Knead dough
- Roll out dough
- Cut out cookies
- Oil pans and baking sheets
- Put cookies on a baking sheet
- Pour batter into baking dishes

Serve and Cleanup
- Wash utensils as meal is being prepared (except for knives and other sharp tools)
- Set table
- Clear table and wash dishes

As kids gain skills they can:
- Use a blender or food processor
- Chop and prepare more ingredients (see Kitchen Safety, page 43)
- Use the stove top to boil, sauté and fry
- Use the oven to bake

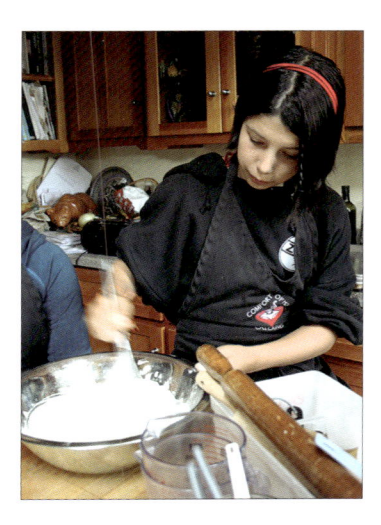

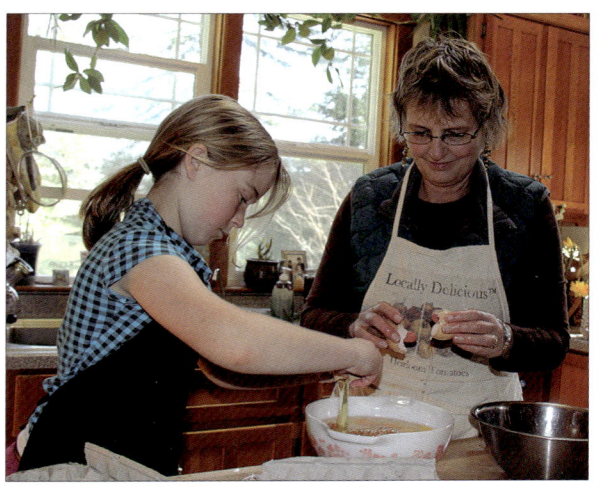

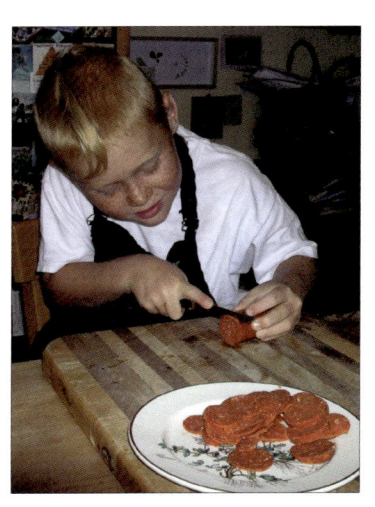

Getting Started Cooking 41

Kitchen Hygiene

Before you begin:
- Wash your hands. And wash them as often as needed during cooking.
- Tie back long hair.
- Wear an apron.

Keep It Clean
- Wash ALL produce before peeling, cutting or eating. Bacteria can linger on the skin of fruit and vegetables and be transported to the inside of the food when it's cut or peeled.
- Keep all surfaces, cutting boards and utensils clean, to prevent food-borne illness.
- Put the sponge into the microwave for two minutes every day and replace it every two weeks. Sponges have the most bacteria of anything in the kitchen.

Handling Meat and Poultry
- Keep meat in refrigerator until ready to use.
- Use separate cutting boards for meat and vegetables.
- Wash hands after handling raw meat.
- Sanitize all surfaces with a mild bleach solution after contact with meat or fish, and particularly after contact with poultry. Use 1½ teaspoons of bleach in 2 cups of water.

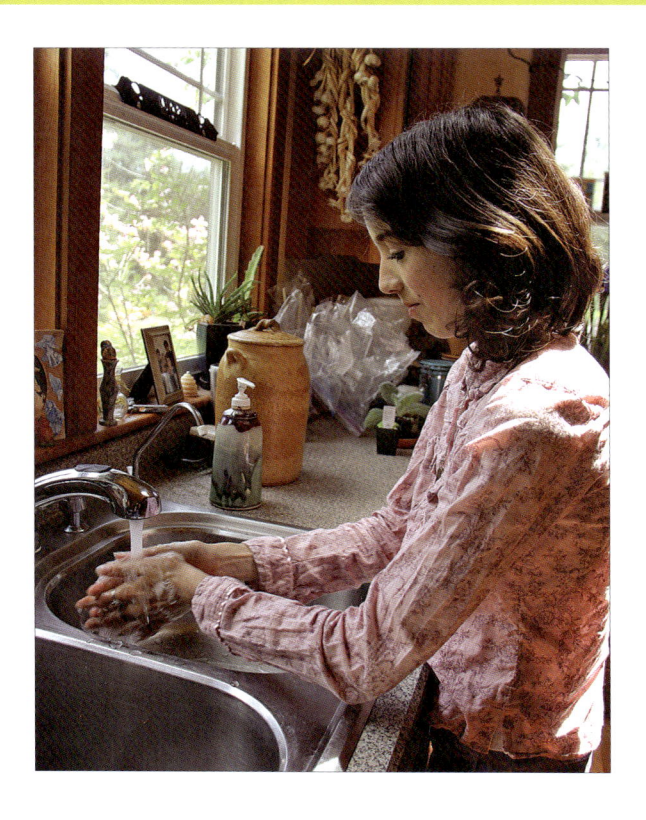

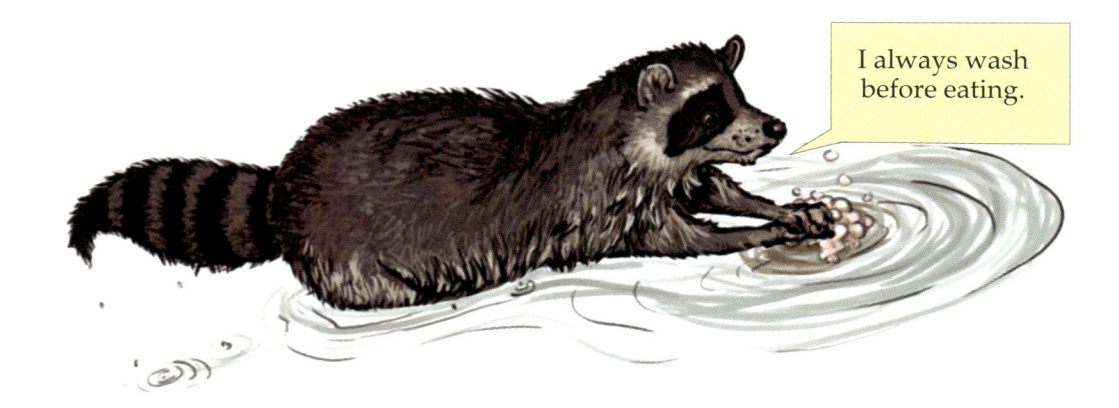

I always wash before eating.

Kitchen Safety

Knife Safety

- Keep knives sharp—a sharp knife is easier to use and safer than a dull one.
- Always use a cutting board.
- Use a knife that fits your hands.
- Hold the knife by the handle (not the blade).
- Always point the knife away from you.
- Hold the item you are cutting with your other hand.
- If the item to be cut is round, cut it in half or cut a little bit from one edge so that it lies flat.
- Curl your fingers under so they don't get cut.

Other Safety Tips

- Have pot holders by the stove.
- Use a dry pot holder to pick up hot pots or pans. A wet one will transmit the heat to your hand and burn!
- If a child is too short to reach the sink or counter, have them stand on a sturdy stool or a chair (with its back against the counter).
- When cooking on a stove top, turn pot handles toward the side of the stove (and not over a hot burner) so you don't accidentally knock the pot off the stove.
- Make sure your hands are dry when you plug or unplug an electrical appliance.

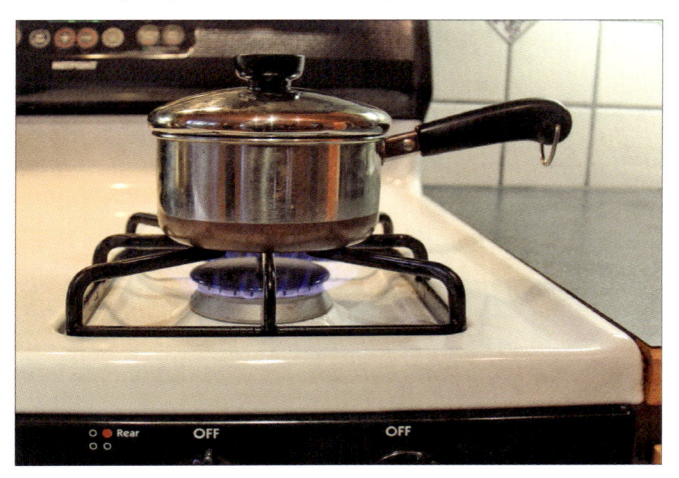

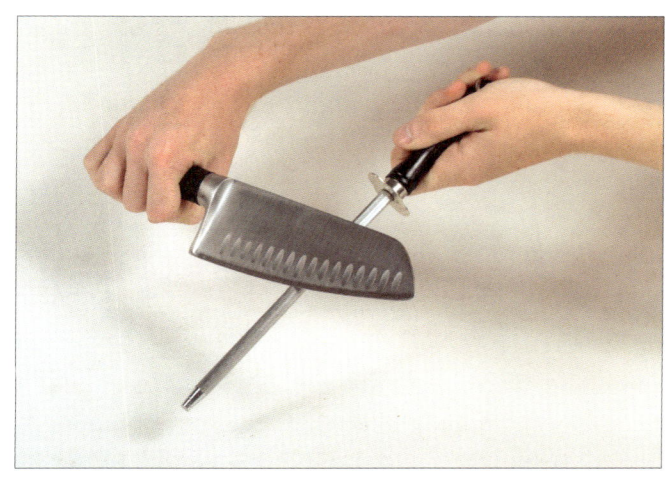

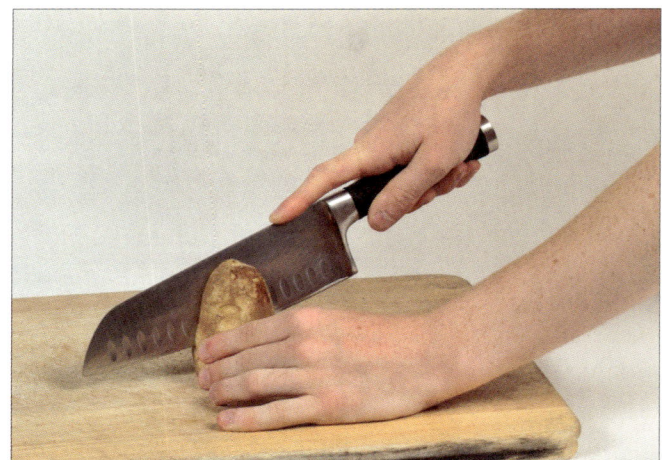

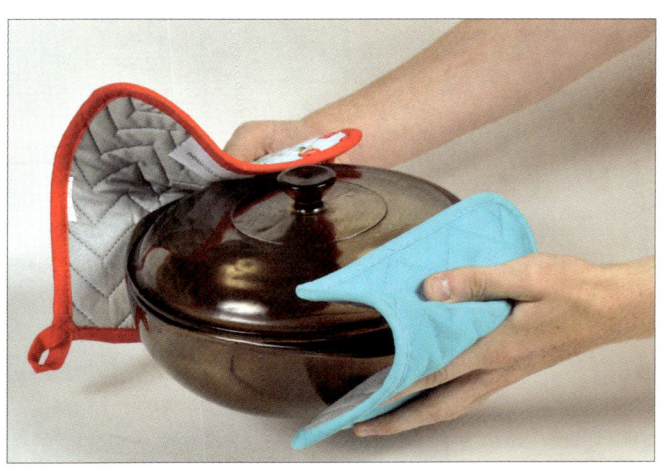

Techniques for Preparing the Ingredients

Knowledge of simple food preparation and cooking techniques is important. Special tools make many techniques easier. Food processors chop, slice, grate and shred. Blenders are useful for soups and smoothies.

Slice

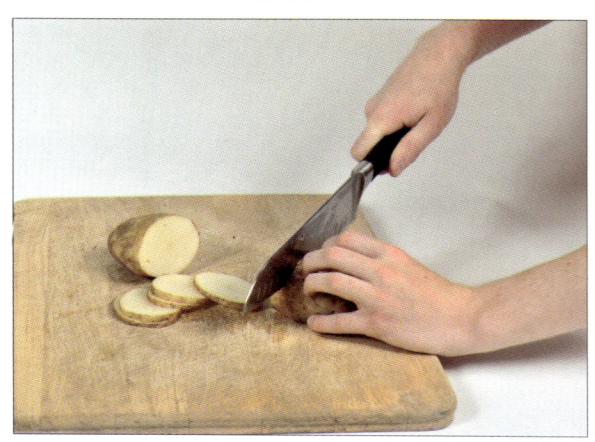

To cut across food in one direction. For larger round objects, it is easier to cut food in half, turn the flat side down, and then slice.

Chop

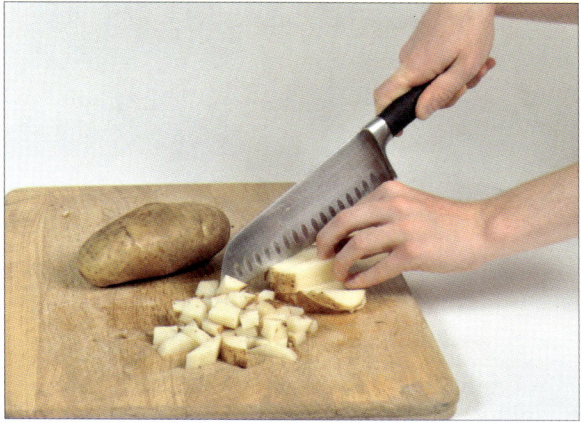

To cut food into approximately equal-sized pieces. Cut in one direction, then crosscut. When foods such as lettuce or cabbage are chopped, it is often called **shredded**. Food chopped into very small pieces is called **diced,** or into tiny pieces it's called **minced.**

Pare or Peel

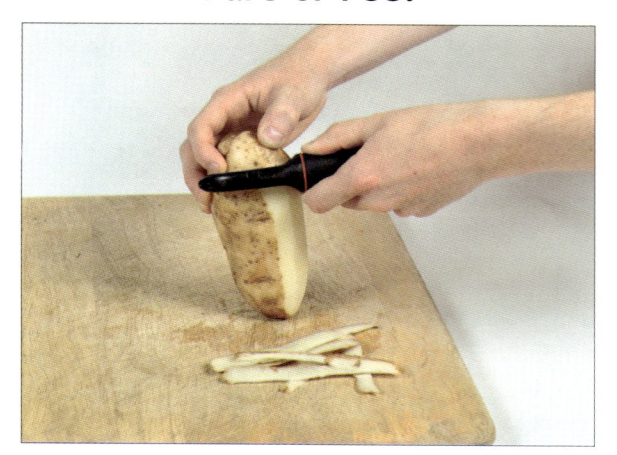

To remove the skin from fruit or vegetable. Do this with a vegetable peeler, moving it away from you.

Grate

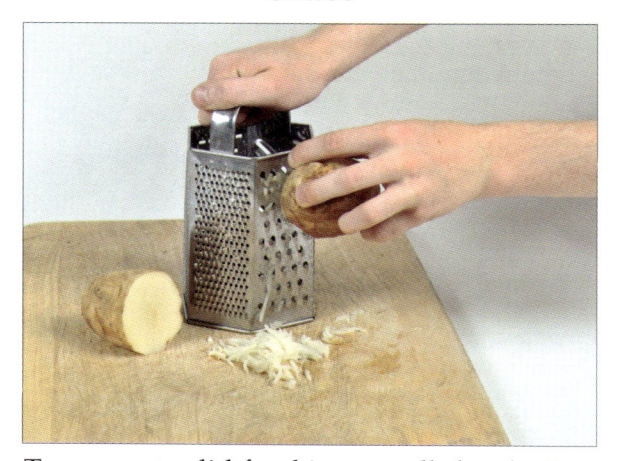

To convert solid food into small shreds. Done with a grater or special food processor disks. Be careful not to scrape your knuckles and fingertips with the grater!

Techniques for Preparing the Ingredients

Whisk

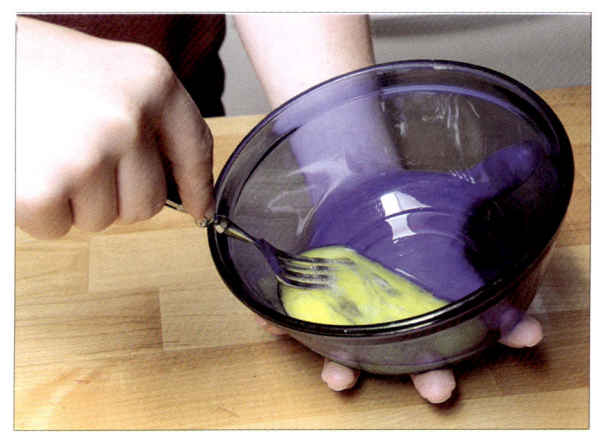

To lightly whip ingredients, using a round-and-round motion. Round whisks incorporate air into eggwhites or cream; flat whisks are used to stir sauces. A fork can also be used to whisk food.

Strain

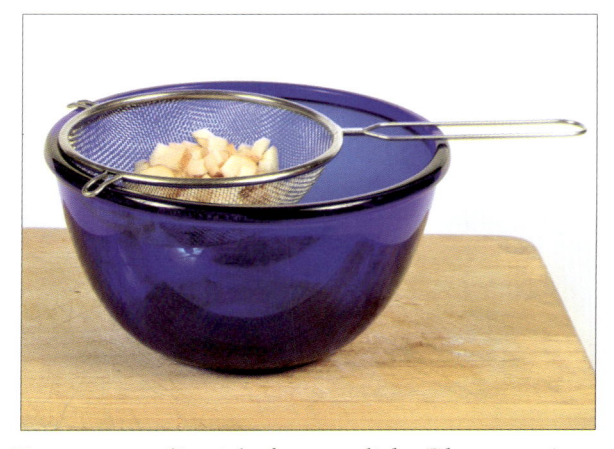

To separate liquids from solids. Place strainer over an empty bowl and pour mixture through the strainer. Sometimes the liquid is kept; sometimes the solids are kept. For larger foods like pasta, a colander is used.

Measure Dry Ingredients

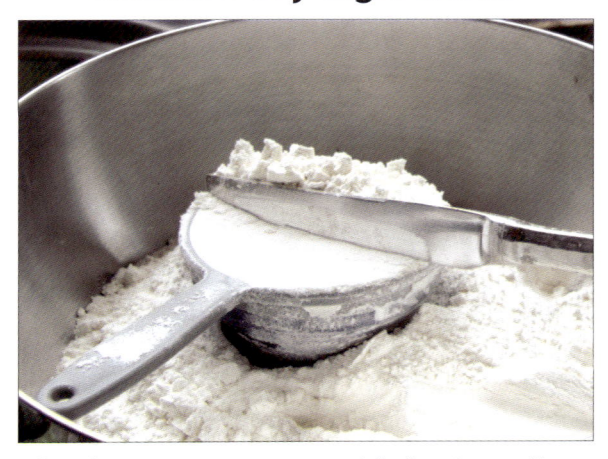

Fill a dry measuring cup with dry ingredient; slide a straight, flat utensil across the top to level. Do not pack (Note: you **do** have to pack brown sugar).

Measure Wet Ingredients

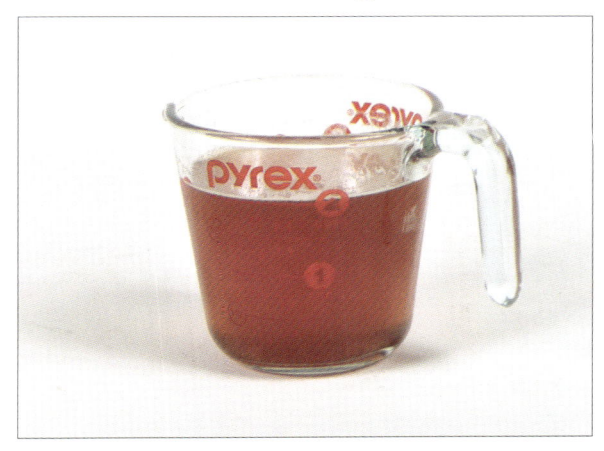

Set a glass measuring cup on counter and fill to the desired level. Hold the cup at eye level and look across the cup to get an accurate measure.

Cooking Techniques

Steam

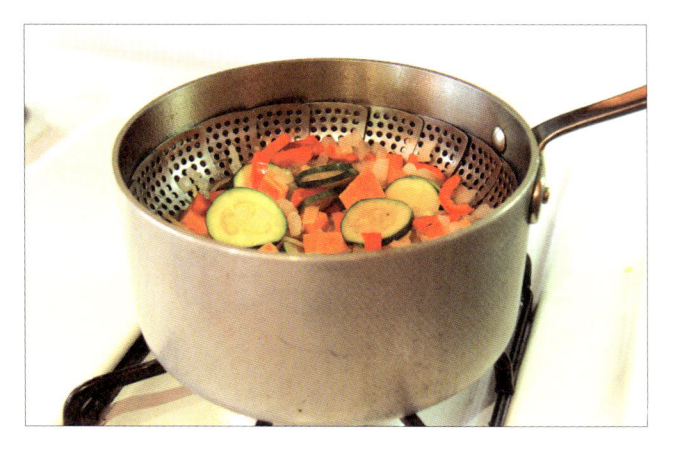

To cook food in a perforated container over a small amount of steaming water. The pot must have a lid to keep in steam. Inexpensive steamer baskets fit into different sized pots.

Sauté

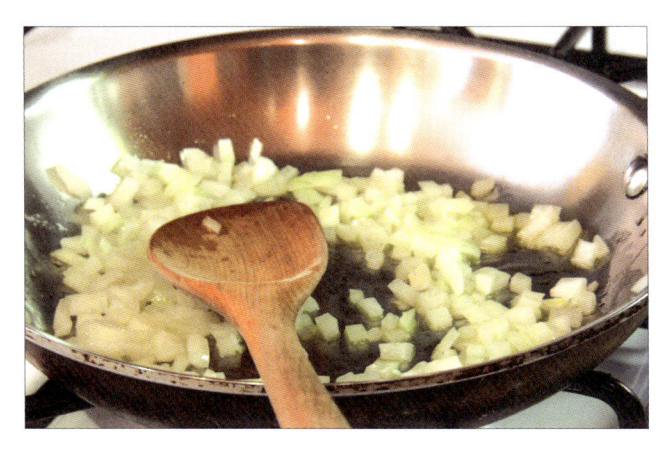

To cook food in a small amount of butter or oil in a skillet.

Simmer

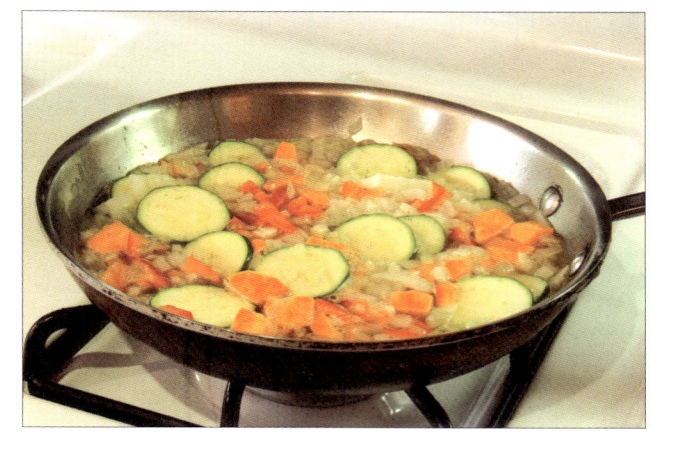

To cook ingredients in liquid over a low heat. The mixture will show slight bubbling.

Boil

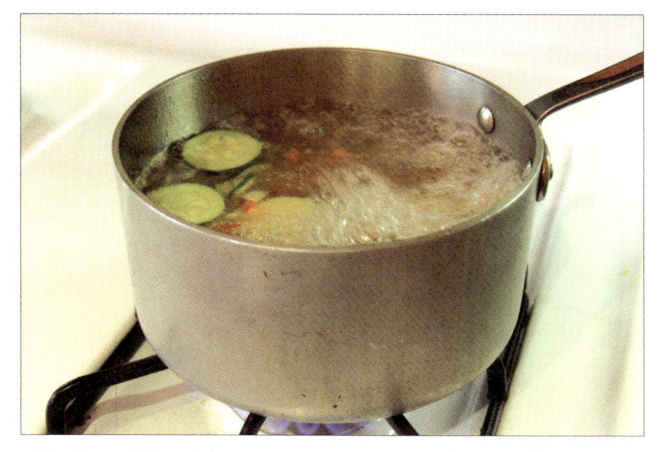

To heat liquid on a stove top or in a microwave oven until it is vigorously bubbling.

Basic Ingredients

Cooking is easier if the kitchen is stocked with basic ingredients and tools.

Staples	Sauces, Oils and Condiments	Baking Ingredients	Dried Herbs and Spices*	Dairy & Eggs
Salt	Olive oil	All-purpose flour	Allspice	Butter
Pepper	Vegetable oil	Whole wheat flour	Basil	Cheese
White sugar	Sesame oil	Baking soda	Bay leaf	Milk
Brown sugar	Vinegar	Baking powder	Chile flakes	Eggs
Bread crumbs	Soy sauce	Baker's yeast	Chile powder	
Rice	Mayonnaise	Vanilla extract	Cinnamon	
Beans	Ketchup		Cumin	
Pasta	Mustard		Ginger	
Peanut butter	Jam or jelly		Nutmeg	
Raisins			Oregano	
Nuts			Parsley	
Tuna, canned			Sage	
Tomatoes, canned			Thyme	
Soup broth or stock			Turmeric	
Garlic				
Onions				

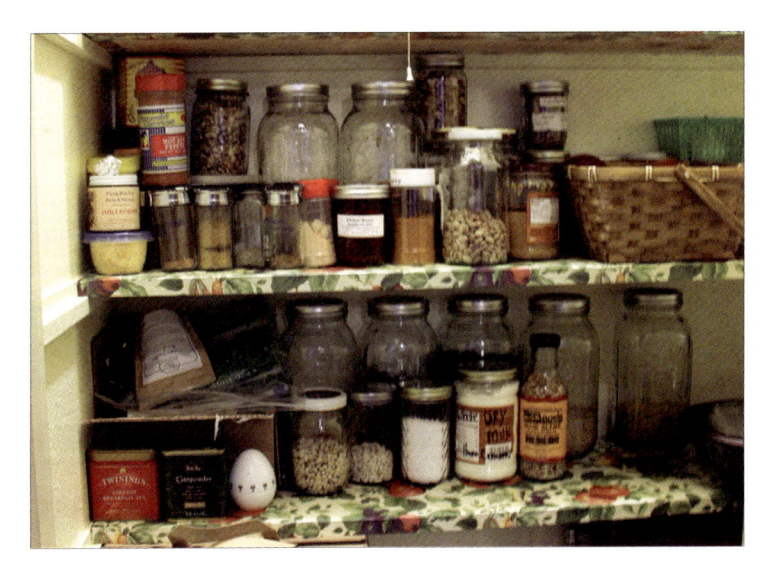

*Instead of buying packages of spice mixes such as taco seasoning, make your own. Buy from bulk bins if possible—the spices are usually fresher. See the spice mixes for Cajun, Mexican, Chinese, Indian, Italian and Thai, page 193.

Getting Started Cooking 47

Basic Cooking Tools

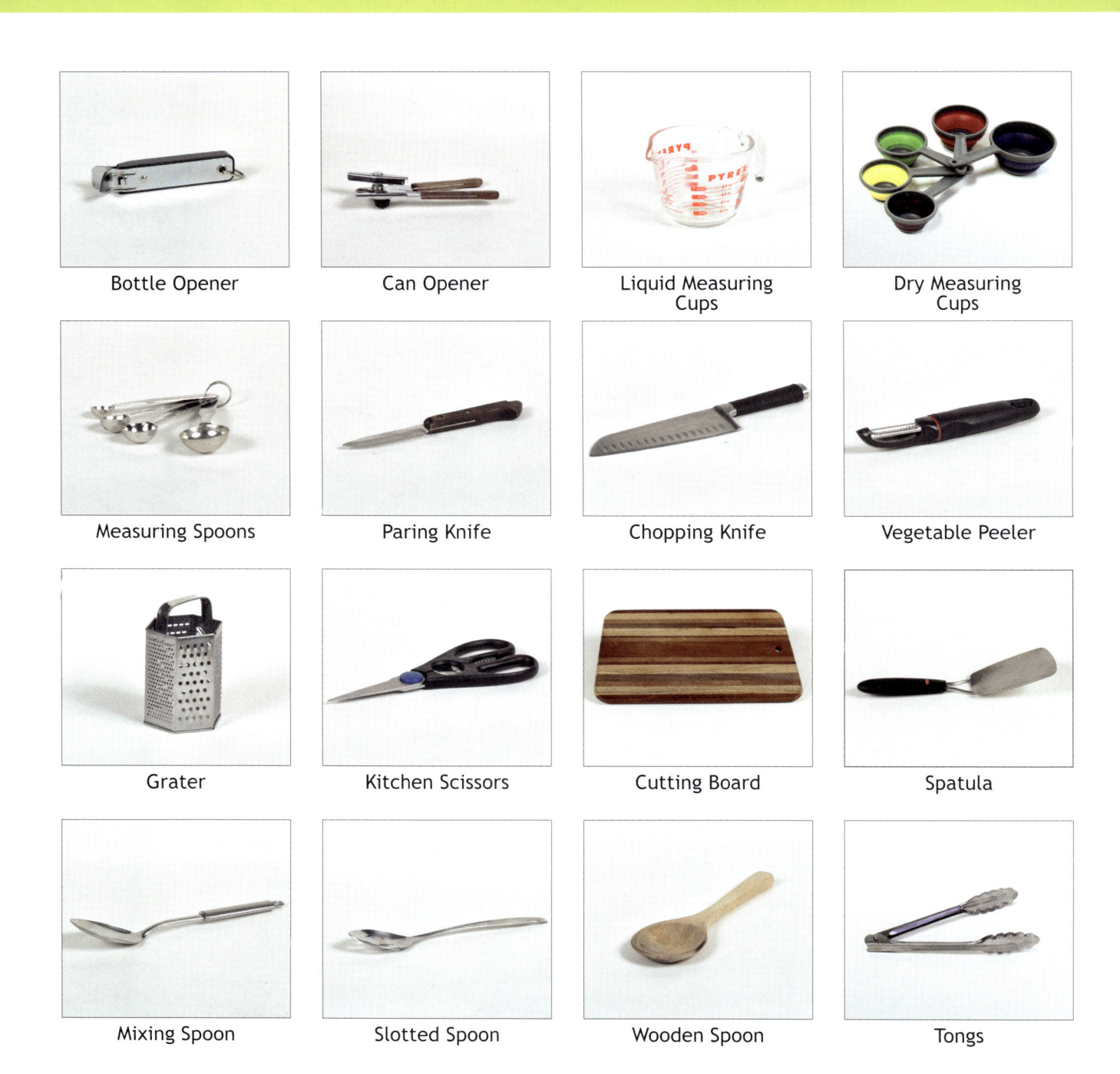

Bottle Opener	Can Opener	Liquid Measuring Cups	Dry Measuring Cups
Measuring Spoons	Paring Knife	Chopping Knife	Vegetable Peeler
Grater	Kitchen Scissors	Cutting Board	Spatula
Mixing Spoon	Slotted Spoon	Wooden Spoon	Tongs

Basic Cooking Tools

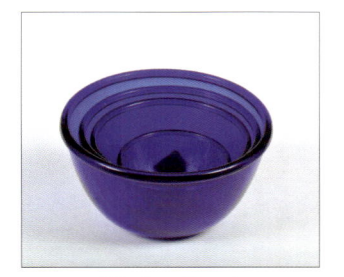

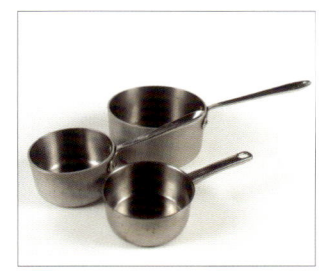

Mixing Bowl	1, 2 and 3-quart Saucepans	8 and 12-inch Frying Pans	10-quart Soup Pot
Steamer	Colander	Strainer with Handle	Loaf Pan
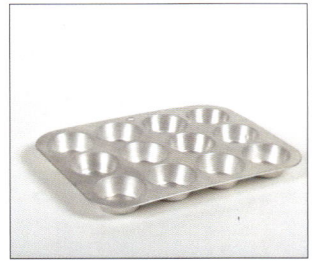 Muffin Tin	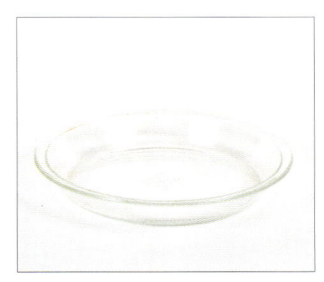 Pie Pan	Covered Baking Dish	9 x 13-inch Baking Pan
8 or 9-inch Square Baking Dish	Rimmed Baking Sheet	Meat Thermometer	Pot Holders

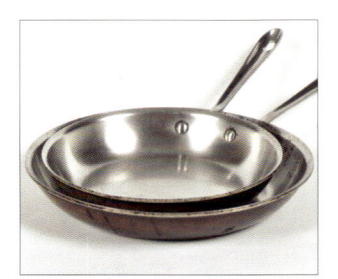

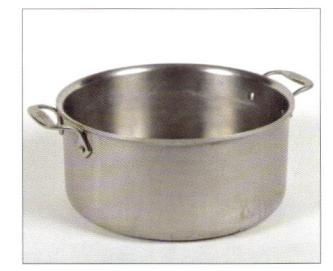

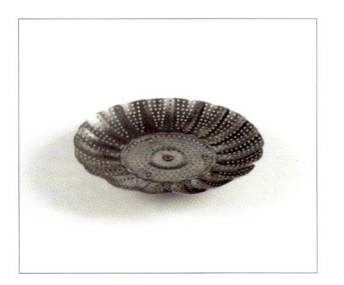

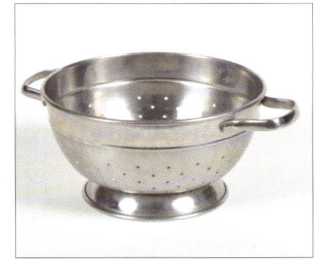

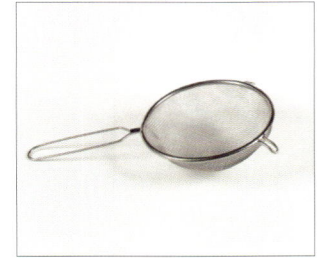

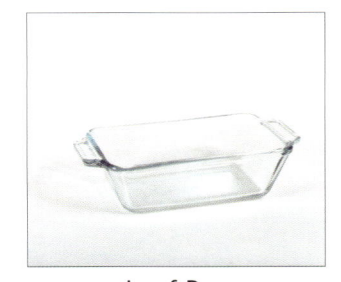

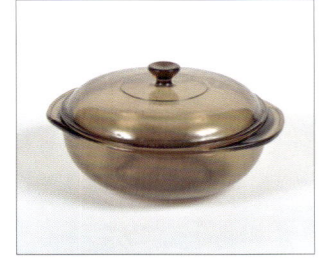

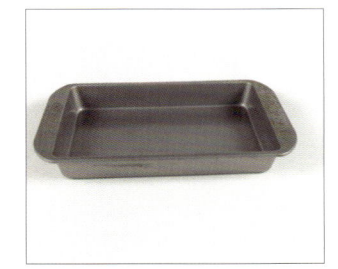

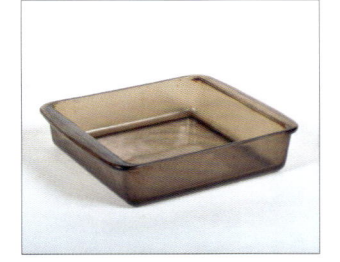

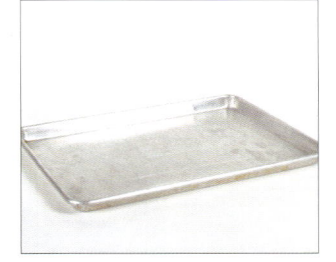

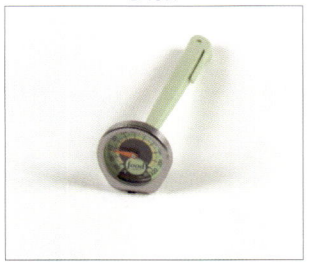

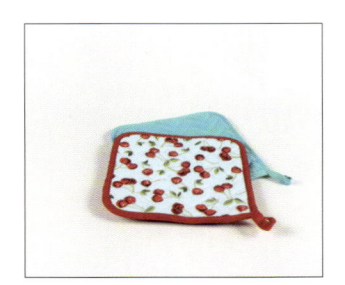

Getting Started Cooking 49

Nice-to-Have Tools

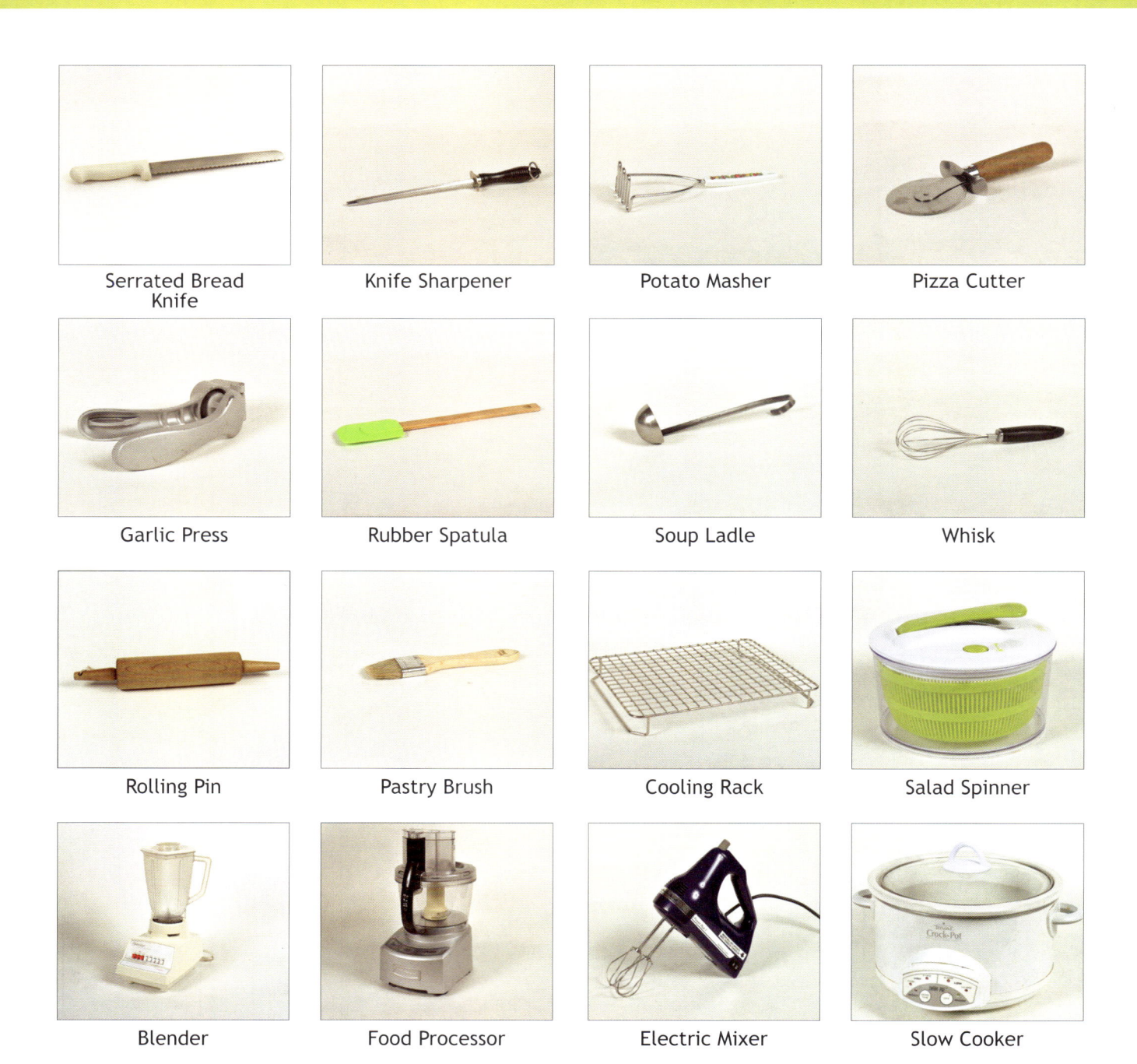

Serrated Bread Knife	Knife Sharpener	Potato Masher	Pizza Cutter
Garlic Press	Rubber Spatula	Soup Ladle	Whisk
Rolling Pin	Pastry Brush	Cooling Rack	Salad Spinner
Blender	Food Processor	Electric Mixer	Slow Cooker

Chapter 5
Recipes

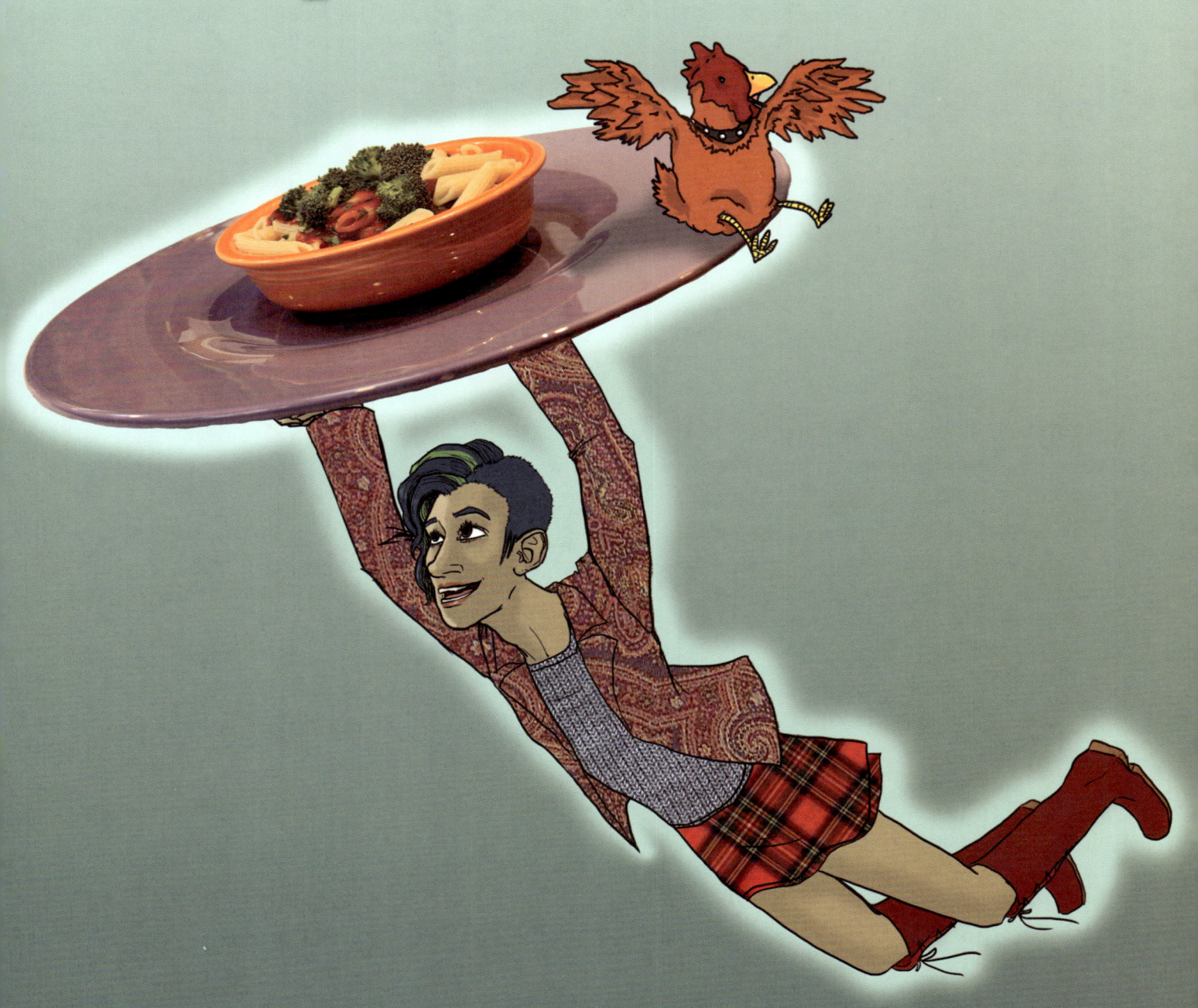

Introduction

Some cooks consider a recipe to be a suggestion; others look at it as the final word. We think of recipes as a starting point. All recipes can be modified to personal taste, seasonality of ingredients, and/or cost and availability of food. *LunchBox Envy* points you in the right direction and you can fill in the gaps. Keep it simple and easy or make it more challenging. The choice is yours.

Recipes are split into **The Main Dish**, **Vegetables**, **Fruits**, **Drinks**, **Treats and Snacks**, and **Dips and Spreads**. All sections after the **Basics** start with a helpful list of lunch components that need little to no preparation. These are quick, healthy items; great for packing in the lunchbox when you are in a rush.

Basics (pages 54 to 66) are foods, such as rice or pasta, that form the base of many of our recipes. Save time by making a double or triple batch of all these ingredients, then freeze them or have them available in the refrigerator for the week. Plan meals around the basics you have already prepared. Most foods are good for a week in the refrigerator or 3 months in the freezer.

Formulas and Recipes

Most sections start with a Formula, which allows a recipe to be adaptable. They are ideas and starting points. Don't limit yourself to the few ingredients we've decided to include. Formulas are guidelines, while recipes are specific instructions.

Skill Level Icons

Recipes have three skill levels, as indicated by the icons below the recipe title. Regardless of age, anyone can be at any level. Just because the recipe has a chef's hat, doesn't mean a beginner can't participate. See page 53.

Freezing Icon

The Freezing icon is to the right of the Skill Level icons. It shows that finished food can be frozen for later use.

MyPlate Icons

MyPlate icons are to the right of the Freezing icon. These show the MyPlate food groups (see page 4).

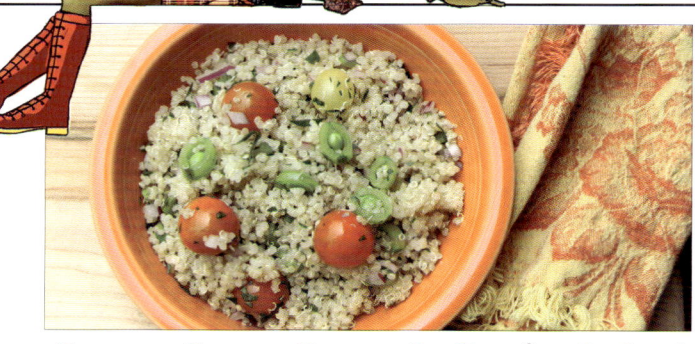

Sugar Snap Peas & Grain Salad

6 servings

Sugar snap peas give a delightful crunch to this salad and little tomatoes add color and sweetness. This salad holds well in the refrigerator for a couple of days.

Salad
- 3 cups cooked pasta, quinoa, or rice
- 2 cups sugar snap peas, cut crosswise
- 1 cup cherry tomatoes
- ½ cup fresh parsley, chopped or (2½ tablespoons dried)
- ¼ medium red onion, chopped (about ¼ cup)

Dressing
- 2 tablespoons olive oil
- 2 tablespoons lemon juice
- ¾ teaspoon salt
- ¼ teaspoon pepper

1. Prepare vegetables. Cook pasta (see page 57), quinoa, or rice (see page 56).
2. Mix dressing ingredients together in a small bowl, or shake in a covered jar. Taste and adjust seasonings.
3. Drizzle dressing on salad; mix well.
4. Refrigerate for one hour before serving.

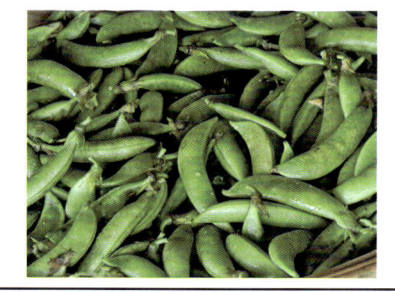

Skill Levels

Levels are based on the following skills:

Beginning
- Pour
- Measure
- Spread
- Mix
- Tear leafy vegetables
- Open cans (be careful of sharp edges)
- Rinse
- Crumble
- Peel with a vegetable peeler
- Easy slicing and chopping such as bananas, cucumbers, summer squash, celery and potatoes

Intermediate
- Pre-cook basic ingredients such as grains, rice, potatoes, beans
- Perform more difficult slicing and chopping tasks, such as onions, cabbage, tomatoes, grapes and citrus
- Peel with a knife
- Grate
- Roll dough
- Use heat—ovens, microwave, toaster oven, stove top
- Handle hot dishes with potholders
- Use blender or food processor
- Use meat thermometer

Challenge Yourself
- Requires sustained attention
- Stir while adding new ingredients
- Bread-making skills—kneading, tucking, folding
- Making more complicated recipes

Mixing Levels - Working Together

Two cooks of different levels working together make cooking easier, faster, and way more fun.

Steps that are for advanced cooks can be done ahead of time, then beginners can attempt the easier steps by themselves. Supervised beginners can complete many intermediate-level recipes all the way up until using the stove or oven.

Basic ingredients (see pages 54-66) that are used as bases can be precooked and saved in the refrigerator or freezer.

Chopped items needing more advanced knife skills (see page 43) can be prepped and stored in the refrigerator.

And of course, the best way to move a beginning cook up a level is to have a more advanced cook supervise while the beginner tries things never before attempted.

Measurements

Dry
Dash = ⅛ teaspoon or less
3 teaspoons = 1 tablespoon
2 tablespoons = ⅛ cup
4 tablespoons = ¼ cup
8 tablespoons = ½ cup
5 tablespoons + 1 teaspoon = ⅓ cup
16 tablespoons = 1 cup
16 ounces = 1 pound

Liquids
1 fluid ounce = 2 tablespoons liquid
8 fluid ounces = 1 cup
2 cups = 1 pint
2 pints = 1 quart
4 quarts = 1 gallon

Cooking Beans

Yield: 2-2½ cups

Beans are the cheapest source of healthy, environmentally responsible protein in the world. Cooking dry beans rather than using canned requires planning, but it saves money, reduces sodium intake and reduces waste. All beans except lentils, split peas and mung beans need soaking first.

    1   cup dry beans
    3-4 cups water for cooking

1. Place beans in a strainer or colander. Remove shriveled beans and small stones. Rinse in cold water.
2. To soak beans:
   - For overnight soak, put rinsed beans in a large pot, cover with two inches of water, and let sit 8 hours or more.
   - For a shorter soak, cover beans with 1-2 inches water and boil for one minute. Turn off the heat, cover, and let sit for at least one hour. To check if the beans have soaked long enough, cut a bean in half. If the center is hard and milky looking, soak beans longer.
3. Drain off the soaking liquid. This liquid contains the starches that give you gas.
4. Add fresh water to about 1 inch above the beans. Do not add salt. Bring to a boil and cook about 15 minutes. Reduce heat to medium-low, cover pot, and simmer until the beans are as soft as you want them (up to 3 hours). Drain off water. Beware: Undercooked beans are harder for the body to digest and cause flatulence (farts). Beans are fully cooked when you can mash them easily with a fork.

Options:
- Use beans immediately or let cool before storing. Store cooled beans in an airtight container in the refrigerator up to 5 days.
- Make a double or triple batch. Scoop beans into freezer-safe containers in 1-2 cup portions with enough liquid to cover beans. Store in freezer up to 3 months, after which they will lose flavor and get mushy.

Reducing Bean Farts

Beans are infamous for their ability to cause our bodies to make gross sounds and smells. Many people aren't affected, but this information is for those who are.

Yogurt or kefir, which contain active probiotics (beneficial bacteria), aid in digestion when eaten along with the beans.

When using **canned beans**, rinse them multiple times.

Although pouring off the soaking liquid helps reduce gas, it also gets rid of many nutrients.

When cooking dry beans:

- Add any of the following herbs to the cooking water, as they help reduce gas: cumin, coriander, caraway, turmeric, epazote (found at most Latino supermarkets) and kombu (found at many Asian markets).
- Cook beans slowly over low heat for a long time—4 to 5 hours. Slow cookers are great tools for this.

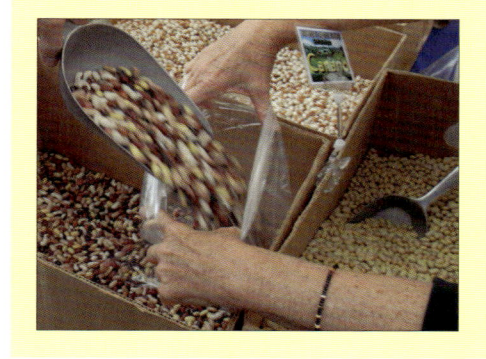

54 Basic Recipes

Scrambled and Hard-cooked Eggs

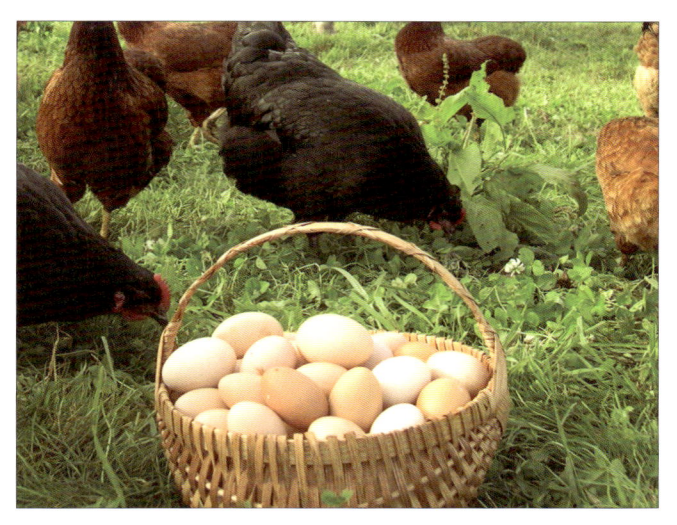

Eggs are a versatile, inexpensive and healthy protein. Scrambled eggs are common to many Asian-inspired lunches, such as Fried Rice (see page 95) or Sushi (see page 80). Whole hard-cooked eggs are great in lunches.

Egg safety: Cook eggs thoroughly, which kills bacteria such as salmonella. Eggs from pasture-raised chickens (see page 31) are less likely to be contaminated with salmonella than factory-farmed eggs.

Suggestion: Hardcook many eggs at a time. Save them in the refrigerator for up to a week.

For Scrambled Eggs:

1. Tap eggs on side of a bowl, then carefully pull the shell apart over the bowl. Whisk with a fork until the white and yolk are combined. Tip: Eggshell sticks to itself. Use a larger shell piece to remove unwanted bits.

2. Heat enough butter at medium heat to coat a skillet. When butter is melted, pour in the eggs.

3. Lower the heat and stir the eggs gently until they're firm but still moist.

Options:

- Make your eggs fluffier by adding a tablespoon of milk or water per egg.

For Hard-cooked Eggs:

1. Choose eggs that are several days old; they are easier to peel.

2. Place eggs in cold water and bring water to a full boil. Turn off heat, cover pot with lid, and leave for 10 minutes.

3. Pour off boiling water. Cover with cold water to stop internal cooking of the eggs. Let cool.

4. Store eggs with the shell on. Mark "H" on the shell to tell hard-cooked apart from raw eggs.

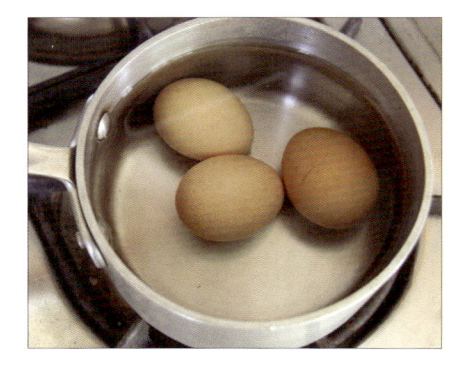

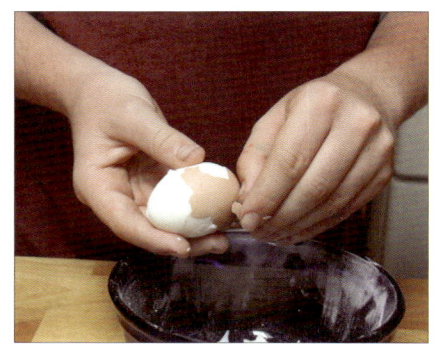

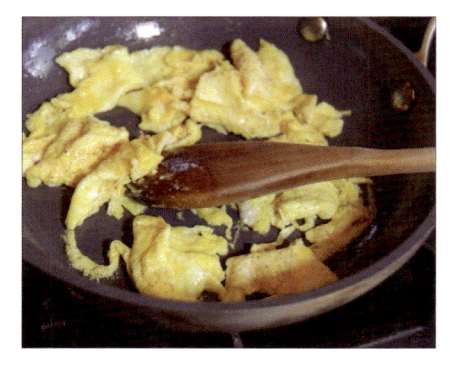

Basic Recipes 55

Rice and Quinoa

Yield: 2 cups cooked rice or quinoa

White rice has been milled; brown rice is the whole rice grain with nothing milled out. Check the bulk bin label or package for specific cooking directions.

Quinoa (pronounced "KEEN-wah") is a seed from the Andes Mountains. It has a higher protein content than any grain. It is a delicious healthy substitute for rice and other grains in many dishes.

Different varieties of rice have slightly different cooking times and yields. Rice and quinoa are forgiving. If you get to the end of the cooking time and the rice isn't cooked, add some more water and cook for a few more minutes.

- 1 cup white rice or quinoa
- 2 cups water

or

- 1 cup brown rice
- 3 cups water

1. Rinse and drain rice or quinoa, to eliminate starch from rice or to remove bitter saponin (outer layer) from quinoa.

2. Add quinoa or rice to a pot with the water. Bring to a rolling boil, reduce heat to low and cover.

3. Simmer 15-20 minutes for white rice or quinoa. Brown rice takes longer, 40-50 minutes. Leave pot covered and don't stir.

4. Check rice or quinoa and continue cooking, if necessary, until tender. Remove from heat. Fluff with a fork.

5. Use immediately or let cool and place in an airtight container. Store in refrigerator up to 3 days.

Options:

- For richer flavor, substitute broth for water.
- Sauté rice, onions or garlic in oil in the pot before adding water.
- Cook rice in the microwave in a covered glass or ceramic dish. Check your microwave instructions for cook time and power level, as microwaves differ.

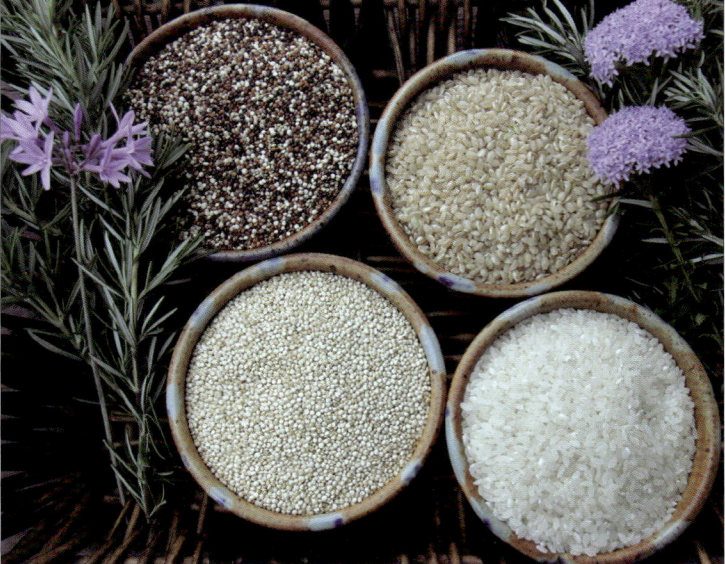

Brown Rice

Brown rice as a whole food is unmilled or partially milled rice that still has the outer layer on it. This outer layer contains healthy fats and vitamins.

Brown rice is nutty, chewier than white, takes a bit longer to cook and has more nutrients than white.

"Enriched" white rice is rice that has been milled and had some of the nutrients added back.

Noodles and Pasta

Yield: 2-3 cups cooked noodles

Cooking times vary for different types and shapes of noodles. Check the bulk bin label or package for specific cooking directions.

1 cup small noodles or pasta, or ¼ pound spaghetti

4 cups water (1 quart)

For Wheat Noodles (most pasta):

1. Bring water to a boil.

2. Pour noodles into the water carefully. Cook for the amount of time stated on package or taste test. Cook until tender, but firm. Drain into a strainer or a colander placed in the sink. Keep your face away from the steam.

3. To save pasta for later, mix in a teaspoon of cooking oil to keep it from sticking together, then let pasta cool to room temperature before storing.

For Rice Noodles:

1. Bring water to a boil and turn off heat.

2. Place noodles in water and let them sit until tender, or for time stated on package.

3. Drain water as above, but rinse immediately with cold water to keep noodles from sticking.

Noodles of the World

Noodles originated in China at least 4,000 years ago. Traders brought them to the Middle East and Europe. Noodles are made out of flour from ground grains or nuts.

"Pasta" is the Italian word for noodles.

Noodles can also be made of:

- wheat - couscous from Northern Africa

    (see Couscous with Peas, page 98)

- buckwheat - soba from Japan
- rice - rice vermicelli or "sticks" from Southeast Asia
- acorn - dotori guksu from Korea

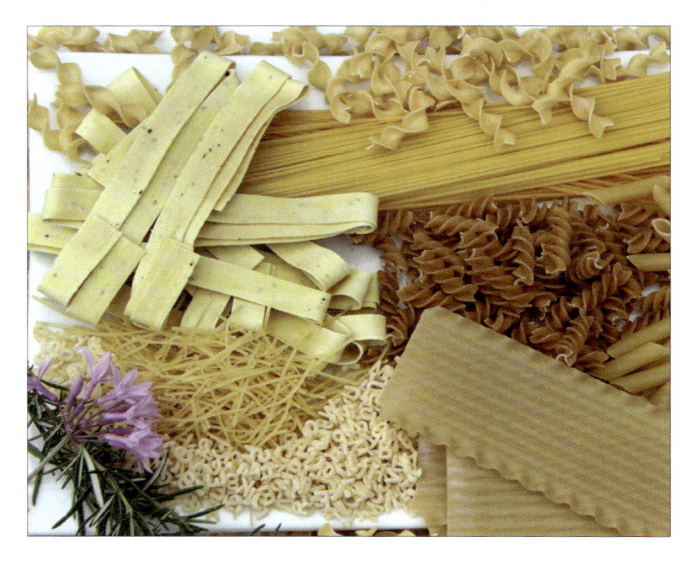

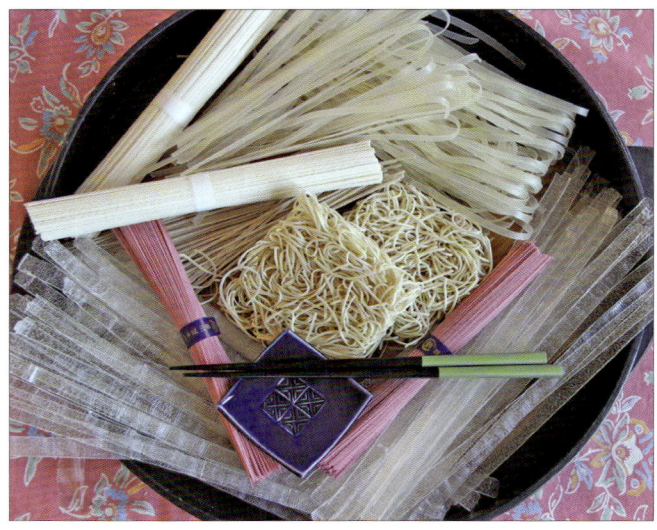

Basic Recipes 57

No-Knead Bread

Yield: 1 Loaf

The easiest homemade bread yet! Any lidded glass or metal oven-safe container will work, but Dutch ovens or enameled pots are best.

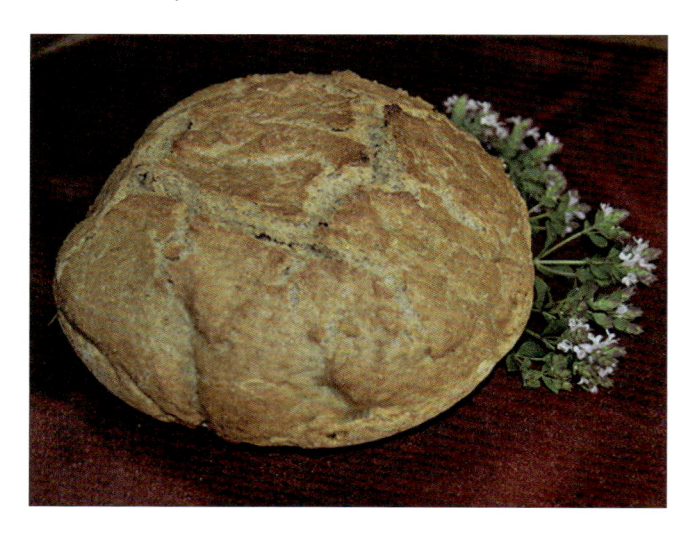

2	cups whole wheat flour
1	cup all-purpose flour
3	tablespoons dry yeast
1	teaspoon salt
1⅝	cup warm water
	Cornmeal

1. Combine flour, yeast and salt in a medium bowl. Add water and stir.

2. Cover bowl with plastic wrap and let sit at room temperature (about 70° is best) until dough has doubled in bulk, about 2 hours. Rising time depends on the temperature of the room.

Preheat oven to 400°

3. Put an oven-safe container with lid into oven and heat it for 30 minutes.

4. Carefully remove heated pot from oven. Sprinkle the bottom liberally with cornmeal.

5. Wet hands with cold water and scoop sticky dough out of bowl. Place carefully into hot pot.

6. Put lid back on, place pot in oven, and bake 30 minutes.

7. Remove lid and bake another 15 minutes.

8. Remove pot from oven. Remove bread and place on a rack to cool.

Options:

- At Step 1, add ½ cup of walnuts, raisins, grated cheese, and/or chopped onion.

Save Money

Save money by making your own high-quality bread. It'll cost about one-third the price of purchased bread of similar quality. The cost will be about $1.50 per loaf, compared to $4.50.

Buy yeast in the bulk department or in jars. The price of individual yeast packages is high.

Only about 10-15 minutes are required to prepare the dough. The dough needs about 2 hours for rising and 45 minutes for baking.

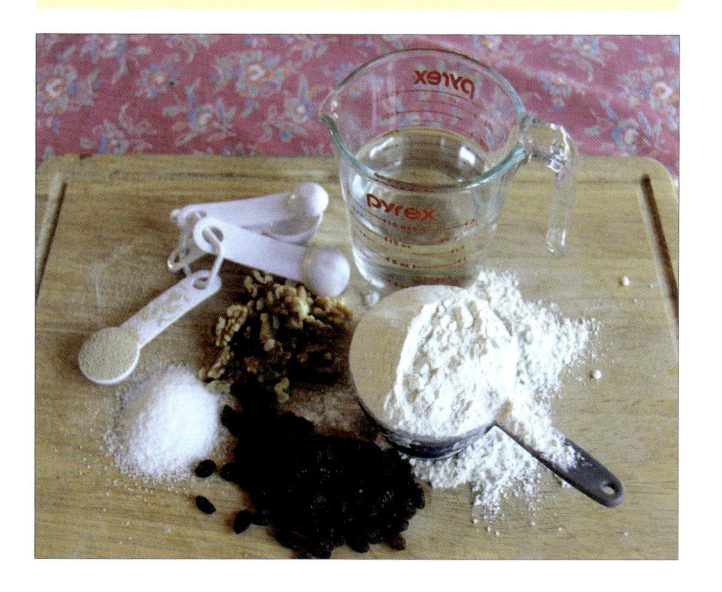

Flour Tortillas

Yield: 8 (7-inch) Tortillas

Wheat flour tortillas are the northern Mexican version of flatbread. They can be used in many kinds of wraps, including Burritos (see page 78), Crunchy Creamy Veggie Wrap (see page 77), and even Sushi (see page 80).

Store tortillas in an airtight container in the refrigerator up to a week. They can be frozen, but place wax or parchment paper in between tortillas to keep them from sticking together when thawed. For a visual guide to kneading, see Simply Scrumptious Scones (page 150) or Pizza Dough (page 65).

- 2 cups all-purpose flour or 1 cup all-purpose flour and 1 cup whole wheat flour
- 1½ teaspoons baking powder
- ½ teaspoon salt
- 2 teaspoons vegetable oil, bacon fat or lard
- ¾ cup water

1. Combine flour and baking powder in a medium bowl.
2. Mix salt, vegetable oil and water in a cup. Add to flour mixture, a little at a time, and stir until the mixture is a workable but sticky dough.
3. Place dough on a lightly floured surface; knead about 2 minutes or until dough holds its shape.
4. Return dough to bowl, cover bowl with a damp cloth, and let rest 15 minutes.
5. Break dough into 8 golf-ball-sized pieces and place on a flat surface, not touching each other. Cover and let rest another 20 minutes.
6. Place dough balls on a flat, floured surface. Hand-shape them into 6- to 7-inch circles, or use a floured rolling pin to roll dough into 7-inch circles.
7. Cook the tortillas on a hot, dry griddle or cast-iron frying pan for about 30 seconds on each side. Tortillas should blister (see below).

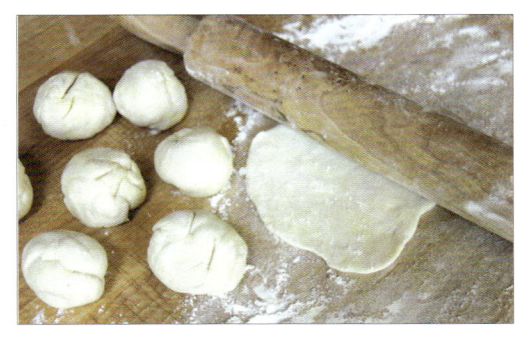

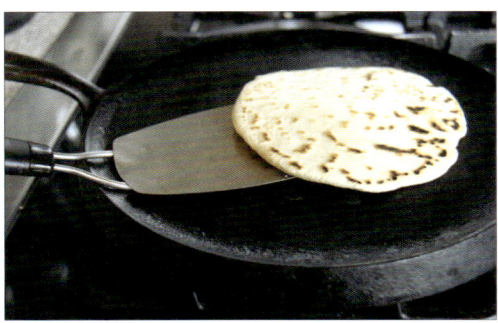

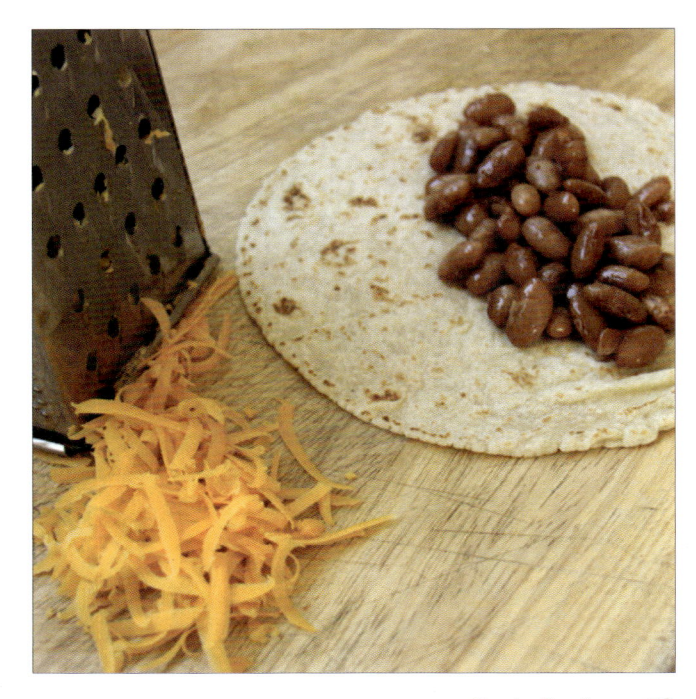

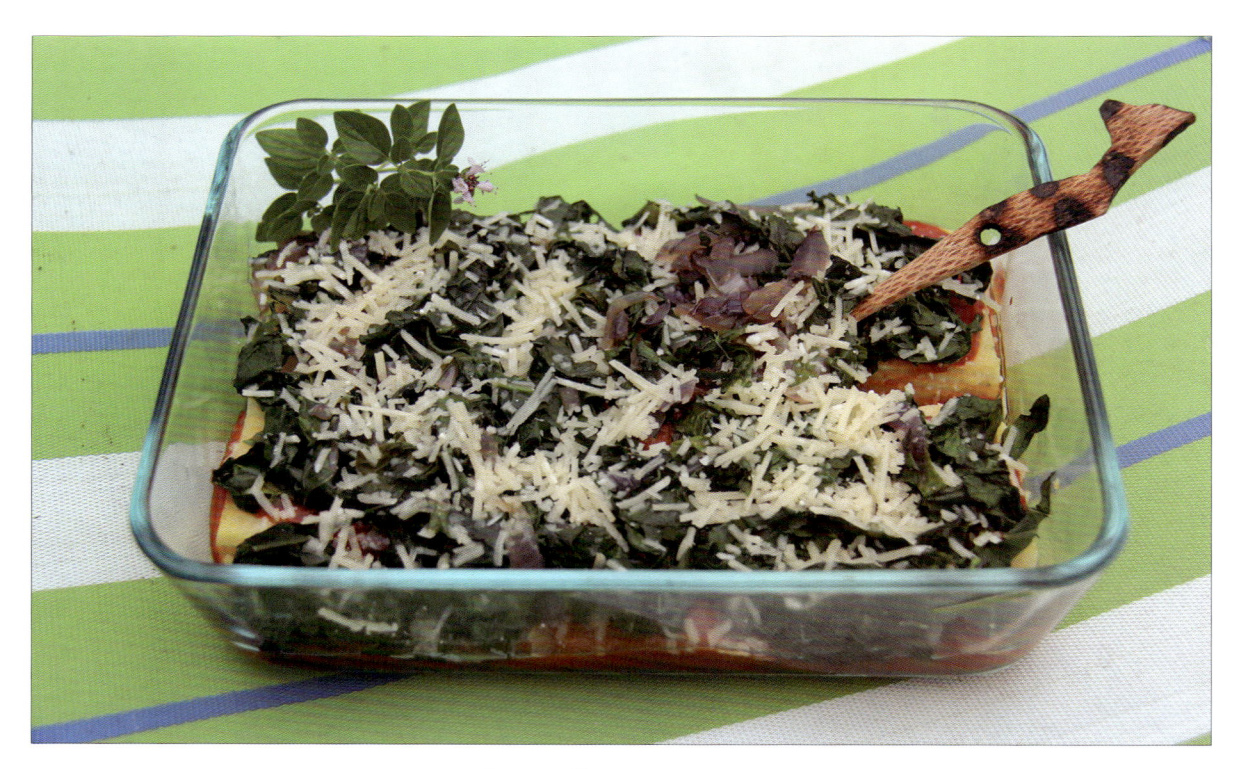

Polenta

Yield: 6-8 squares or 1 crust for Quiche

This recipe can be made into squares or used as an alternative crust for Quiche (see page 103). Whatever you choose, polenta is inexpensive, delicious and gluten free. A wooden spoon works well for stirring polenta.

- 1 cup cornmeal
- 1 cup cold water or broth, or ½ cup milk and ½ cup water
- ½ teaspoon salt
- 2 cups boiling water
- 1 tablespoon melted butter or oil

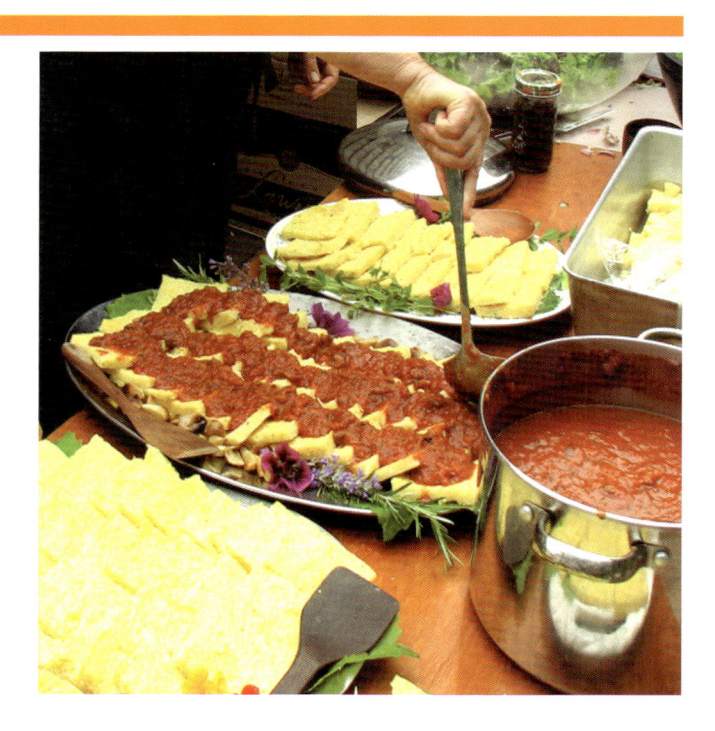

1. Mix the cornmeal and 1 cup cold water or broth in a 2-cup measuring cup—this is called a "slurry." Set aside.

2. Add the salt to the 2 cups boiling water. Pour the slurry into the rapidly boiling water while stirring continuously. This will prevent clumping.

3. Cook over low heat, stirring occasionally to avoid sticking, until the polenta pulls away from the edge of the pot (about 10-15 minutes).

For Squares:

1. Pour cooked polenta into greased baking pan and spread evenly. Polenta should be 1-2 inches thick.

2. Cool and invert onto a clean countertop by flipping over the pan. Cut into squares.

Options:

- Sprinkle grated cheese over squares and put in broiler or toaster oven to melt cheese.
- Pour warm tomato sauce over cut squares.

For Quiche Crust:

Preheat oven to 350°

1. Lightly oil a pie pan. Spread thickened polenta on bottom and sides of the pan with a spatula. Cover top with melted butter or olive oil.

2. Bake until crust is crisp but not burned. Check progress at 30 minutes. Cool slightly before adding the quiche filling. Bake according to Quiche recipe (see page 103).

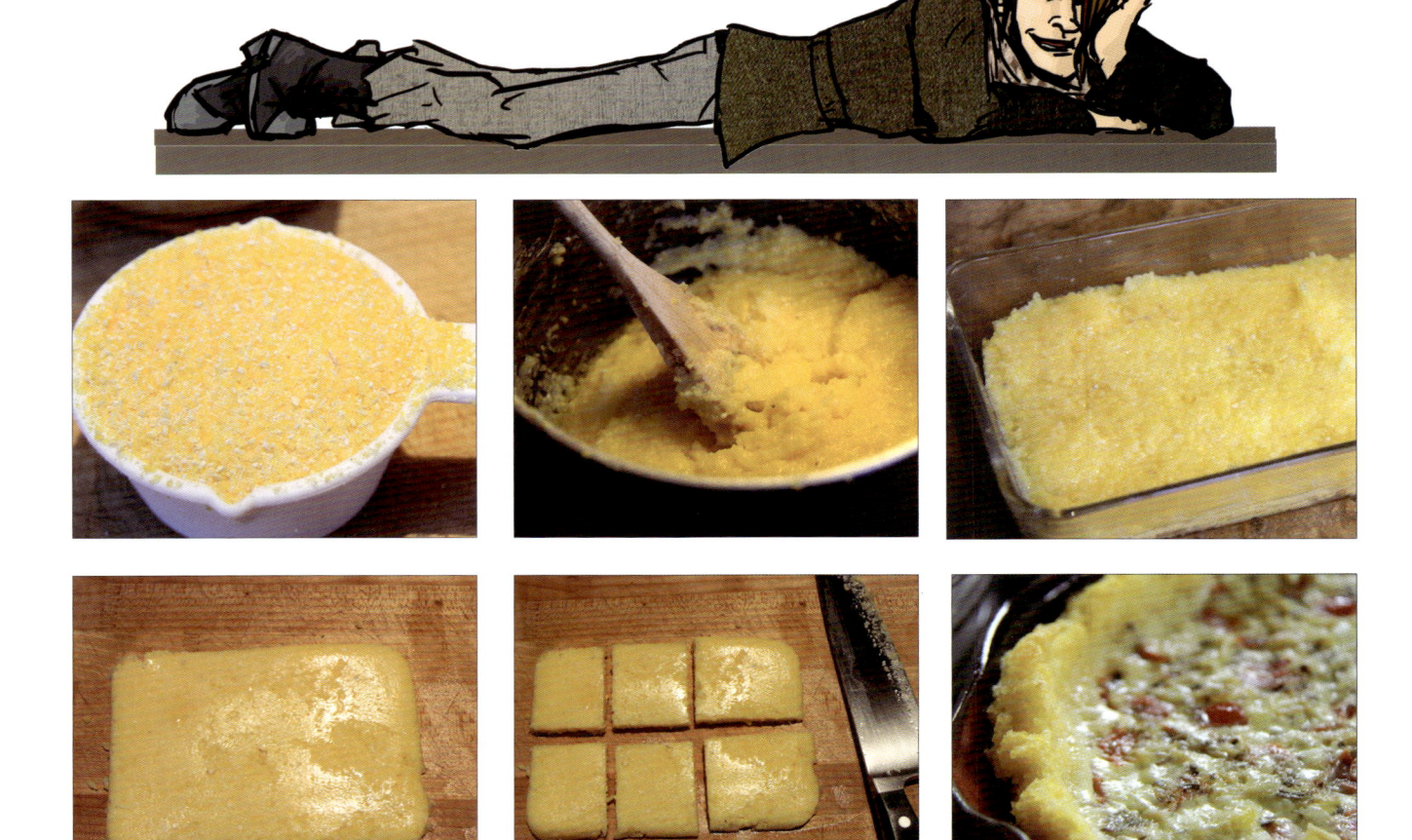

Basic Recipes

Broth

Yield: 8 cups

Good food that is normally wasted, such as leftover meat bones and juices or vegetable peelings, can be transformed into a delicious base for soups and other dishes. Homemade broth is much less expensive than purchased broth.

Chicken and other meat can be used separately or combined. Double the vegetable ingredients and leave out meat for a vegetable broth.

The key to homemade broth is saving meat and vegetable scraps in the freezer. Every time you go to throw away bones, juices, cuttings, peelings or ends, put them in a freezer-safe container instead.

1	chicken carcass, or similar amount of meat odds and ends such as leftover chicken, turkey, pork, or beef, pan drippings, bones, raw meat pieces*
1	onion, chopped, or onion skins and scraps*
1-2	carrots, scrubbed and chopped*
1-2	stalks celery or celery tops and scraps,* washed
1	cup clean vegetable scraps and peelings (about 1 cup)*
	Water

*Note: These amounts and ingredients can vary. Use what you have; that's the point of this broth.

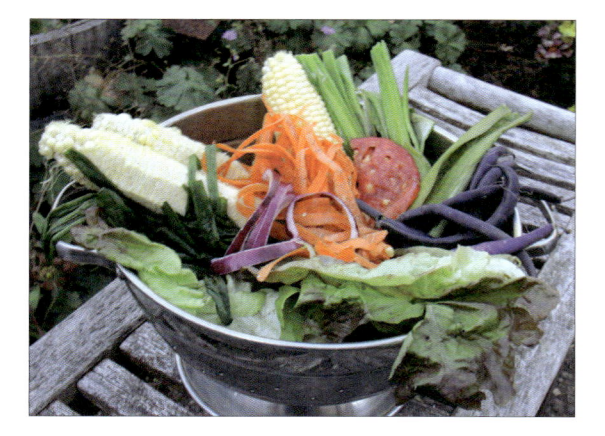

1. Put raw and cooked meats, bones, juices, and all vegetables into a large pot.

2. Add twice as much cold water as ingredients. Cover partially with lid.

3. Bring pot to a rolling boil, then reduce heat and simmer 2 hours.

4. Drain broth into another container, using a large strainer or colander to remove bones and vegetables. Use immediately or cool before storing.

Options:
- Season to taste with salt, pepper, and herbs.

Storing:
- If using within a week, store in refrigerator, leaving the layer of fat that forms on top to keep broth fresh; remove fat layer before using.
- To freeze, pour cooled broth into freezer-safe containers in portions, leaving a 1-inch space at the top. Write date on containers and freeze.

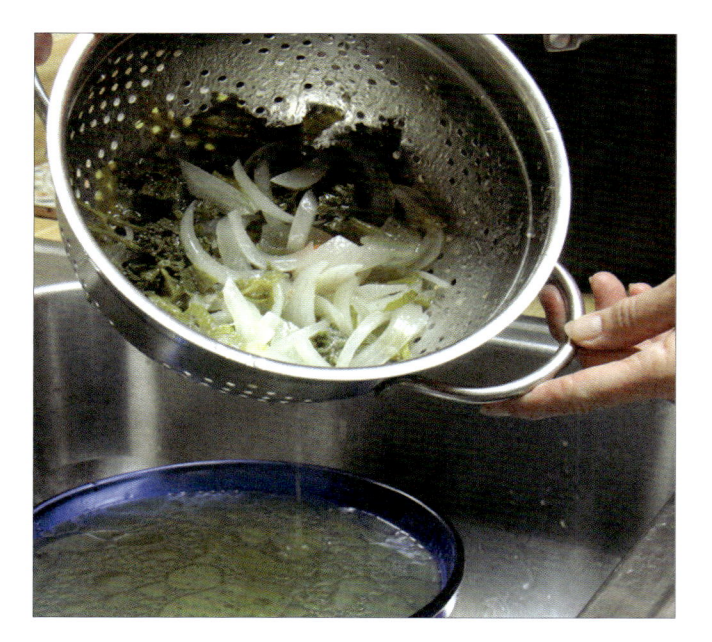

Pie Dough

Yield: 2 (9-inch) pie crusts

This is an easy pie dough recipe to make. Be sure to have well-chilled butter sticks before you start. Purchased pie dough is twice as expensive as homemade. Use this dough for Empanadas (see page 86), Quiche (see page 103) and, of course, pie.

- 2 cups all-purpose flour
- ½ teaspoon salt
- ¾ cup butter, chilled (1½ sticks)
- 4-5 tablespoons cold water

*Note: Humidity and the type of flour used affect the amount of water needed.

1. Mix salt and flour in a medium-sized bowl. Using a cheese grater, grate the chilled butter into the dry ingredients and combine well. Refrigerate 10-15 minutes.

2. Remove mixture from refrigerator. Sprinkle in cold water, one tablespoon at a time. Toss mixture lightly with a fork until dough has no dry spots and will press together into a ball.

3. Shape dough into a 5-inch-wide disk; wrap and refrigerate at least 30 minutes.

4. Divide dough into two equal pieces. Shape each half into a ball and flatten. Working from the center outward, roll dough until it is two inches larger than the diameter of pan. As you work, rotate dough in quarter turns. This makes for even rolling and avoids sticking.

Options:

- Save half the dough. Wrap it so that it's airtight, then freeze. Thaw dough before rolling it out.

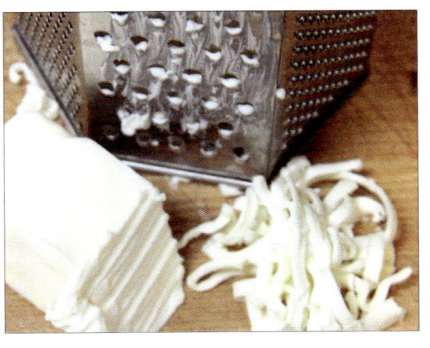

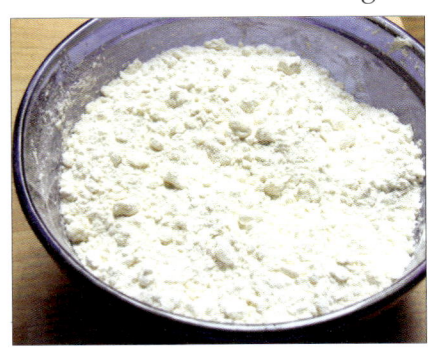

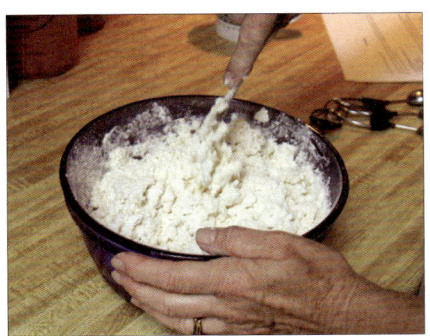

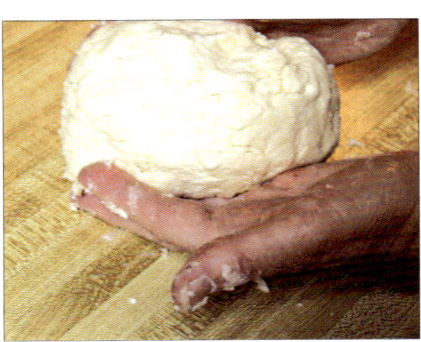

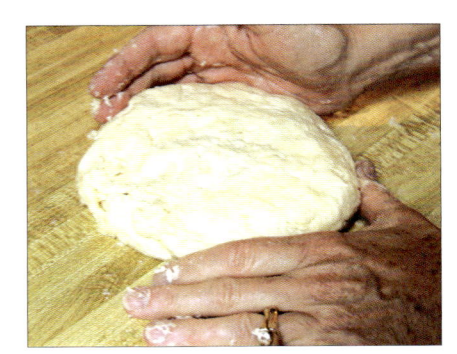

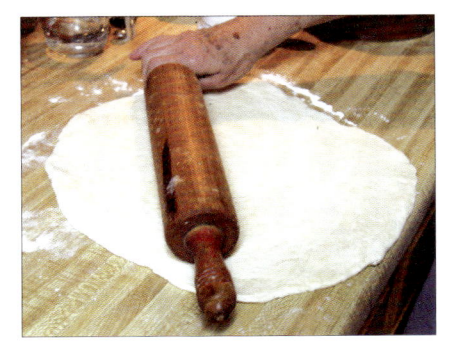

Basic Recipes 63

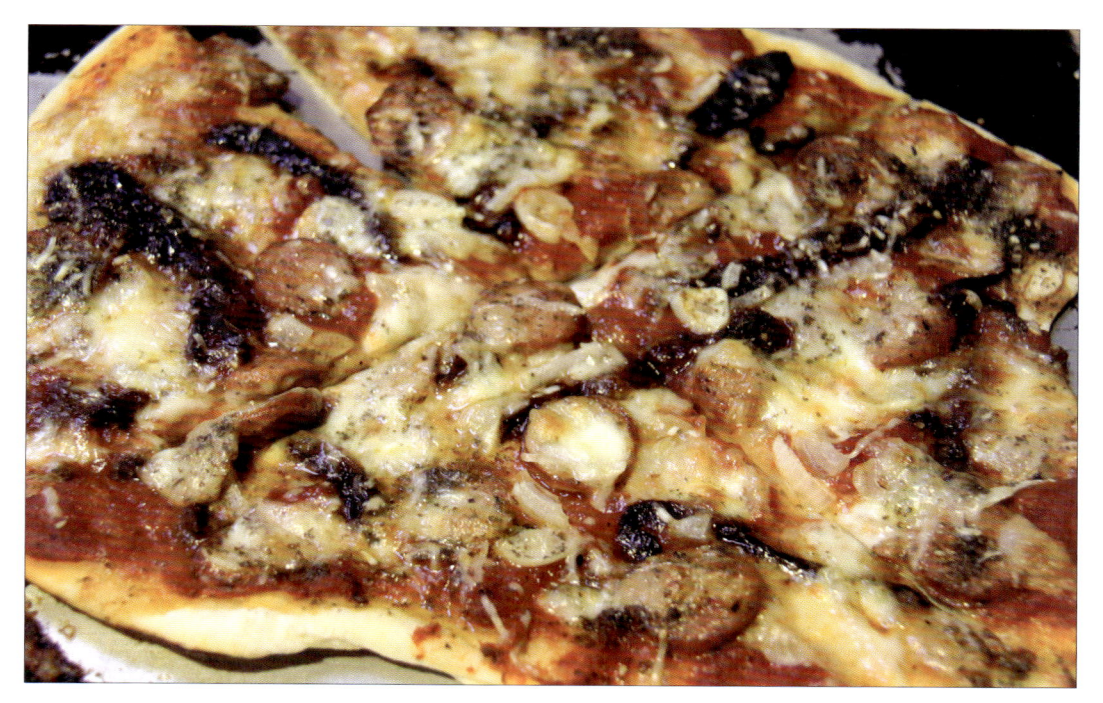

Pizza Dough

Yield: 3 dough balls

Homemade pizza not only smells good, it tastes good! You can add whatever toppings you want. See Pizza Formula (page 82) for ingredient ideas and directions on making pizza.

This dough recipe can also be used for Pita Bread (see page 66) or Calzones (see page 84). Freeze extra dough balls for future use.

1½	cups warm water (115-120°)
1	tablespoon dry yeast (1 package)
3	cups all-purpose flour
2	tablespoons vegetable or olive oil, divided
½	teaspoon salt
1	tablespoon cornmeal

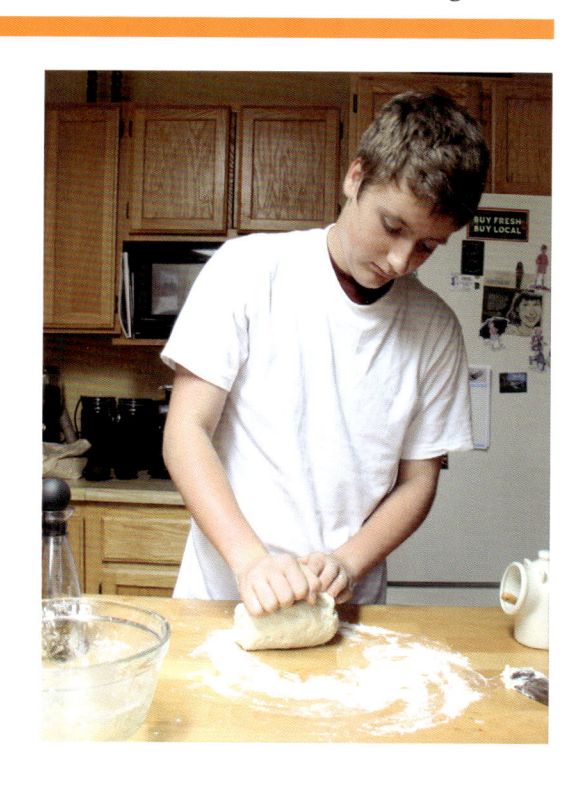

64 Basic Recipes

1. Mix yeast and 1 cup flour in a large bowl; stir in water. Wait 5 minutes to let yeast foam and do its work. (See page 66, about yeast.)

2. Add the remaining 2 cups of flour, 1 tablespoon oil and salt into mixture. Turn dough onto a floured surface and knead until smooth and elastic, 8-10 minutes.

3. Grease bowl with remaining oil. Place dough in bowl, turning once to grease the top. Cover bowl with plastic wrap or a damp dish towel. Let dough rise in a warm place until doubled in size, 45-60 minutes, depending on how warm an area is available.

4. Punch down dough, divide into three equal balls and let rise, covered, 15-20 minutes. If freezing for later use, see **Options**, next column.

For Pizza:

Preheat oven to 425°

1. Cover two of the dough balls to keep them from drying out. Roll the third one into a circle 12-18 inches in diameter, depending on size of pan. If you're using a baking sheet, it can also be a rectangle.

2. Use a pastry brush and oil to grease the surface of your baking sheet. Sprinkle sheet with cornmeal. Move dough to pan and top with other ingredients. See Pizza Formula (page 82).

3. Bake 18-20 minutes or until dough is lightly browned.

4. Use the two remaining dough balls for more pizzas or freeze for later use.

Options:

- Substitute 2 cups all-purpose flour and 1 cup whole wheat flour for 3 cups all-purpose flour.
- To freeze unused balls of dough, dust balls with flour after the second rising, wrap in plastic wrap or place in freezer-safe bag or container.
- Use a pizza stone for a crispier crust.

Simple Tomato Sauce

Use for pizza, calzones or with pasta.

- 2 15 ounce cans tomato sauce (4 cups)
- 1 tablespoon Italian herbs (basil, oregano, rosemary)
- 2 tablespoons olive oil
- 1 clove garlic, minced
- 1 small onion, minced

1. Sauté onions and garlic for 5 minutes.
2. Add spices, sauté for 1 minute.
3. Add tomato sauce, simmer for 20 minutes.

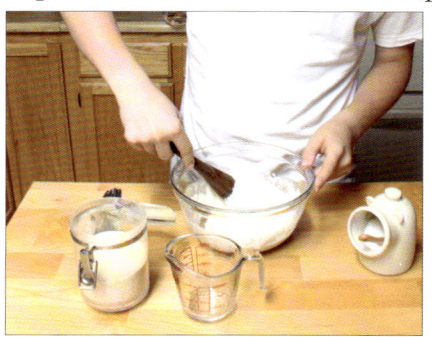

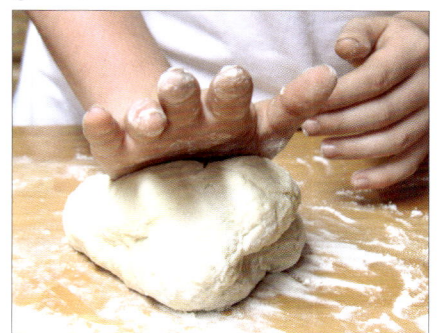

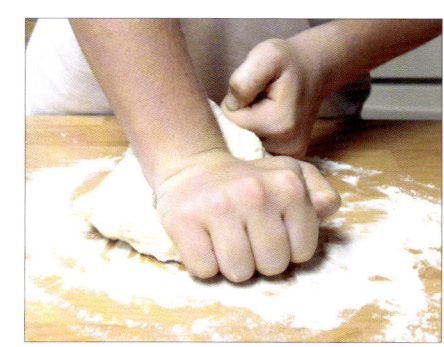

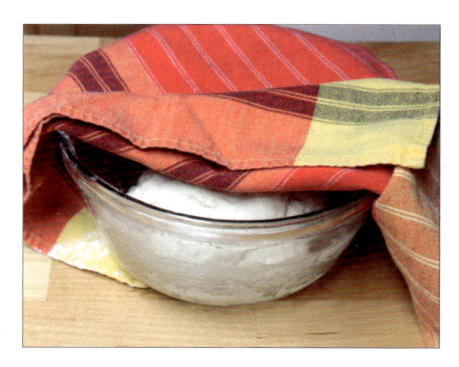

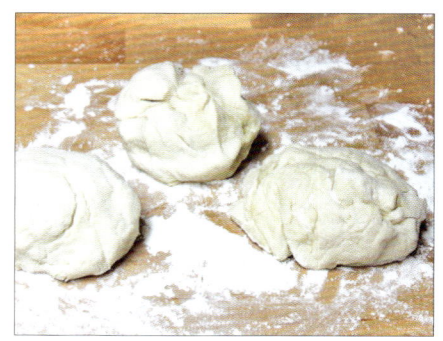

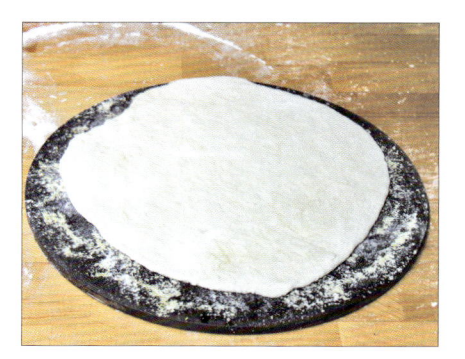

Basic Recipes 65

Pita Bread from Pizza Dough

Yield: 6 pockets

Pita bread is a Middle Eastern flatbread that uses the same recipe as pizza dough. It puffs up when baked, making little pockets to fill with good stuff such as a main-dish salad, roasted or grilled meats and vegetables, or to serve on the side with a dip like Hummus (see page 167) or the Black or White bean spread (see page 163).

1   Pizza Dough recipe (see page 64)

Preheat oven to 425°

1. Using pizza dough recipe, pinch off a piece of dough the size of a your fist. Flatten the dough into a circle 4-5 inches in diameter and ¼-inch thick.

2. Place on an ungreased baking sheet. Bake 8-10 minutes, until lightly browned. The circles will puff up.

3. Wrap finished pita bread in a dish towel for 10 minutes to keep bread soft until ready to use.

4. To use, cut ½ inch from one side. Separate the sides from each other and leave the edges together.

5. Store unused pita bread in plastic bags.

Options:

- Freeze unused pita bread.
- Use any salad—chopped, vegetable, fruit or main-dish— as a filling. (See Main Dish Salads, pages 110-115.)

Yeast

Yeast is a one-celled organism. It will work for you to make your bread fluff up if you give it a warm, wet place to grow and something sweet to eat.

As it eats, yeast gets gassy. By the process of fermentation, yeast converts food (sugar) into alcohol and carbon dioxide. These gasses get trapped inside the dough, making small bubbles that force the dough to stretch and rise. When the dough is baked, the heat of the oven evaporates the alcohol, leaving behind empty spaces where the alcohol had been. These air pockets are what create the texture we see when we cut into anything that has been made with yeast.

Some people don't like working with yeast because of its finicky nature. With proper care and an understanding of how yeast works, it will be more than happy to do your bidding.

Use bakers' yeast for baking. Save money by buying in bulk or in large packages. Individual packets can be expensive.

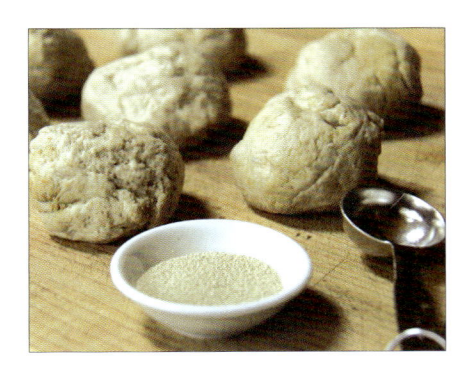

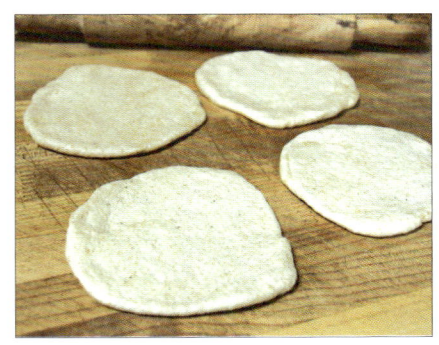

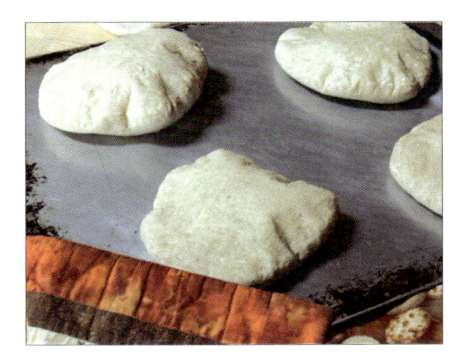

The Main Dish

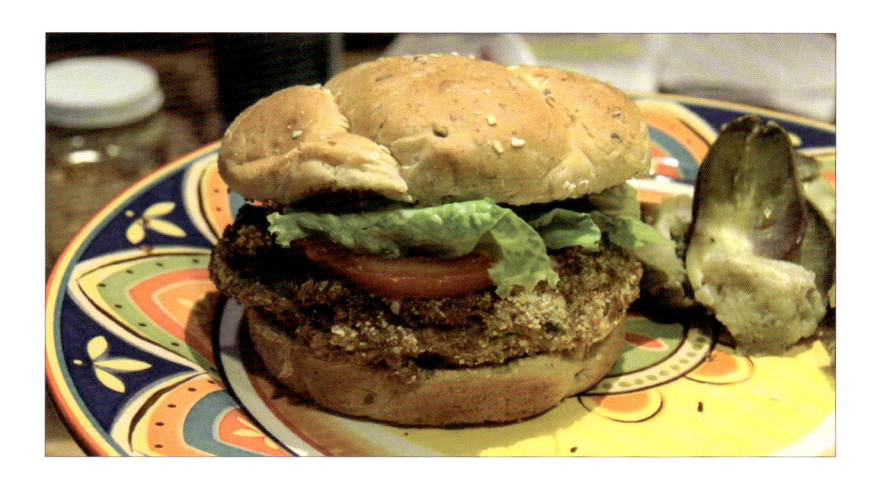

The Main Dish often combines MyPlate components and almost always includes protein. Since protein comes in many forms, such as cheese, meat, or nuts, the Main Dish is an adaptable part of lunch. In this section of recipes you'll find:

Sandwiches & Wraps (pages 68-87)
Grains & Noodleds (pages 88-99)
Egg-Based Dishes (pages 100-107)
Main-Dish Salads (pages 108-115)
Soups (pages 116-124)

No-Prep Main Dishes

Before you make anything for lunch, think about last night's dinner leftovers. Check the refrigerator.

Online Recipes

Searching for recipes on the Internet is a great way to find a recipe with the exact combination of ingredients that you have on hand, as well as to get new ideas.

Look in your refrigerator and cupboard, then search for the combined items as key words. For example, there is a rapidly aging zucchini, leftover pasta, yogurt and a chunk of cheese in your refrigerator. When searched, many sites show these items will combine to produce creamy baked pasta recipes.

Bookmark your favorite online magazines and cooking blogs.

Some useful sites are:

- **Yummly.com** - include or exclude specific ingredients in recipe searches for picky eaters or those with allergies.

- **Gluten-free recipes**: elanaspantry.com or glutenfreegoddess.blogspot.com

Leftovers
- Pasta dishes
- Chicken drumstick or wings
- Grain or pasta salads
- Soup
- Meatloaf

Low-prep
- Cottage cheese and fruit
- Yogurt with fruit
- Hard-cooked eggs
- Cubed tofu
- Garbanzo beans
- Nuts

← Mix 'n' Match →
- Cheese
- Sliced roasted meat
- Nut butters
- Spreads
- Bread
- Crackers
- Rice cakes
- Vegetable chips

Sandwich and Wrap Formula

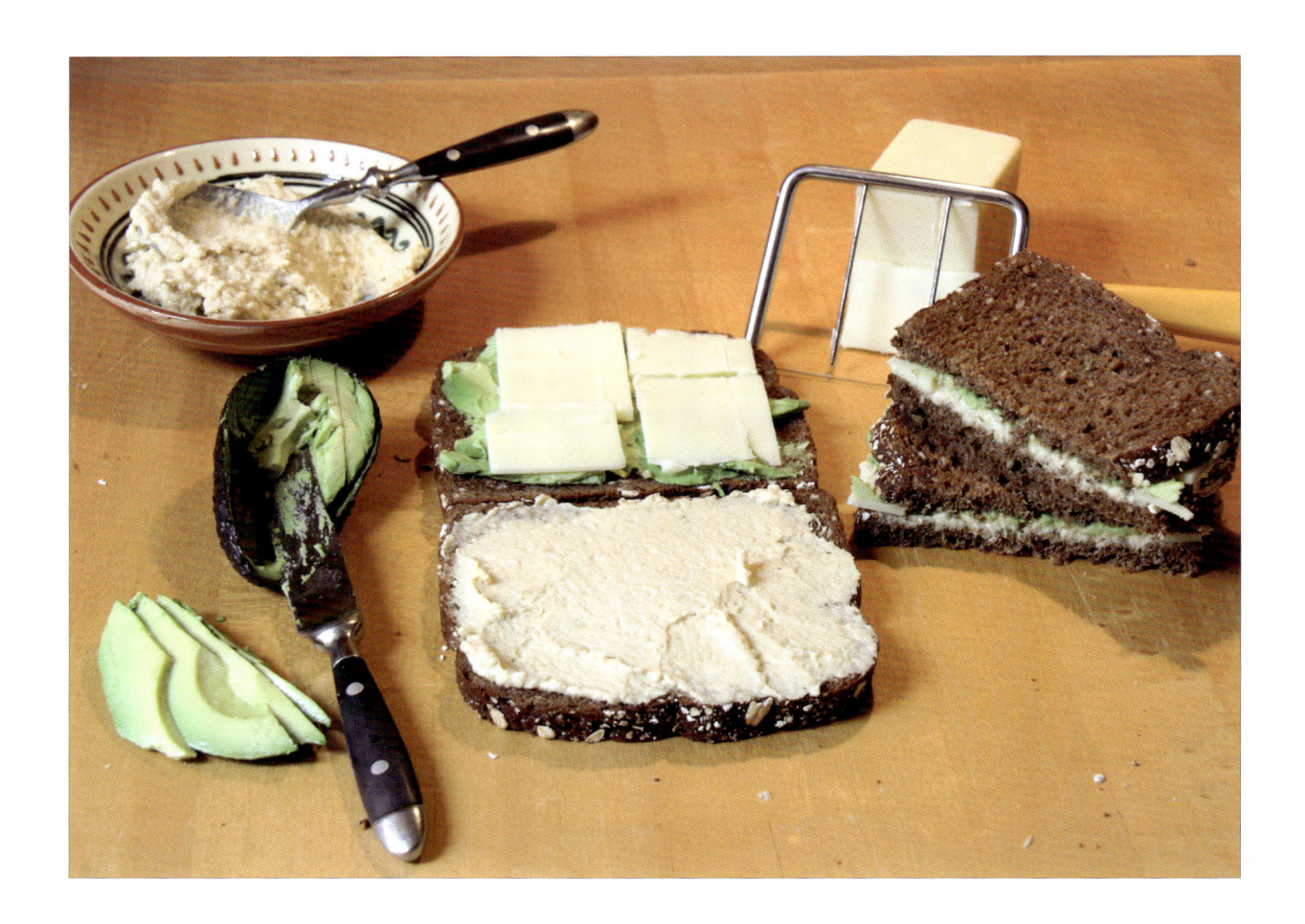

1. Smear your spread of choice on one side of a piece of bread or a wrapper.

Leave some space around the edge of the wrapper so that the filling doesn't leak out.

2. Layer or spread your protein filling.

3. Add extras.

4. If using bread, place second piece on top. If using a tortilla, a wrap, or a lettuce leaf, fold it around filling. For folding technique, see Burrito recipe, page 78.

Ingredient Ideas

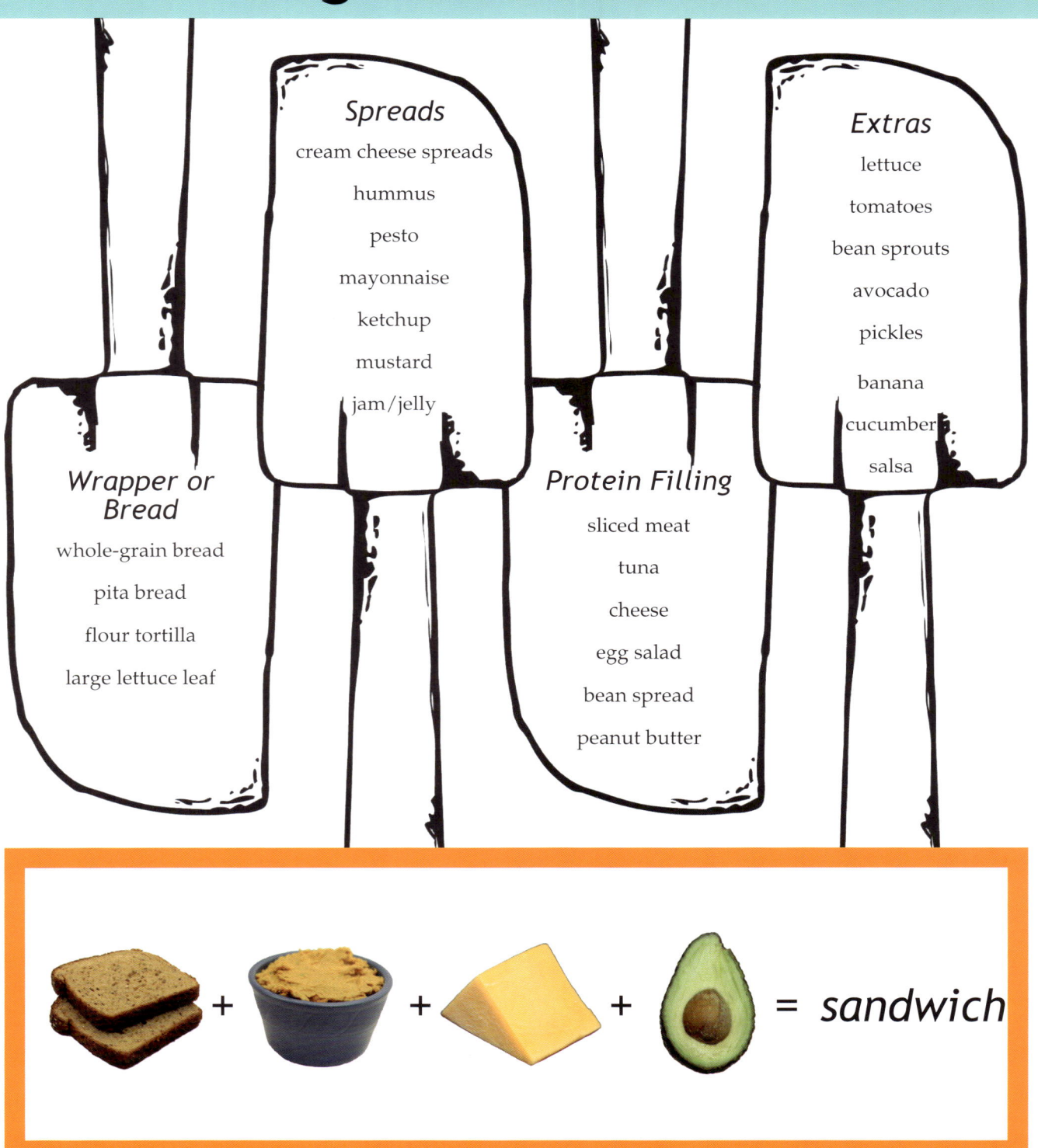

Wrapper or Bread
whole-grain bread
pita bread
flour tortilla
large lettuce leaf

Spreads
cream cheese spreads
hummus
pesto
mayonnaise
ketchup
mustard
jam/jelly

Protein Filling
sliced meat
tuna
cheese
egg salad
bean spread
peanut butter

Extras
lettuce
tomatoes
bean sprouts
avocado
pickles
banana
cucumber
salsa

+ + + = *sandwich*

Stackable Sandwiches

Yield: 12 tiny sandwiches

Kids go crazy for stackable food that can be made into sandwiches at school. Make your own healthy, tasty version. Using a cookie cutter and stacking are fun activities that can involve children of any age.

3-4	slices of deli meat or sliced home-roasted meat
3-4	slices of Cheddar or Jack cheese
½	cucumber, sliced
3-5	slices of bread, or 12 crackers

1. Cut meat, cheese and bread into slices no more than ½ inch thick.
2. To make different shapes, cut them from larger slices of of meat, bread and cheese, using a knife or small cookie cutter.
3. Slice cucumber and other vegetables to same size as meat.
4. Stack in a container.

Options:

- Add sliced bell peppers, tomatoes, lettuce leaves, sautéed or roasted summer squash, or baked sweet potato.
- Choose home-roasted meats that are soft enough to cut with a cookie cutter or knife but won't fall apart, such as ham, pork loin, beef pot roast and turkey breast.
- Save meat and vegetable scraps for other dishes or Broth *(page 62)*. Save bread scraps for making Strata *(page 104)*.

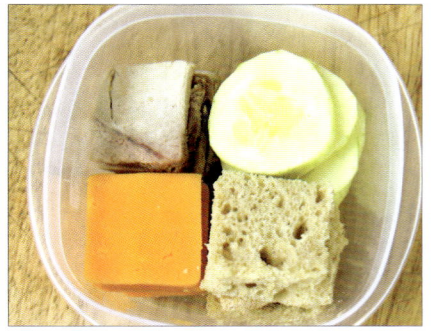

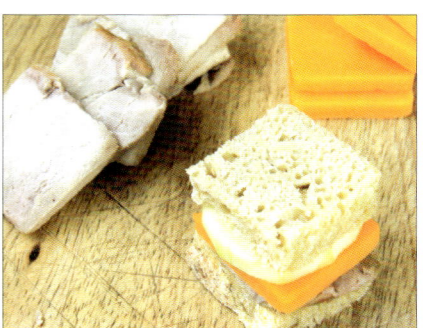

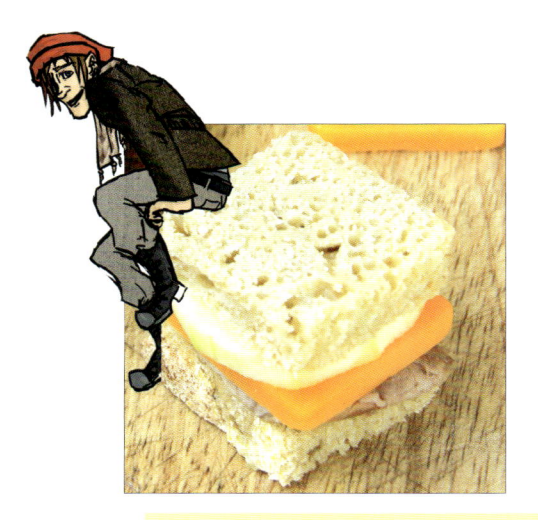

Roasting Meat

To save money on sandwich lunch meat, reduce packaging waste, avoid additives, and take care of other meals at the same time, roast your own.

Beef pot roasts, ham, or whole chickens can be cooked and eaten for dinner, then stored in the refrigerator for the next few days.

Slice off thin portions throughout the week for sandwiches.

Finally done? Don't throw out the bones, make broth! (see page 62)

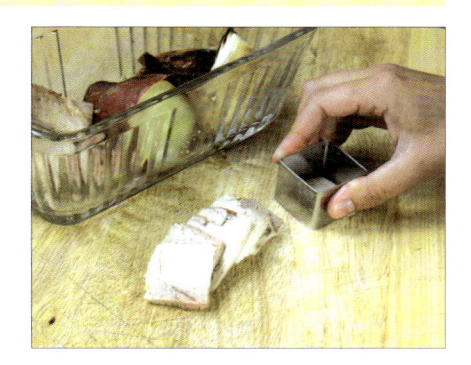

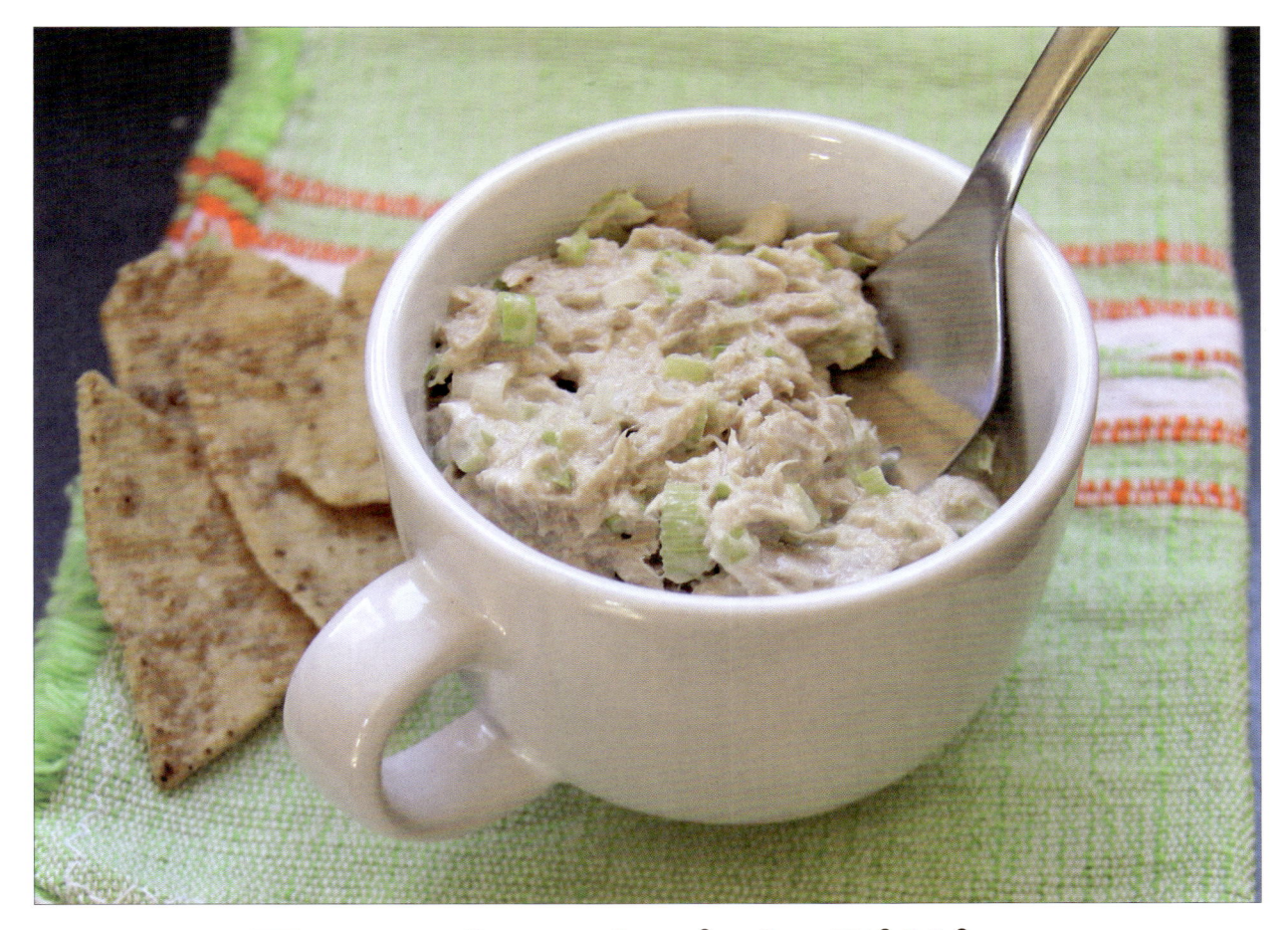

Tuna Sandwich Filling

Yield: Filling for 2 sandwiches

This is a basic chopped salad recipe. Substitute chopped chicken or turkey or hard-cooked eggs for the tuna.

- 1 6-ounce can tuna, well drained
- 3 tablespoons mayonnaise
- 1 green onion, chopped
- 1 tablespoon chopped celery

1. Drain tuna well and place in a bowl.
2. Add green onion, celery and mayonnaise to tuna and mix well.
3. Cover and refrigerate any leftover mixture.

Options:

- Substitute 1 tablespoon finely chopped red onion for green onion.
- Add seasonings of your choice (see page 193) for more flavor.

PBJ Pinwheels

Yield: 8 Pinwheels

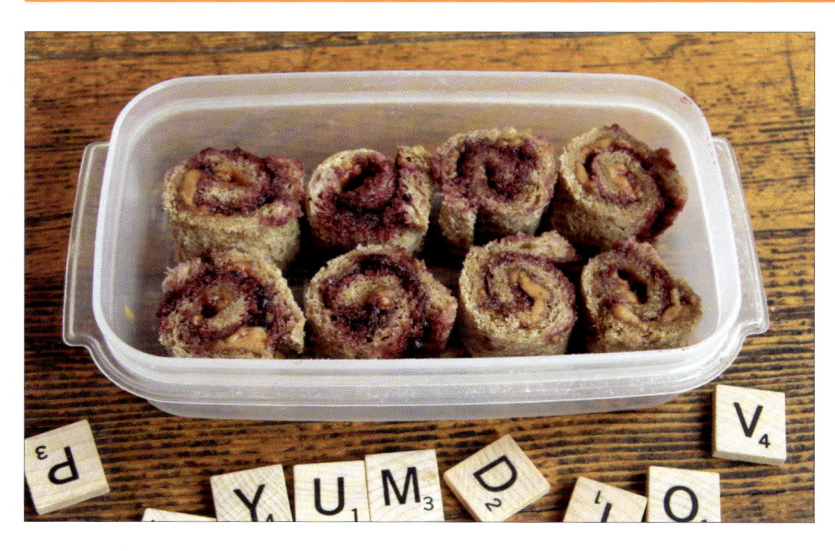

Peanut-butter-and-jelly sandwiches (PBJs) are a classic kid lunch item in the U.S. Here is a creative way to turn them into bite-size pieces.

- 2 slices of bread
- 2 tablespoons peanut butter
- 2 tablespoons jelly or jam

1. Cut the crusts off the bread. Compress bread slices with a rolling pin, large can, or bottle.

2. Spread peanut butter evenly on bread, then spread jelly or jam on top of the peanut butter.

3. Roll up bread into a tight spiral.

4. Slice roll into four pieces. Use a bread knife to make cutting easier.

Options:

- Roll and slice any sandwich that uses squishable ingredients. Replace the jelly with mashed banana slices, or use bean dip (see page 163) and avocado. Spread should be sticky enough to hold the bread together.
- Substitute other nut butters for peanut butter.
- Save bread crusts for making Strata (see page 104).

Peanut Butter

Peanut butter is a kid favorite, but most major brands are full of additives like salt, sugar, oil, preservatives and emulsifiers that keep the peanut butter blended. Check the ingredients. The healthiest peanut butters have the fewest ingredients. Some have just one: peanuts. Some stores let you buy and grind your own peanuts. See Chapter 3, page 28, for a comparison of ingredients.

Combining peanut butter with cocoa powder and honey makes plain peanut butter into a sweet treat.

Chocolate Peanut Butter Spread

- ½ cup creamy peanut butter
- ¼ cup cocoa powder
- 2 tablespoons warmed honey

1. Heat honey to thin liquid consistency. **On stove top:** Place honey in a glass container. Heat the container in 2 inches of water, until honey is thin. **In microwave:** Heat honey in a glass container until thin. Start with 15 seconds of cooking time. Don't use plastic containers in the microwave.

2. Mix ingredients together.

3. Use in a sandwich with bananas or as a special dip for fruit and vegetable slices.

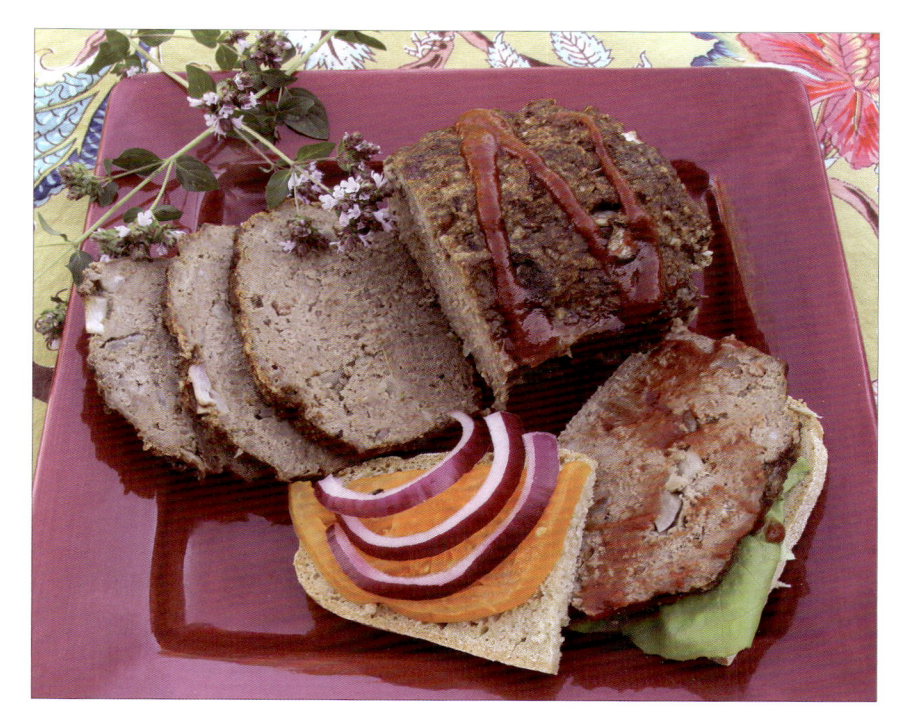

Meatloaf

Yield: 1 Meatloaf

Every family probably has their own way of making meatloaf by adding specific herbs or fillings, but this one will certainly fulfill any craving for a good meatloaf sandwich. Use this recipe to make a meatloaf for dinner, then use the leftovers in sandwiches for the next day.

- ½ teaspoon oil
- 2 pounds ground beef, pork, turkey or chicken, or a combination of meats
- ½ teaspoon salt
- 1 tablespoon Italian Spice Mix (see page 193) or combination of dried thyme, oregano and rosemary
- ½ teaspoon pepper
- 1 tablespoon Worcestershire sauce
- ½ cup bread crumbs
- 1 egg, beaten
- 2 tablespoons ketchup, for topping

Preheat oven to 350°

1. Coat an 8-inch loaf pan with the oil.
2. Combine all ingredients, except ketchup, in large bowl.
3. Spread meat mixture into the coated pan and smooth the top.
4. Bake 30 minutes or until the top is browned.
5. Spoon or squeeze ketchup on top of loaf and bake an additional 5 minutes.
6. Remove from oven, let sit 5 minutes, then slice and serve.

Option:
- Grate 1 carrot or zucchini into meat mixture.

Main Dish ☞ Sandwich and Wrap Recipes

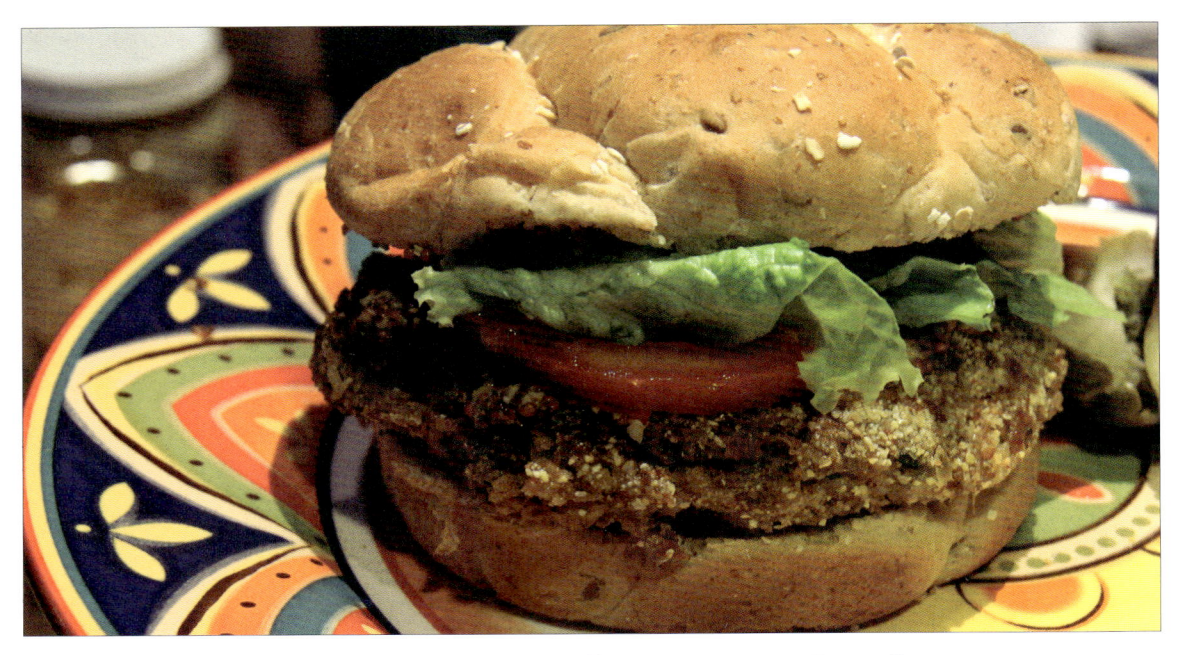

Black-Eyed Pea Cakes

Yield: 8 Pea Cakes

Black-eyed peas are a New Year's tradition for some cultures. These cakes can be mild or spicy. Size the cakes to fit a hamburger bun, and add a slice of tomato, lettuce, and a touch of ketchup or mayonnaise. For bite-size snacks, make them smaller.

- 2 tablespoons olive oil, divided
- ½ small onion, chopped (about ¼ cup)
- ½ teaspoon grated lemon rind
- 1½ teaspoons chopped fresh thyme (or ½ teaspoon dried)
- 1 garlic clove, minced
- 4 cups cooked black-eyed peas (2 cups dried or two 14.5- to 16-ounce cans)
- 1 egg
- 1 cup bread crumbs (plain or panko)
- 1 tablespoon chopped fresh parsley (or 1 teaspoon dried)
- 2 teaspoons Dijon-style mustard
- ½ teaspoon salt
- ½ teaspoon black pepper
- ¼ cup cornmeal

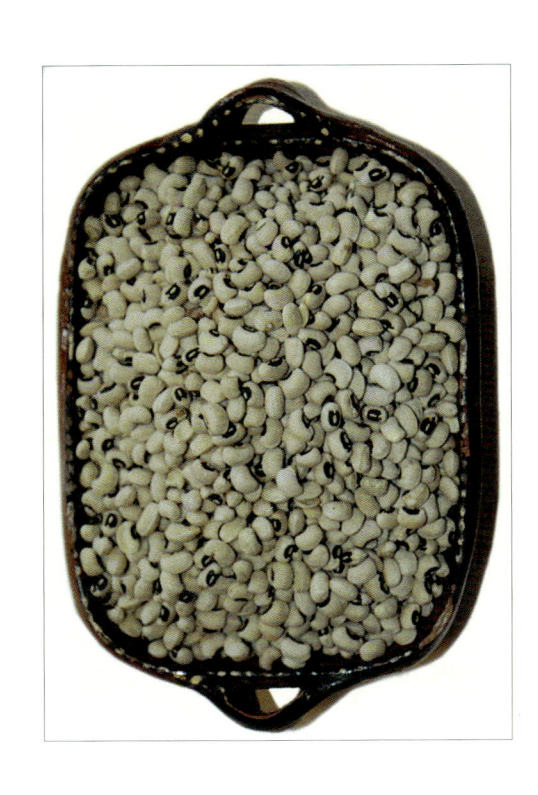

1. Prepare vegetables and lemon rind. Cook dry peas or rinse and drain canned peas.

2. Heat 1 tablespoon olive oil in a large frying pan over medium heat.

3. Add the onion, lemon rind, thyme and garlic. Sauté for one minute.

4. Place all ingredients except cornmeal in a 2-quart bowl and mash with a potato masher, or place in a food processor and blend.

5. Divide the mixture into 8 portions and flatten into ½-inch-thick cakes.

6. Place the cornmeal in a flat dish or pie pan. Coat both sides of cakes in cornmeal. Place cakes on a cookie sheet and refrigerate 15 minutes.

7. Heat 1 tablespoon olive oil in the frying pan over medium heat and cook cakes about 2 minutes per side or until brown.

Options:

- At Step 4, add 1 cup minced, sautéed mushrooms, ½ cup roasted tomatoes, or 1 cup steamed or roasted vegetables.
- At Step 4, add ½ cup toasted walnuts or pecans, chopped, and/or 2 teaspoons hot pepper paste.

Cost Comparison: Beans

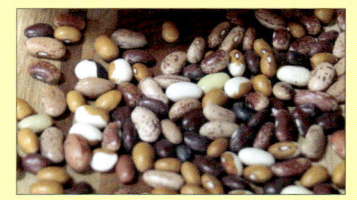

Bulk, dry
9.1¢ per ounce
22¢ per cup, cooked

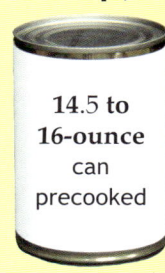

14.5 to 16-ounce can precooked

11.3¢ per ounce
79¢ per cup, cooked

*Prices vary. Estimate based on nationwide chain grocery store generic brands, 2012

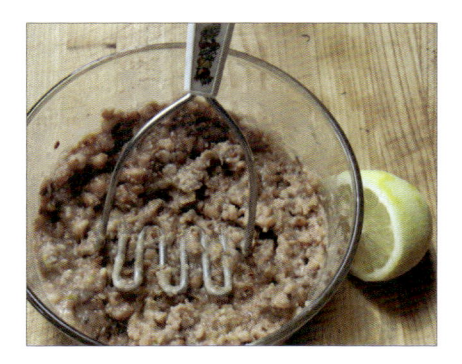

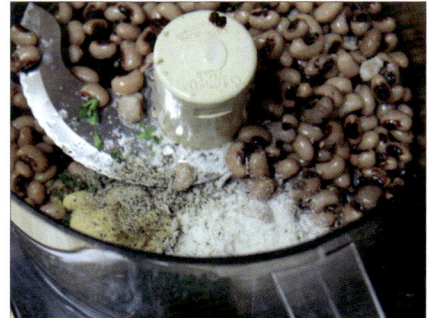

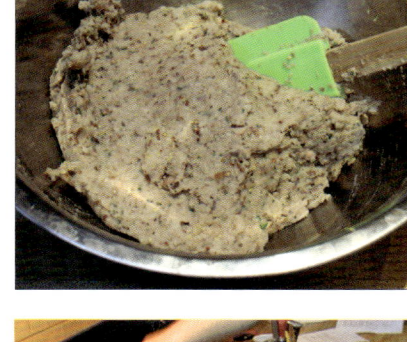

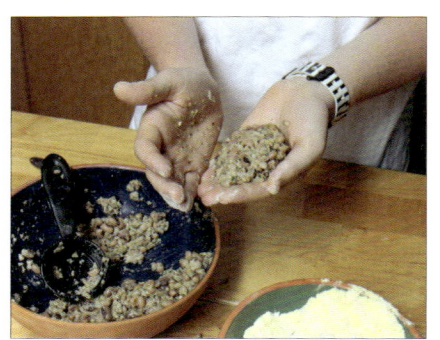

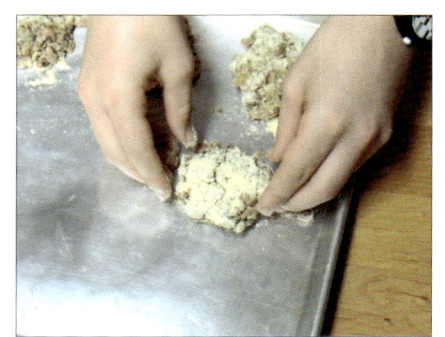

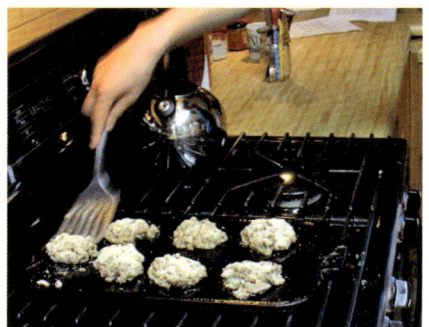

2-in-1 Chicken & Fruit "Saladwich"

3-6 servings

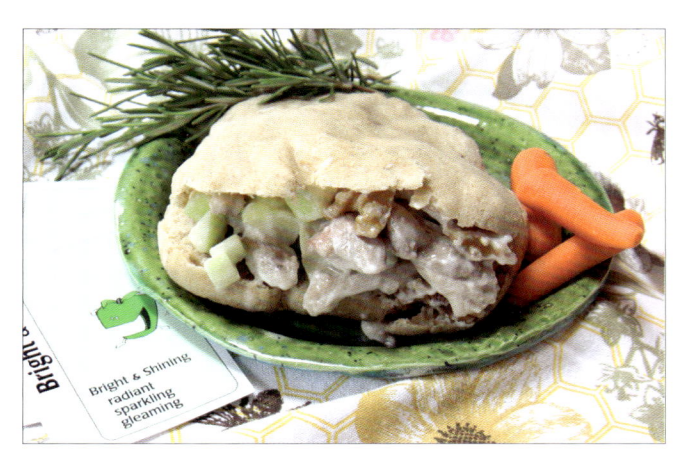

Here's a time-saver! Make a chicken and fruit salad, then use leftovers as filling for a pita sandwich the next day. Lemon juice in the dressing adds a tangy flavor and keeps the fruit from turning brown.

Salad
- 1 tablespoon vegetable or olive oil
- ½ pound chicken breasts, cut into thin strips, or ½ pound cooked chicken strips
- 1 medium apple, cored and chopped (about 1 cup)
- 2 celery stalks, chopped (about ½ cup)
- ¼ cup chopped walnuts, almonds or pecans
- 3 pitas, purchased or homemade (see page 66), and cut in half

Dressing
- 1 cup plain yogurt
- 1 teaspoon warmed honey or 1 tablespoon apple juice
- 1 tablespoon lemon juice

1. Prepare apple, nuts, and celery. Juice lemon. Cut pita bread in half.

2. Cut chicken into strips and cook thoroughly in hot oil. Remove from heat and cool.

3. Combine cooled chicken strips, apple, celery and nuts in a bowl.

4. Mix together yogurt, lemon juice and warmed honey or apple juice. Pour over ingredients and toss. Cover and refrigerate.

5. Fill a small container with the chicken and apple mixture for a school lunch. Wrap pitas separately. Scoop filling into pita pockets just before eating.

Options:
- Substitute 1 cup fresh fruit, chopped, or ¼ cup chopped dehydrated fruit (page 137), cranberries, raisins, or dates, for the apple.
- Substitute a can of tuna, well drained, for the chicken.
- At Step 3, add 1 teaspoon garam masala seasoning or curry powder.

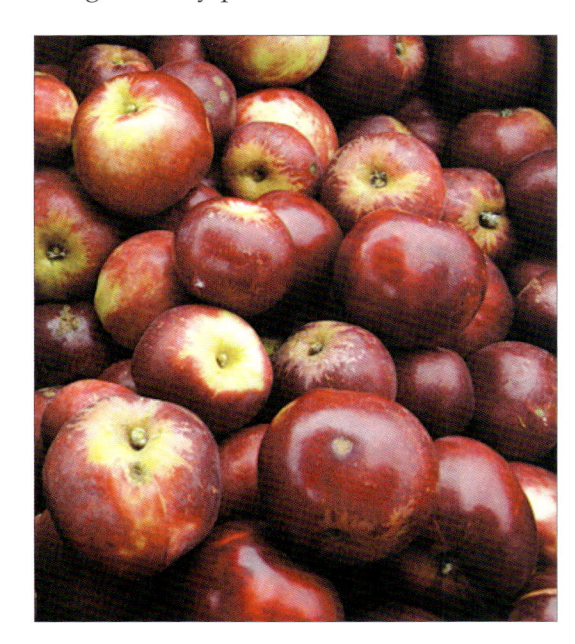

76 Main Dish ☞ Sandwich and Wrap Recipes

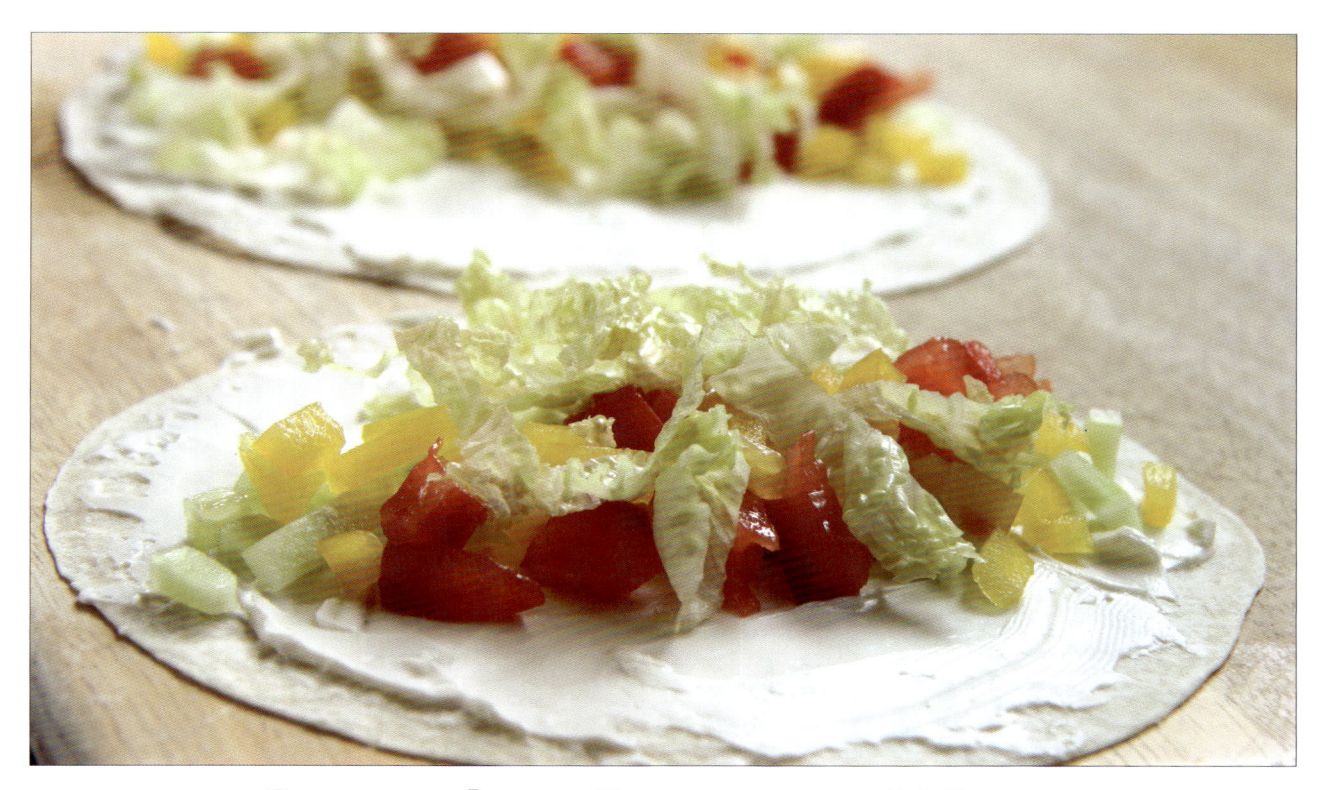

Crunchy Creamy Wrap

1 Serving

This is a fresh version of a wrap (see Sandwich Formula on page 68). Substitute or leave out specific fillings, based on availability or your preference.

    1 flour tortilla
1-2 tablespoons cream cheese
    1 medium tomato, chopped
    2 slices cucumber, chopped
    2 slices bell pepper, chopped
    6 fresh spinach leaves, chopped
    4 olives, drained and sliced
    1 tablespoon chopped nuts

1. Bring cream cheese to room temperature. Spread evenly on tortilla.

2. Chop tomato, cucumber, pepper and spinach leaves. Slice olives.

3. Spread vegetables out evenly over cream cheese.

4. Roll up tortilla with fillings, or fold it like a burrito (see page 79).

Options:

- Substitute lettuce for the spinach leaves.
- Substitute low- or non-fat cream cheese for cream cheese or choose a different spread.
- Substitute other crunchy vegetables like cabbage, jicama, or bean sprouts for vegetables listed.

Main Dish ☞ Sandwich and Wrap Recipes

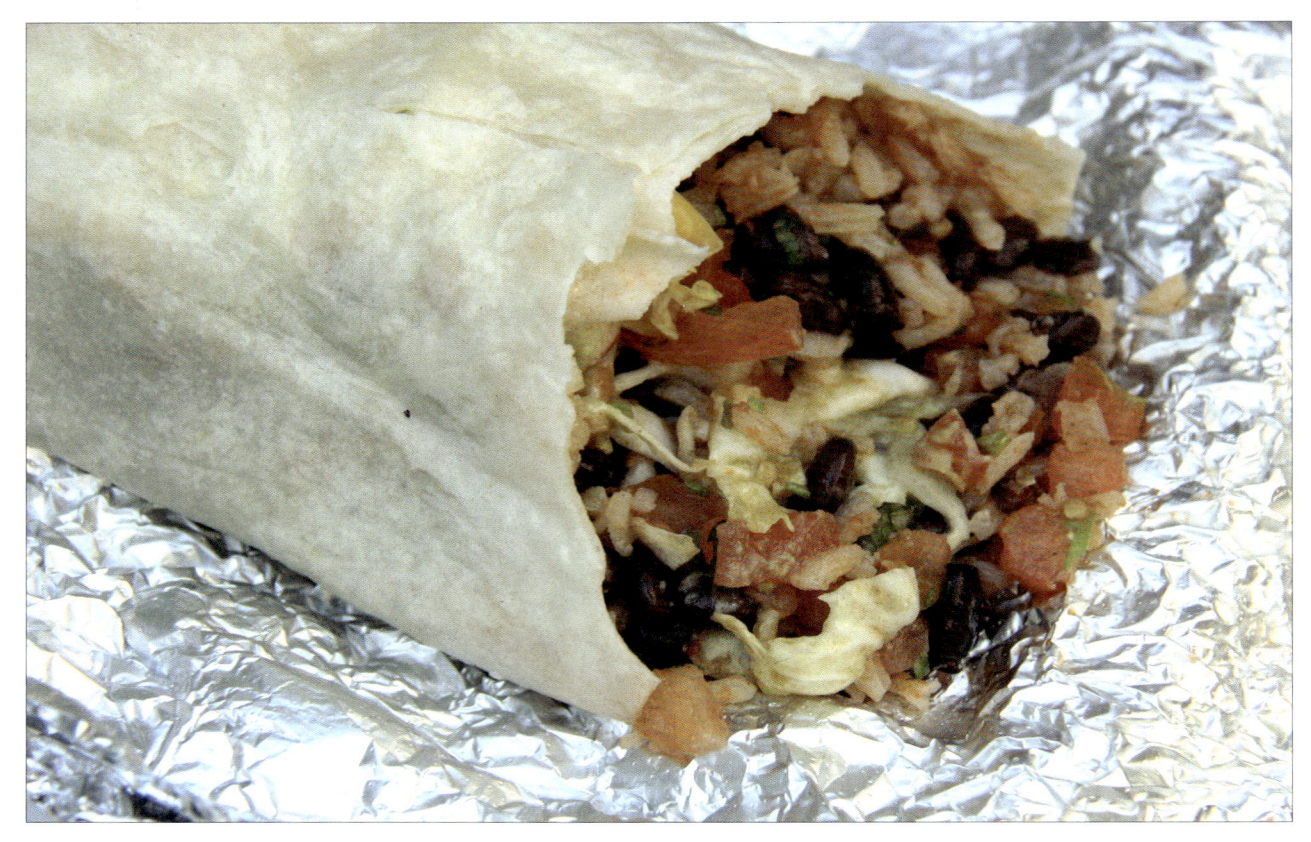

Burritos

Yield: 4 Burritos

Burrito *is Spanish for "little donkey." If you pack your "little donkey" just right, it'll carry a whole, delicious lunch for you. These wraps were developed in Mexico and in Native and Mexican-American communities in the U.S. For your first attempt at rolling, use a little less filling than you think you want. The more stuffing, the trickier it is to roll up.*

- 2 tablespoons vegetable oil
- 1 small onion, chopped (about ½ cup)
- 1 garlic clove, finely chopped
- 1 cup cooked black, pinto or red beans (½ cup dried or half a 14.5- to 16-ounce can)
- 1 small tomato, chopped
- 1 tablespoon Mexican Spice Mix (see page 193) or a combination of your favorite Mexican spices. Try 1 teaspoon each of cumin, oregano, chile powder, ½ teaspoon salt and ⅛ teaspoon pepper to start.
- 2 cups cooked rice (1 cup uncooked)
- 1 cup grated cheese
- 1 cup lettuce, chopped
- 4 10 to 12-inch flour tortillas (see page 59)
  Salsa or guacamole to taste

1. Clean and prepare the vegetables. Grate the cheese. Cook the rice (see page 56) and beans (see page 54) if necessary. Rinse and drain beans if canned.

2. Place oil in a 10-inch frying pan over medium-low heat. Add onion and garlic and sauté until onion becomes translucent, about 5 minutes.

3. Mix in the beans and tomato; add seasoning. Cook 2 to 3 minutes. Stir occasionally.

4. Spread ¼ of the bean mixture down the center of each tortilla, sprinkle with ¼ of the rice, ¼ of the cheese and some greens.

5. Roll the burrito up following the pictures below. Tuck sides, pull bottom up and tuck edges under contents. Roll.

6. Wrap in foil and place in a sealable bag. To reheat at school, take the burrito out of the foil wrap.

Options:

- Substitute finely sliced cabbage or other leafy greens for the lettuce.
- At Step 2, add finely sliced or chopped tofu, scrambled egg, or leftover meat.

Beans

Beans are a central part of diets worldwide. They are the rock stars of inexpensive, healthy eating. Common beans include black, pinto, kidney, red, garbanzo/chickpeas, black-eyed peas, lentils, edamame/soy, lima and fava. Beans are in the same legume family as peas.

For sandwiches and wraps, you can use whole beans, chopped tofu (soybeans), Hummus (see page 167), or Black or White Bean Spread (see page 163).

Cooking dried beans yourself is the cheapest way to go, and allows you to lessen the bean's most notorious result: making people fart! (see page 54).

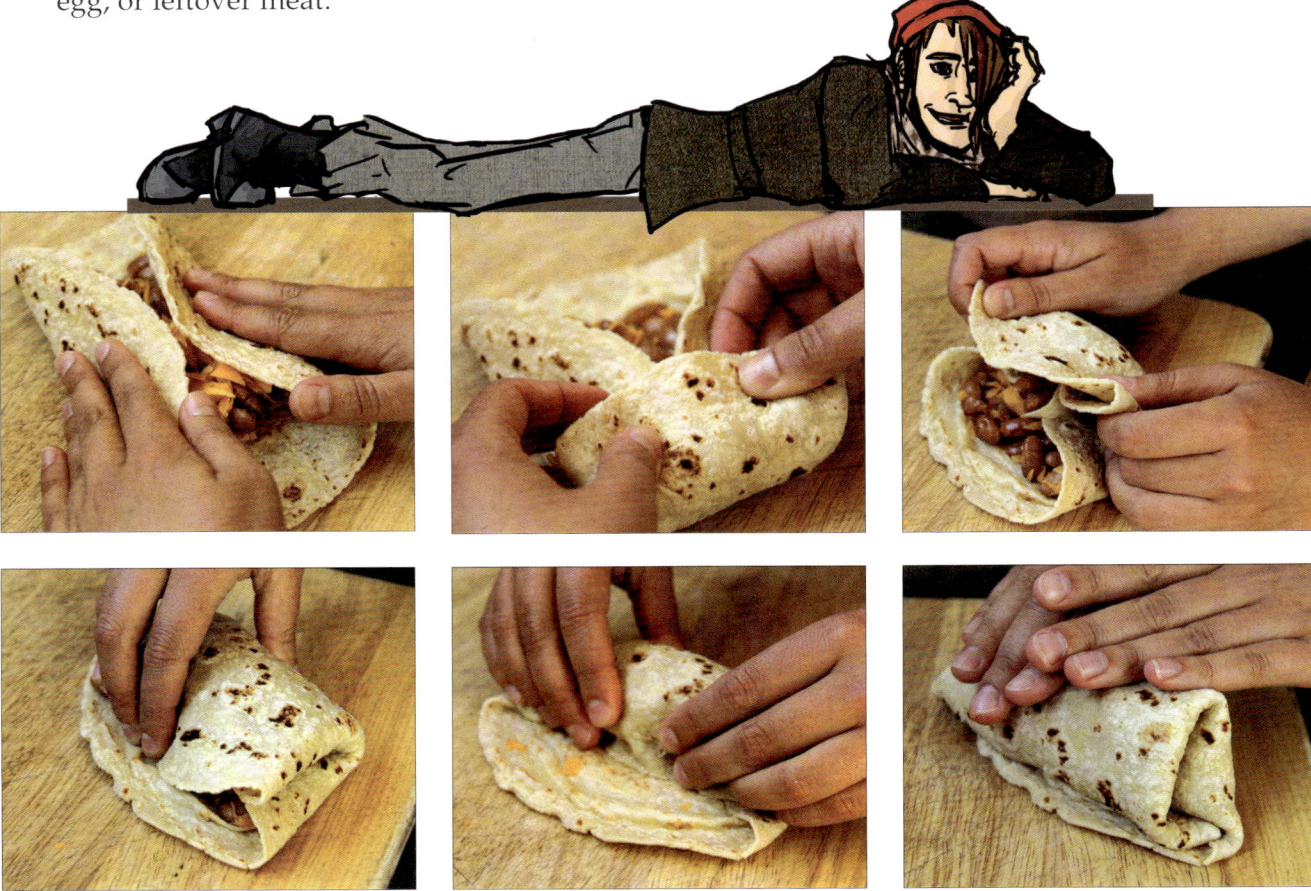

Main Dish ☞ Sandwich and Wrap Recipes

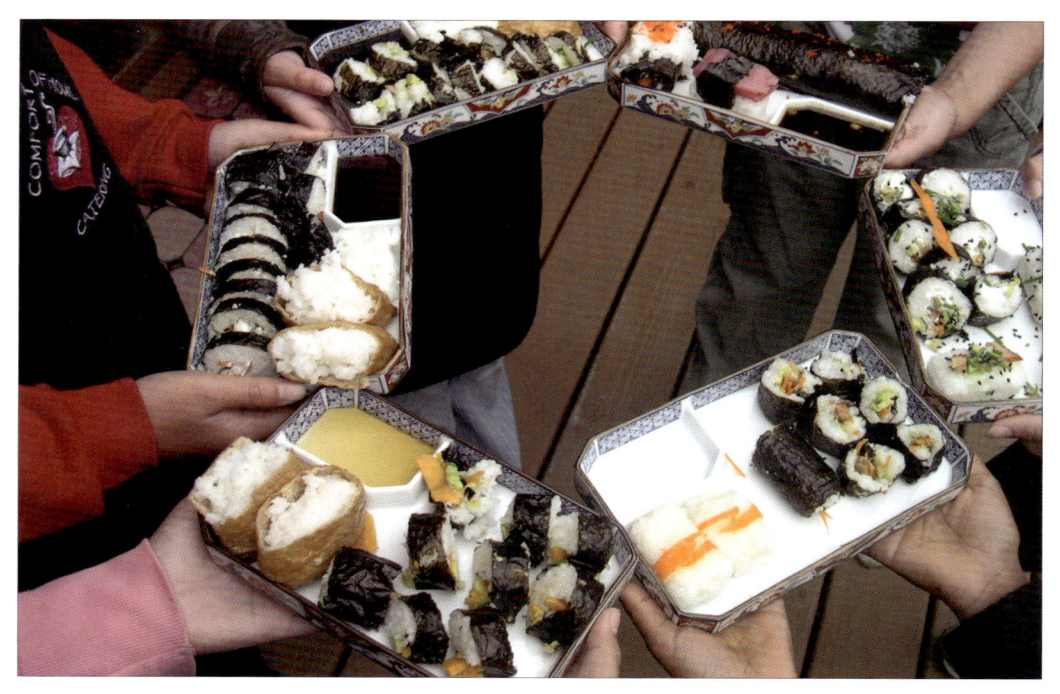

Sushi

Yield: About 30 pieces

This recipe is fun to play with. Choose any fillings you know you like, or try some new ones. Sushi is a high-value trading item in the cafeteria.

- 4 nori wrappers
- 2 cups cooked rice (1 cup uncooked, see page 56)
- ¼ cup rice vinegar
- ½ teaspoon salt
- 1 teaspoon sugar
- 8-12 thin matchstick-like slices of fillings including avocado, cucumber, carrot, bell pepper, cabbage, kale
- 4 ounces baked tofu (see page 145), smoked salmon, chicken, or tuna
- 4 ounces baked sweet potato, cream cheese or peanut butter

Soy sauce or tamari for dipping

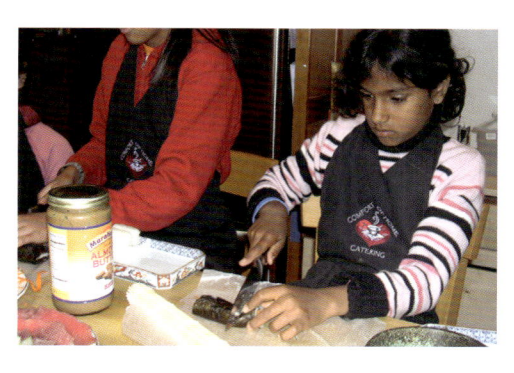

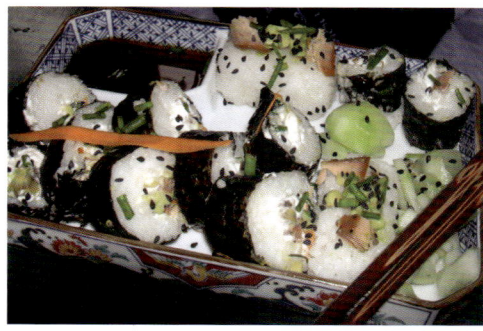

1. Cook rice (see page 56) if necessary.
2. Mix vinegar, sugar and salt. Stir into rice. Let cool.
3. Clean, prepare and lay out vegetables and other fillings.
4. Lay out nori with the short side closest to you. Spread ½ cup cooled rice over ⅔ of the nori.
5. Place 2-4 filling items over the rice. Extend the filling to the edge of the nori.
6. Pull nori up and over the fillings. Roll tightly to the end of the rice (see photos, below).
7. Dip your finger in a bit of water and dampen the top edge of the nori. Continue rolling. The dampened nori should stick to the roll, making a tight closure.
8. Using a sharp knife, cut the roll into 1-inch slices. Serve with soy sauce.

Options:
- Substitute flour tortillas for nori. (See page 59.)
- Serve with peanut sauce, chile dipping sauce, pickled ginger pieces and/or wasabi and put in individual containers. Watch out—that wasabi stuff is hot!
- Use of a sushi mat makes rolling easier.

Nori Snacks

Nori is dried seaweed used as the wrapper for sushi. It comes in packs of oblong sheets, which can be found at many grocery stores.

Other sea vegetables are eaten in many parts of Eastern Asia, and are now popular in the U.S. Sea vegetables are high in important vitamins, minerals and oils.

Making nori snacks at home saves money and reduces waste.

Tear or cut up plain nori sheets into smaller pieces or brush large sheets with curry paste, wasabi, or soy sauce. Bake in an oven on low heat until nori is crisp, then break up into pieces for snacks. Keep nori crunchy by storing in an airtight container.

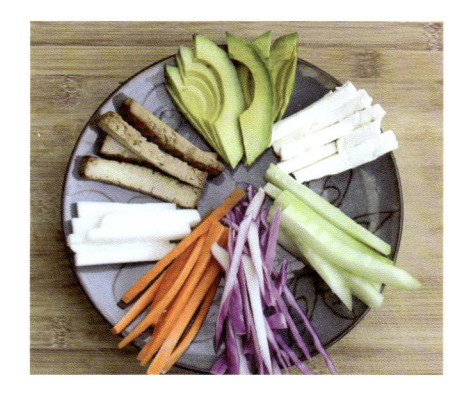

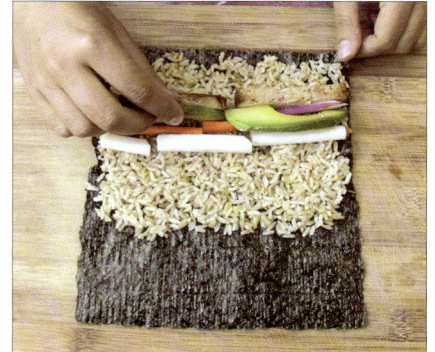

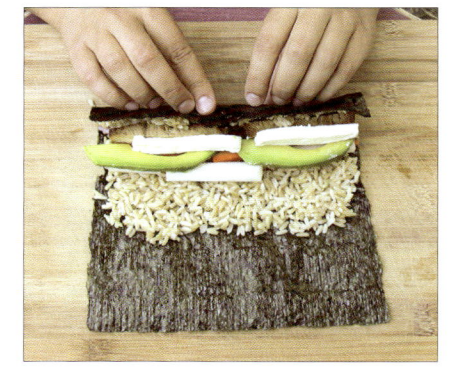

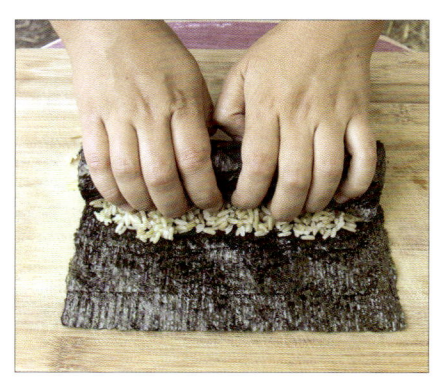

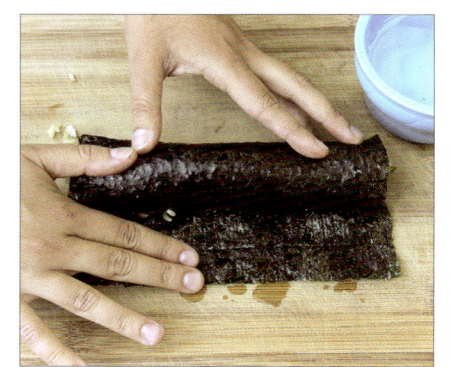

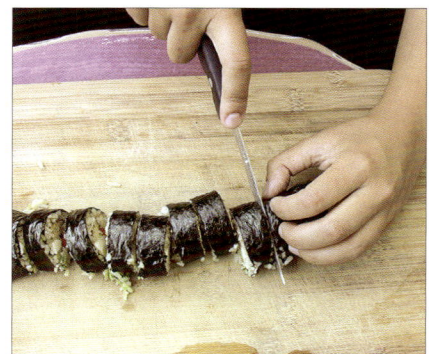

Pizza Formula

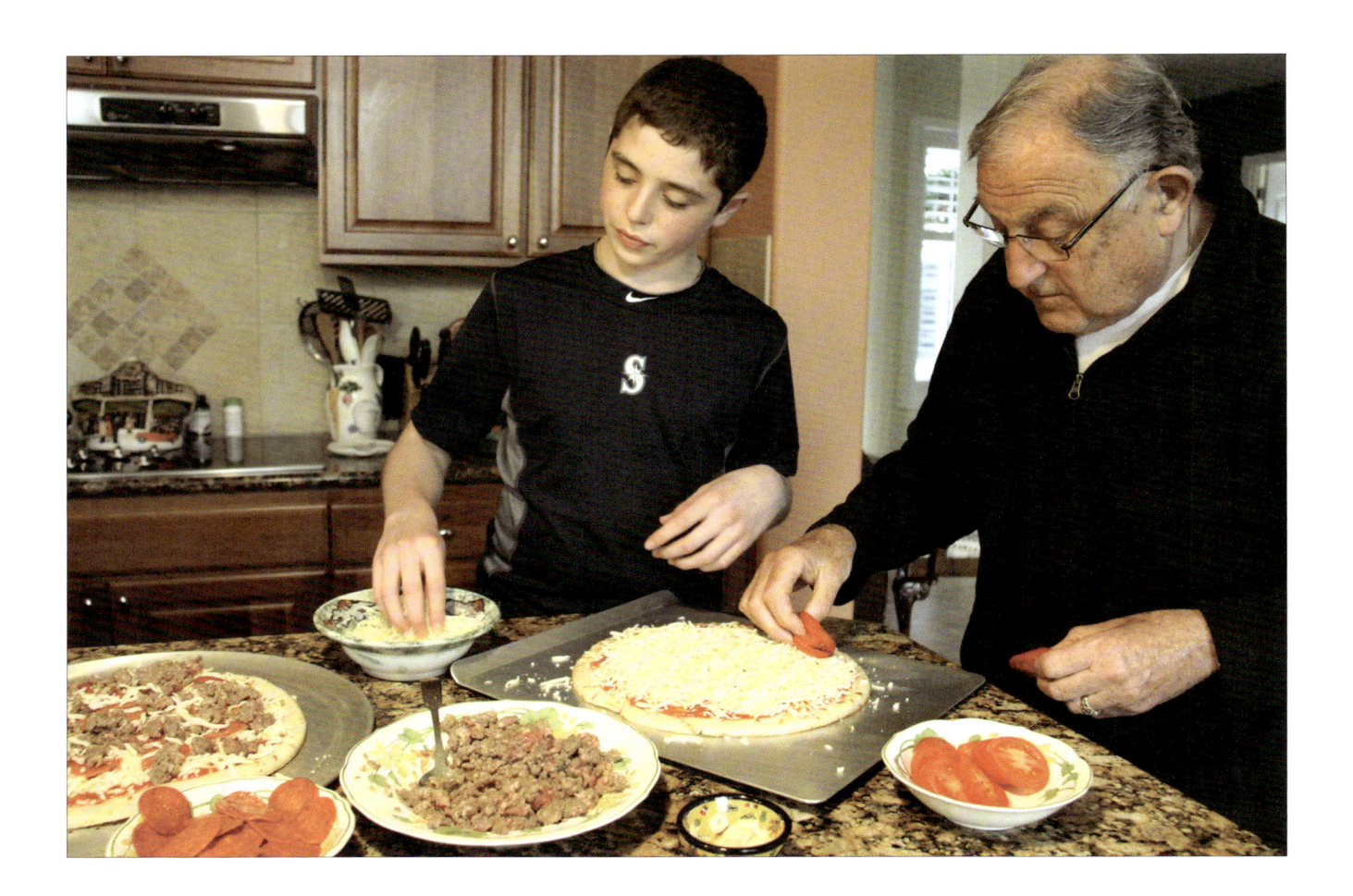

1. Preheat oven to 425°. Choose a crust on which to build your pizza.

2. Lightly oil a baking sheet or sprinkle it with cornmeal. Place crust on baking sheet.

3. Spread sauce on the base.

4. Spread grated cheese over the sauce.

5. Spread toppings over all. Some vegetables may need precooking.

6. Bake pizza until cheese is melted and base is crisp.

Ingredient Ideas

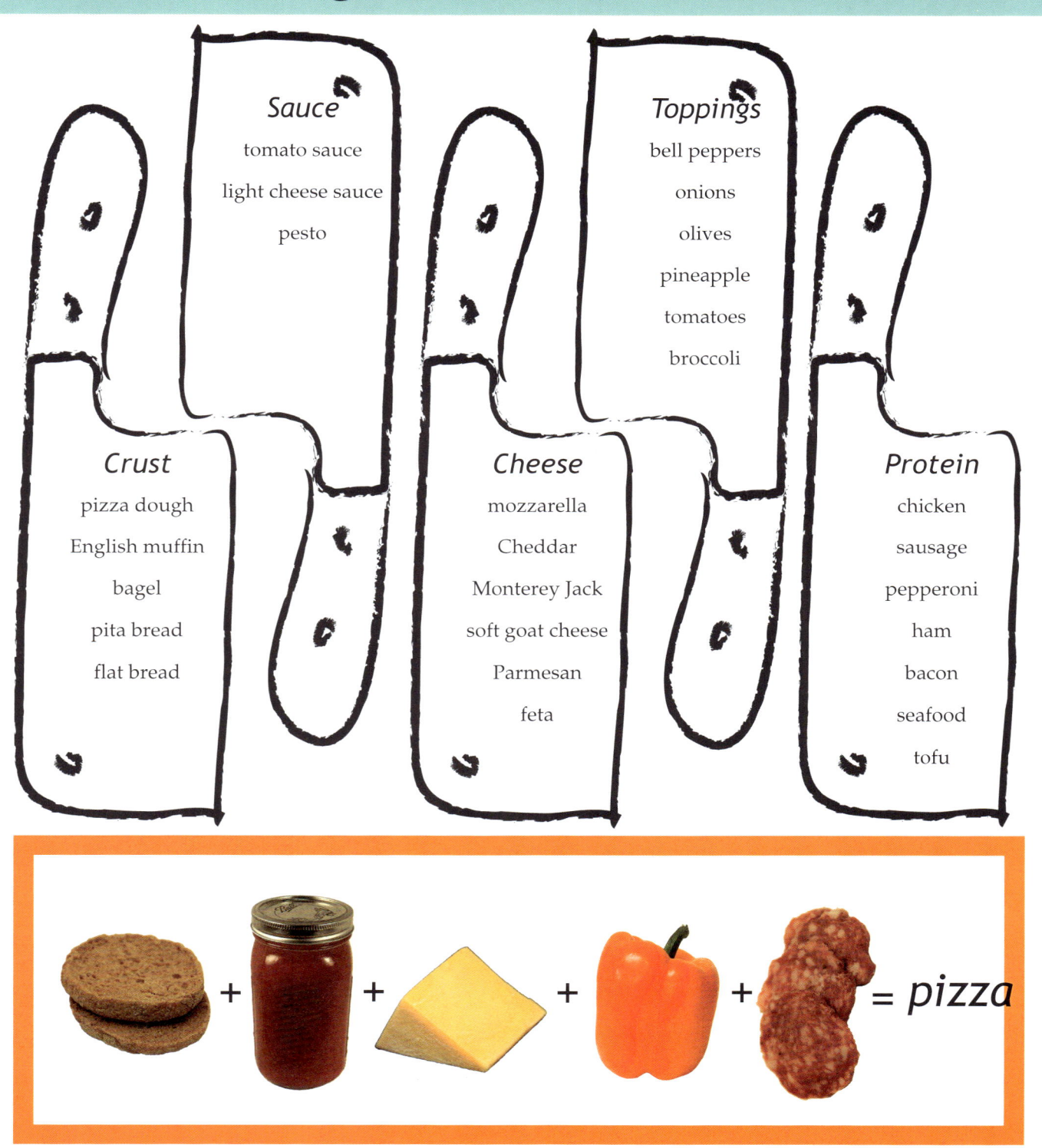

Crust
pizza dough
English muffin
bagel
pita bread
flat bread

Sauce
tomato sauce
light cheese sauce
pesto

Cheese
mozzarella
Cheddar
Monterey Jack
soft goat cheese
Parmesan
feta

Toppings
bell peppers
onions
olives
pineapple
tomatoes
broccoli

Protein
chicken
sausage
pepperoni
ham
bacon
seafood
tofu

+ + + + = *pizza*

Main Dish ☞ Sandwich and Wrap Recipes

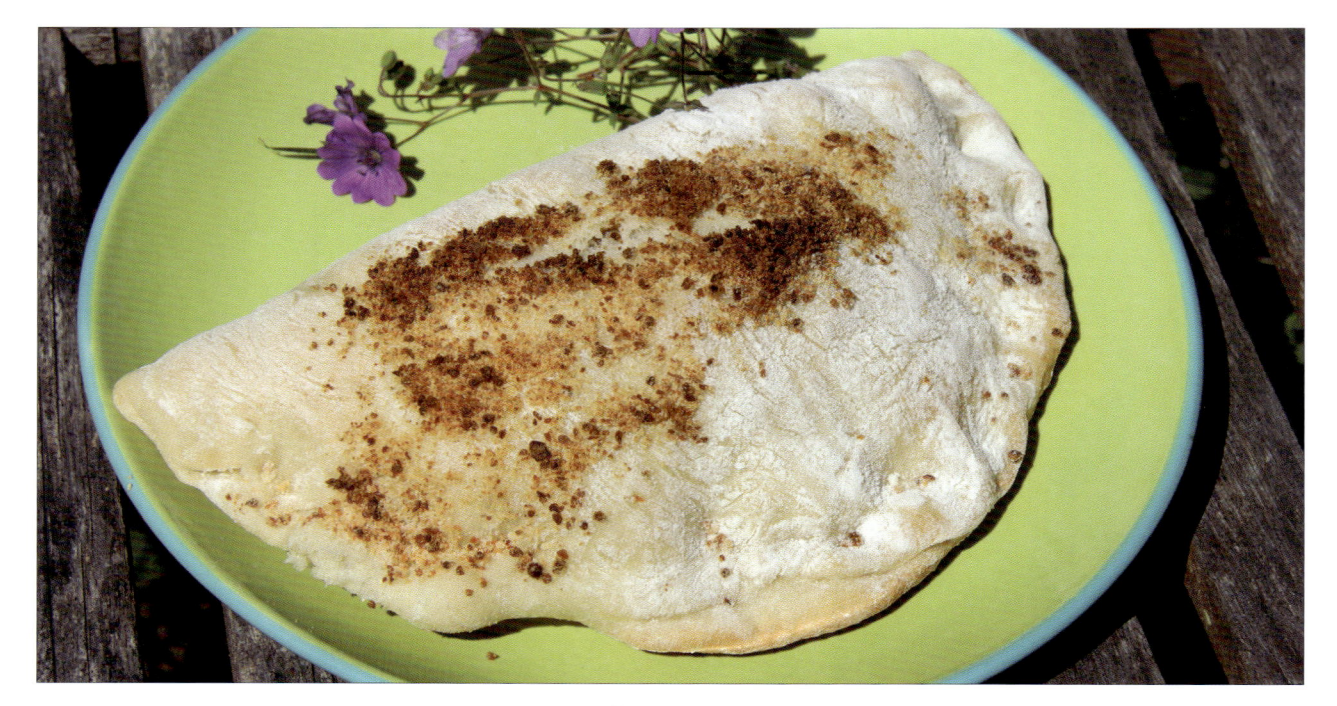

Calzones

Yield: 6 Calzones

Calzones are a covered pizza. Simply fold dough in half and bake ingredients inside, rather than on top of the crust. Make the calzones either family- or single-serving sizes.

- 2 tablespoons flour or cornmeal, for rolling dough
- 1 recipe Pizza Dough (see page 64)
- 15 ounces tomato (see page 65) or other sauce (about 2 cups)
- 1 cup chopped filling. Choose from pepperoni, salami, Canadian bacon, chicken, pineapple, mushrooms, olives, onions, red or green pepper, zucchini, tomato
- ½ cup grated Parmesan cheese
- Cornmeal for baking sheet
- Olive or vegetable oil

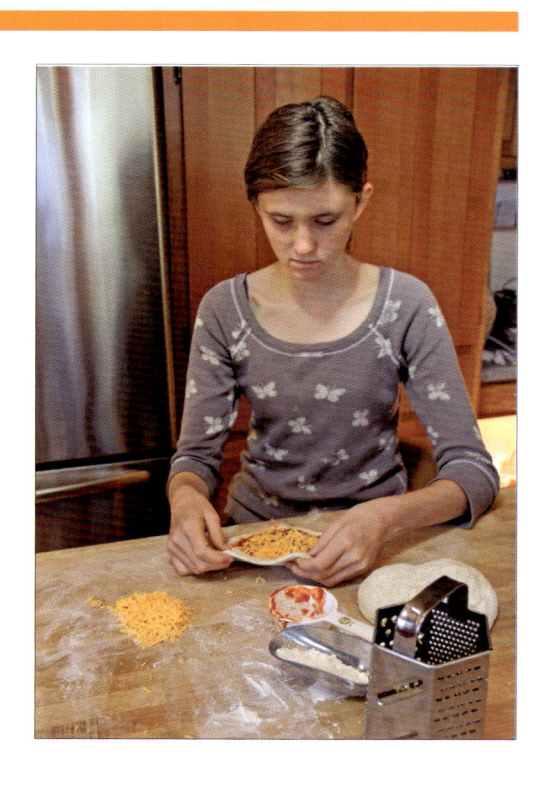

84 Main Dish ☞ Sandwich and Wrap Recipes

Preheat oven to 425°

1. Prepare pizza dough and divide into six equal pieces. Sprinkle flour or cornmeal on a clean counter surface. Roll each piece into a 7-inch circle.

2. Prepare the fillings.

3. Spread the sauce evenly over the dough. Leave a ¼-inch edge all the way around.

4. Place ⅓ cup filling along with 2 tablespoons cheese on half of dough circle.

5. Use water to moisten ¼-inch around the edge of each circle of dough. Fold the dough in half to enclose the filling. Crimp the moistened edges together with fingers or by pressing with a fork. Seal edges so the filling doesn't leak out.

6. Lightly sprinkle a baking sheet with cornmeal and place the calzones on the baking sheet about 2 inches apart.

7. Brush tops lightly with oil and sprinkle with remaining cheese if desired.

8. Bake until golden brown, 15-20 minutes. Let cool slightly before removing from pan.

Pockets of the World

Fillings inside of baked or fried dough are found all over the world.

Calzones are an Italian pocket, and Empanadas (see page 86) are found in Spanish-influenced regions.

Other pockets include:

- **Pierogis** from Eastern European countries and the U.S. Midwest
- **Samosas** from India and Southeast Asia
- **Pasties** from the UK
- **Gyoza** from Japan
- **Boa** from China

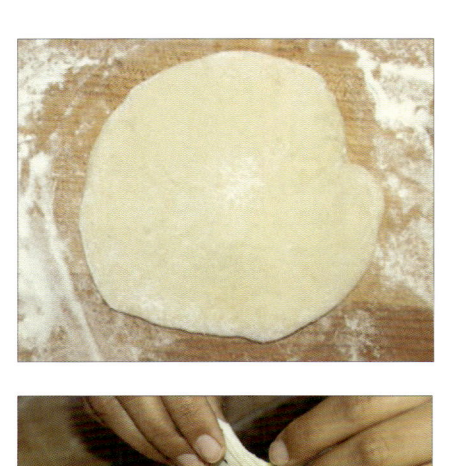

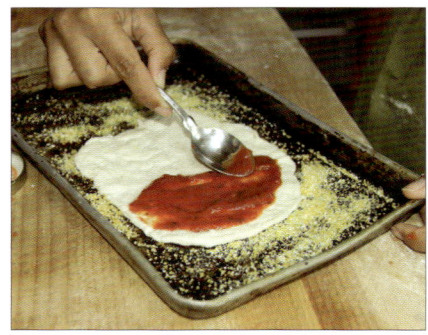

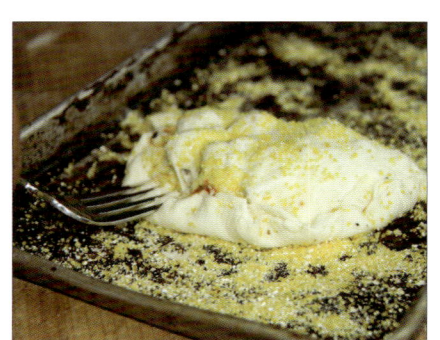

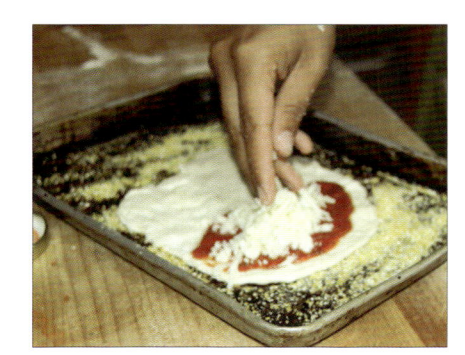

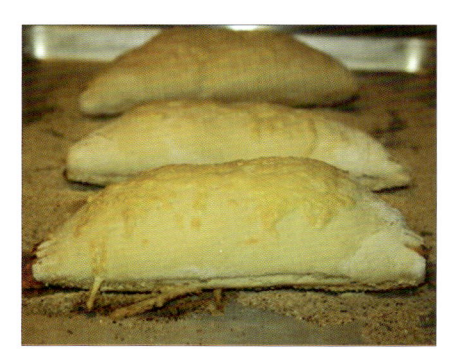

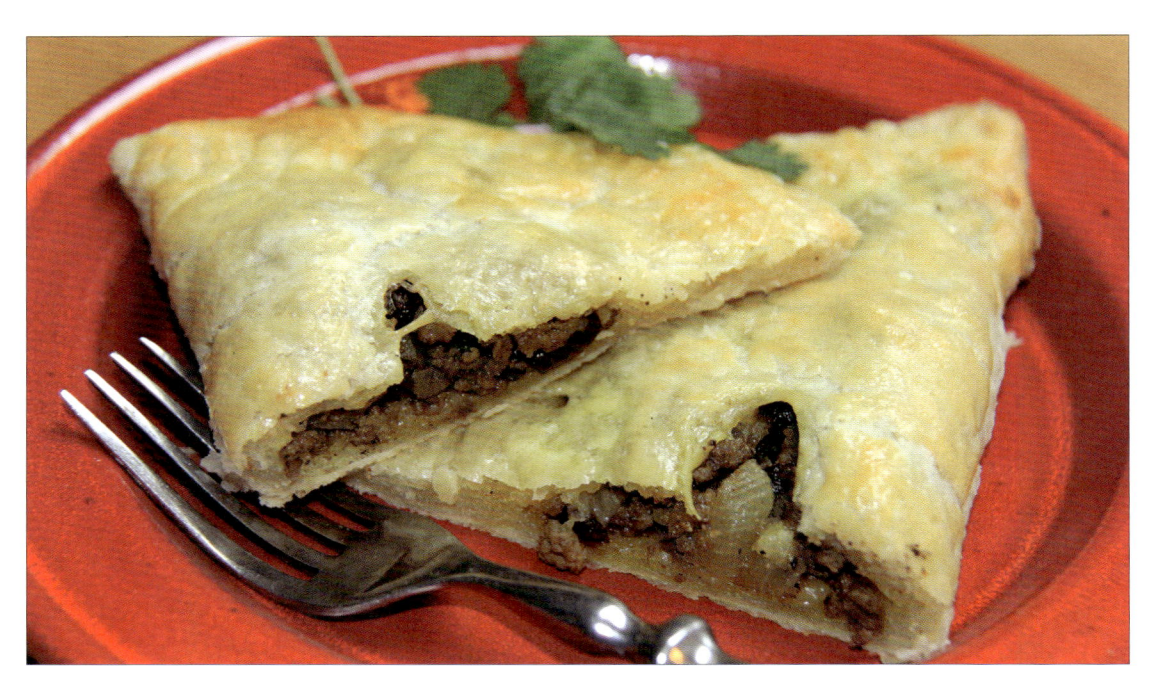

Empanadas

Yield: 8-12 Empanadas

In Spanish, empanar *means "to bake in a bread-like cover." Empanadas are meals wrapped in dough. There are many options for empanadas. You'll find these flavorful pockets in Spain, across Central and South America, the Caribbean, Southeast Asia and parts of West Africa. To prepare them for quick lunches for 1-2 weeks, make a double or triple batch.*

- 1 recipe pie dough (see page 63)
- 1 cup warm water
- ½ cup raisins
- 2 tablespoons olive oil, vegetable oil or butter
- 1 large onion, chopped (about 1½ cups)
- 1 pound ground meat (pork, beef, turkey, chicken)
- 1 teaspoon Mexican Spice Mix (see page 193) or try 1 teaspoon each of cumin, oregano, chile powder, ½ teaspoon salt and ⅛ teaspoon pepper to start.
- 1 egg
- 1 cup water

Prepare Dough

For Filling:

1. Add water to raisins in a small bowl. Let soak while you cook the filling.

2. Wash and prepare vegetables.

3. Add oil or butter to skillet over medium heat. Add onions; sauté until translucent, 3-5 minutes.

4. Add the meat to the onions. With a spatula, break meat into smaller pieces. As meat and onions cook, add 2 teaspoons of spice to mixture. Cook until meat is no longer pink. Taste. Add more spice as needed.

5. Drain raisins, add to filling.

6. Whisk the egg in a small bowl and set aside.

Assemble and Bake the Empanadas:

Preheat oven to 350°

1. Lightly oil baking sheet.

2. Whisk egg in a cup or small bowl.

3. For homemade dough, divide dough into four even pieces and roll ¼ inch thick, about 6 inches in diameter. For purchased dough, cut out 6-inch circles. Combine and re-roll excess into another round.

4. Spoon 2 tablespoons of filling on one side of a round. Use a brush or your fingers to wet edges of dough.

5. Fold dough in half to cover filling. Crimp moistened edges together with fingers or by pressing with a fork. Poke top of the empanada with fork to make holes for steam to escape.

6. Place empanadas on oiled baking sheet. Brush each lightly with whisked egg.

7. Bake about 25 minutes, or until golden brown.

Options:

- Use packaged rolled pie dough instead of making your own.
- Alternate fillings: Use ½ pound meat and 1 cup cooked beans. Try tuna, black beans, or cooked winter squash, pumpkin, sweet potatoes, yams, potatoes, carrots or corn; try hard-cooked egg, black olives, fruit, or 3 small summer squashes, chopped.
- Cook, freeze, and re-heat: Bake and let cool. Wrap in small groups or individually and put in freezer. Remove empanadas from freezer the night before and defrost in the refrigerator. Bake in toaster oven for a few minutes in morning so the empanadas aren't soggy at lunchtime.
- Prepare and freeze for later use: Omit egg glaze and freeze individually wrapped, raw empanadas. Remove from freezer and bake 30-35 minutes, according to Step 6.

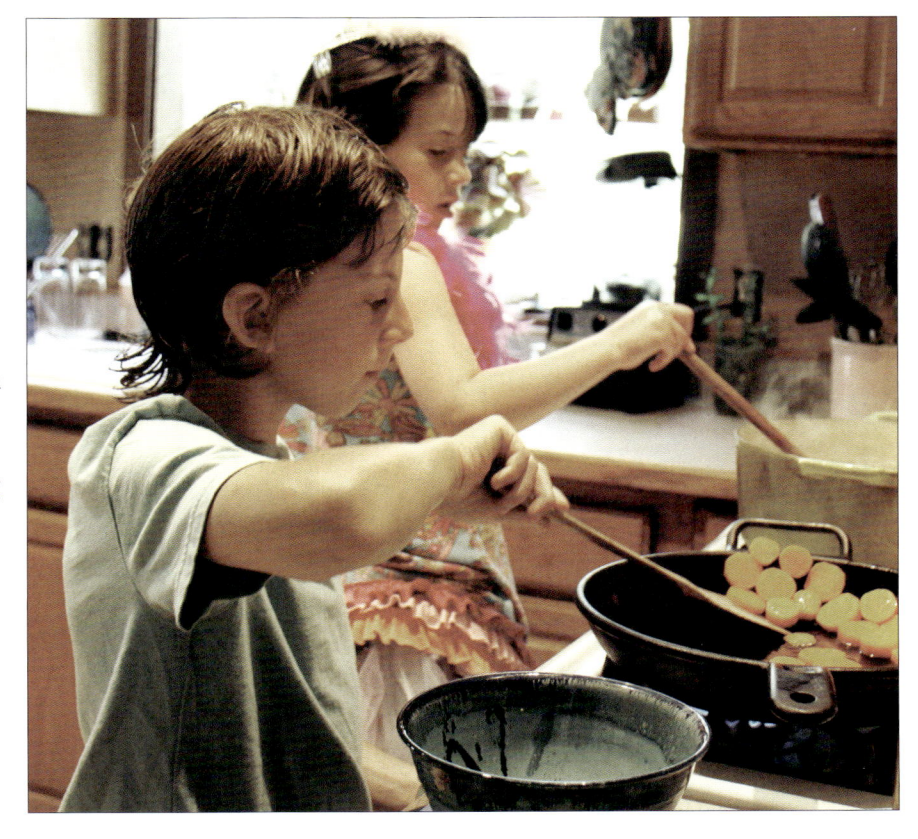

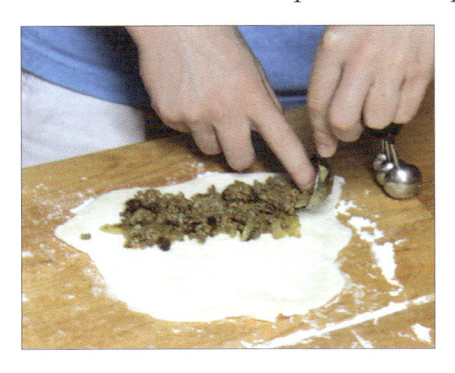

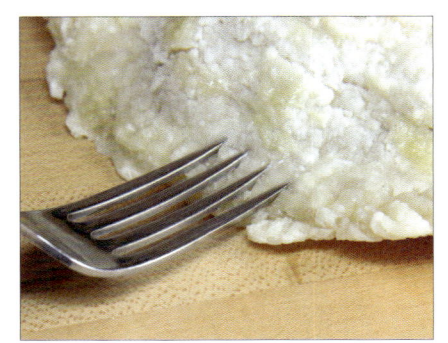

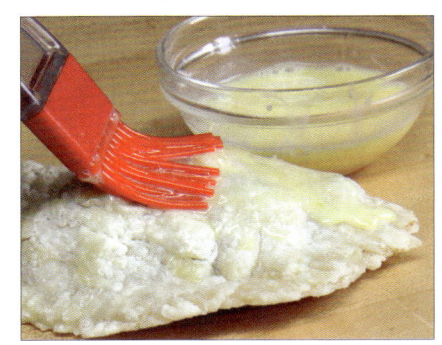

Main Dish ☞ Sandwich and Wrap Recipes

Italian Pasta Formula

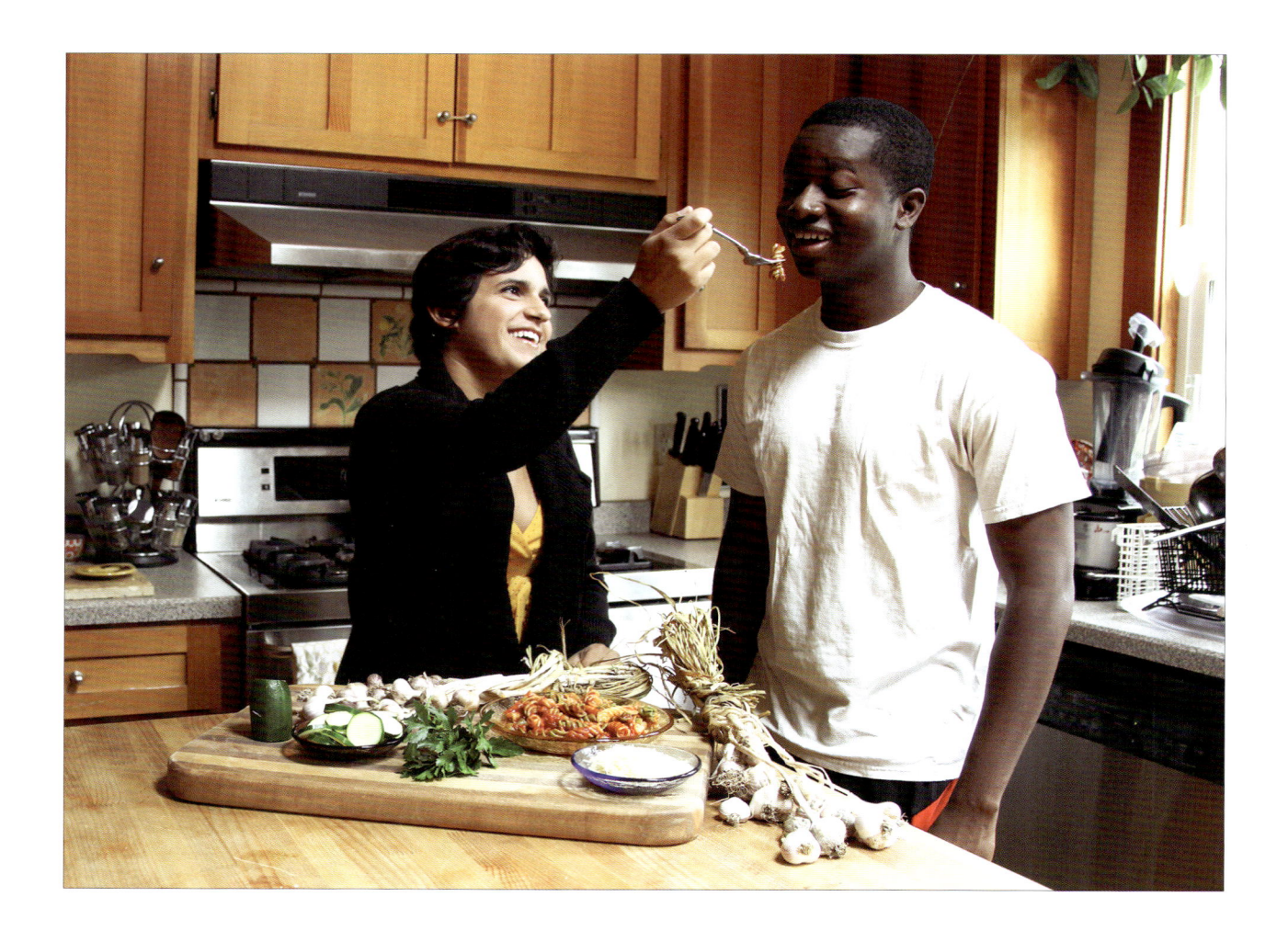

1. Fill 2-quart pot halfway with water. Bring to boil, then add pasta carefully. Cook (see page 57).

2. Sauté, steam, grill, or roast raw mix-ins. Set aside.

3. Prepare or heat sauce while pasta is cooking.

4. Pour cooked pasta through a colander set over the sink, to drain off the water.

5. Combine mix-ins, sauce and noodles. Sprinkle with toppings.

Ingredient Ideas

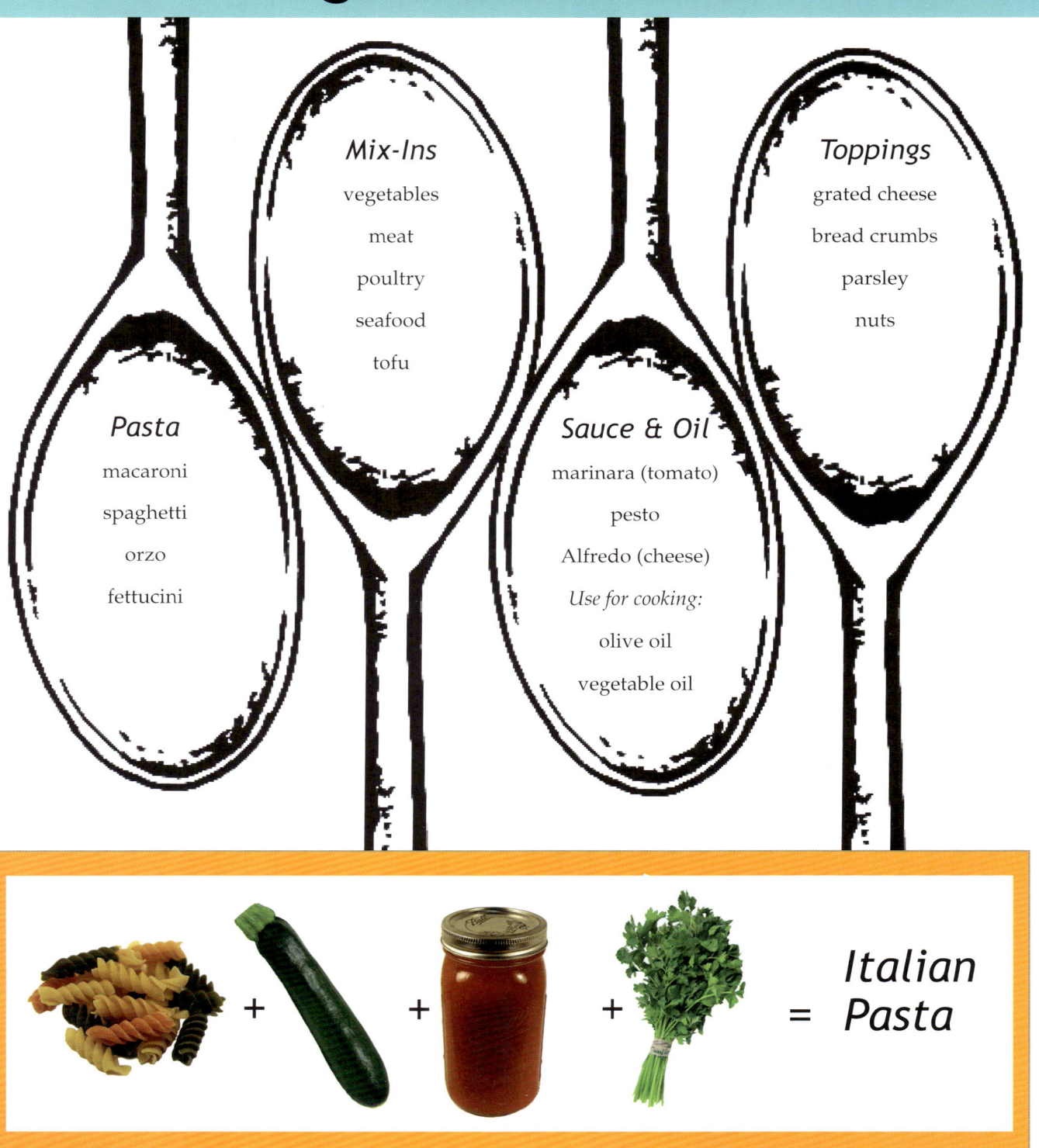

Pasta
- macaroni
- spaghetti
- orzo
- fettucini

Mix-Ins
- vegetables
- meat
- poultry
- seafood
- tofu

Sauce & Oil
- marinara (tomato)
- pesto
- Alfredo (cheese)

Use for cooking:
- olive oil
- vegetable oil

Toppings
- grated cheese
- bread crumbs
- parsley
- nuts

pasta + zucchini + sauce + parsley = *Italian Pasta*

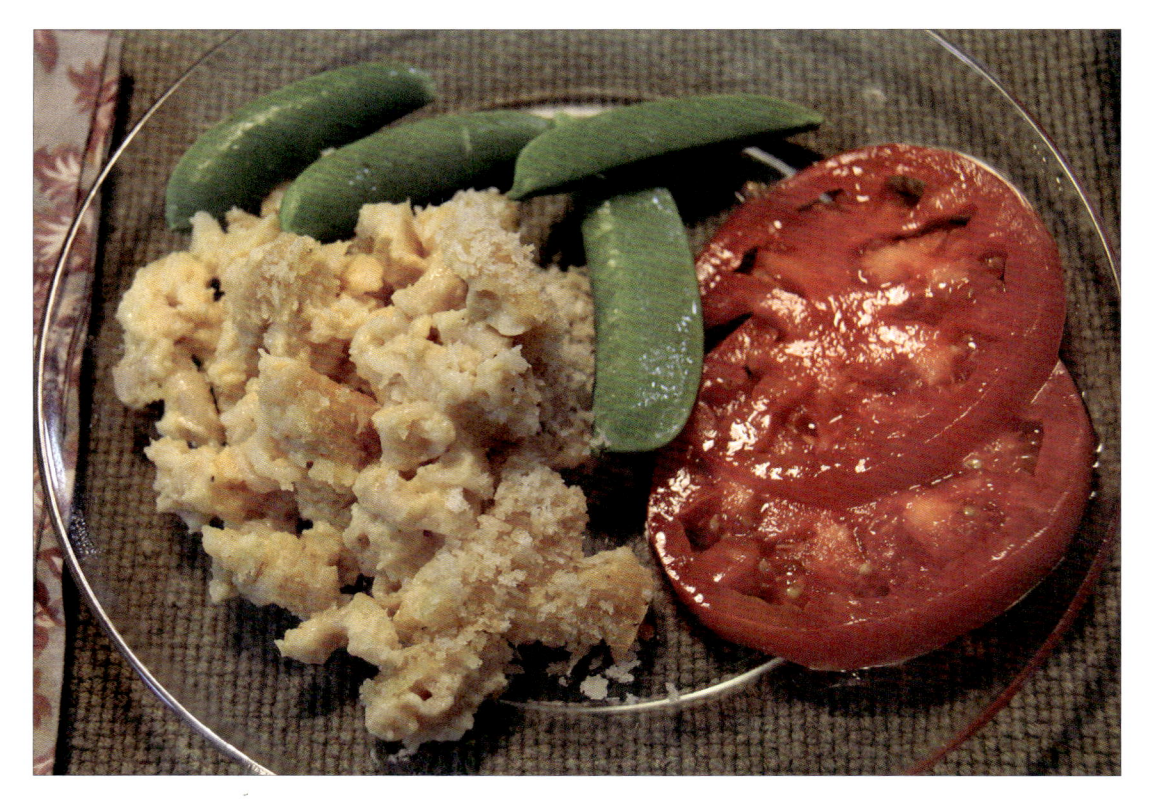

Mac & Cheese

6-8 servings

Mac and cheese from the box sure is easy, but nothing compares to the richness of homemade or to the fun of making it. This version is the favorite of two young experts, the nephews of one of the authors of this book (the boys in the photos). Mix in favorite vegetables as a great way to make this cheesy dish even healthier.

- 4 quarts water
- 1 pound macaroni
- 1 quart milk (4 cups)
- 1 stick unsalted butter (8 tablespoons), divided
- ½ cup flour
- 1½ teaspoon salt
- 2 cups grated sharp Cheddar cheese (10 ounces)
- ½ teaspoon pepper
- ½ teaspoon nutmeg
- 1 cup bread crumbs or panko flakes

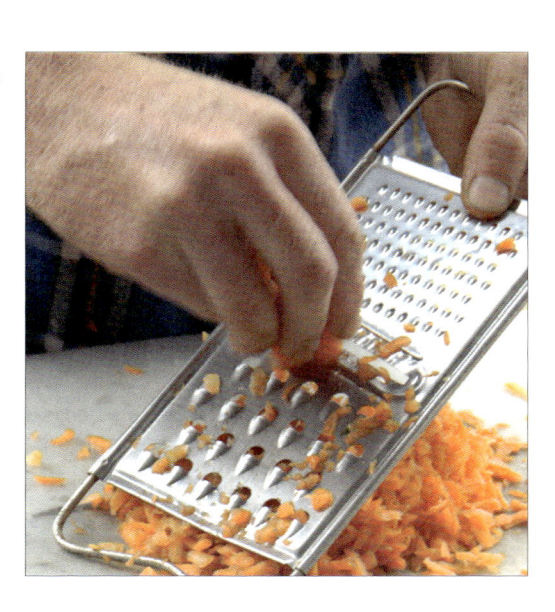

90 Main Dish ☞ Grain and Noodle Recipes

Preheat oven to 375°

1. Oil a 3-quart baking dish.

2. Bring water to a boil in large pot. Carefully add macaroni and cook (see page 57). Drain.

3. While macaroni is cooking, bring milk to a simmer in small pot or microwave. Grate cheese.

4. In 5-quart pan, melt 6 tablespoons butter over low heat. Whisk until flour and butter are incorporated, about 2 minutes. This is called a *roux* (see Tomato Soup, page 120 for photos).

5. Continue whisking and slowly add hot milk. Cook, stirring, until sauce is thick and smooth, 5-7 minutes. Remove from the heat. This is called a *white sauce*.

6. Add salt, Cheddar cheese, pepper and nutmeg to white sauce. Add cooked macaroni to pan and stir until well coated with sauce.

7. Pour into oiled baking dish.

8. Melt 2 tablespoons of butter and combine with panko flakes or bread crumbs. Sprinkle over pasta and sauce.

9. Bake 30 minutes or until bubbling and browned on top.

Options:

- At Step 6, substitute multiple kinds of cheese, including 2 cups Swiss and ½ cup Jack, for the Cheddar. Try different combinations, but don't add more Jack cheese, as it will make the sauce too greasy. Mix in vegetables that won't get mushy, such as frozen peas, carrots, cauliflower or broccoli.

- At Step 8, top with ¼ cup Parmesan cheese.

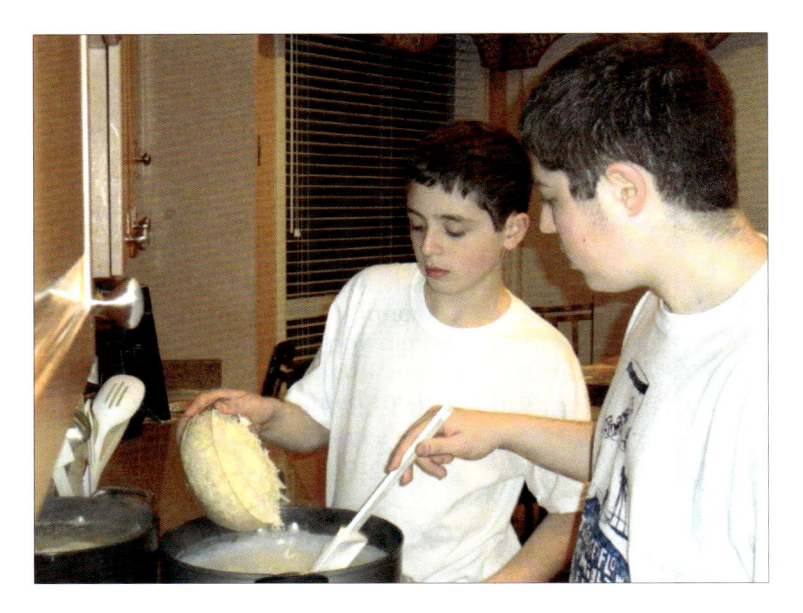

Bread Crumbs

Making your own bread crumbs from dry bread is far cheaper than purchased versions.

Homemade Bread Crumbs:

1. Save bread odds and ends in a sealed bag in the freezer until needed.

2. Lay out bread on baking sheet and dry it in a 300° oven, 10-15 minutes. Turn bread over after about 6 or 7 minutes.

3. To crumble, place bread in sealable bag and roll with a rolling pin or bottle, or chop in a food processor into course bits.

4. Season with salt, pepper and herbs, or leave plain.

Panko is the Japanese version of bread crumbs. These are crunchier, lighter and crispier than other bread crumbs. They're excellent for breading or for meatballs as a filler. The flakes have a large surface area, which absorbs seasoning well. Panko stays crisp longer than other bread crumbs and absorbs less grease.

Gluten-free panko variation

1. Place puffed rice cereal in a plastic bag.

2. Use a rolling pin or a bottle to crush the cereal.

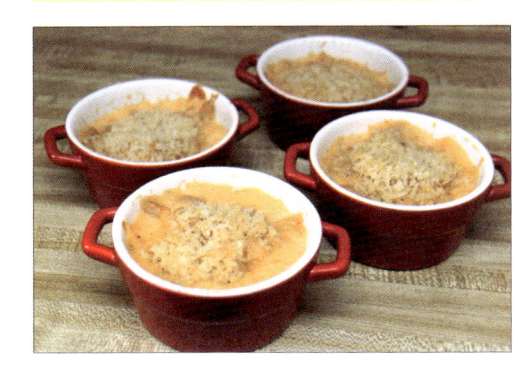

Asian Noodle Formula

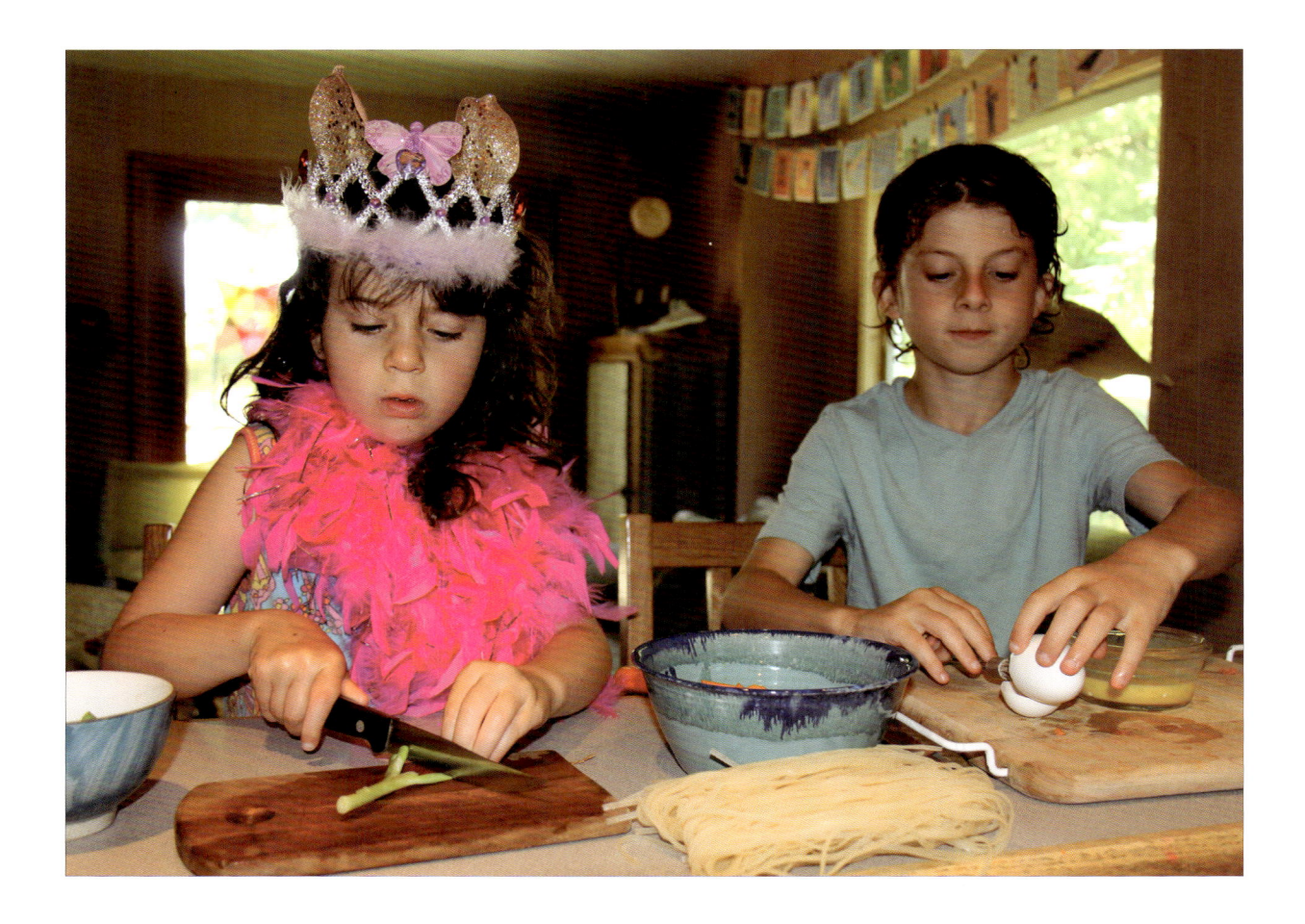

1. Fill large pot halfway with water. Bring to boil. Carefully add noodles. For wheat noodles: Simmer over medium heat. For rice noodles: Turn off heat, let soak until tender (see page 57.)

2. Steam raw mix-ins or sauté them in oil in large sauté pan.

3. When noodles are cooked, pour into colander set over the sink. Rinse and drain. Pour away from you to avoid being burned by steam.

4. Add noodles and sauce to sautéed mix-ins. Stir occasionally to avoid sticking.

5. Serve hot or portion into insulated containers and add toppings.

Ingredient Ideas

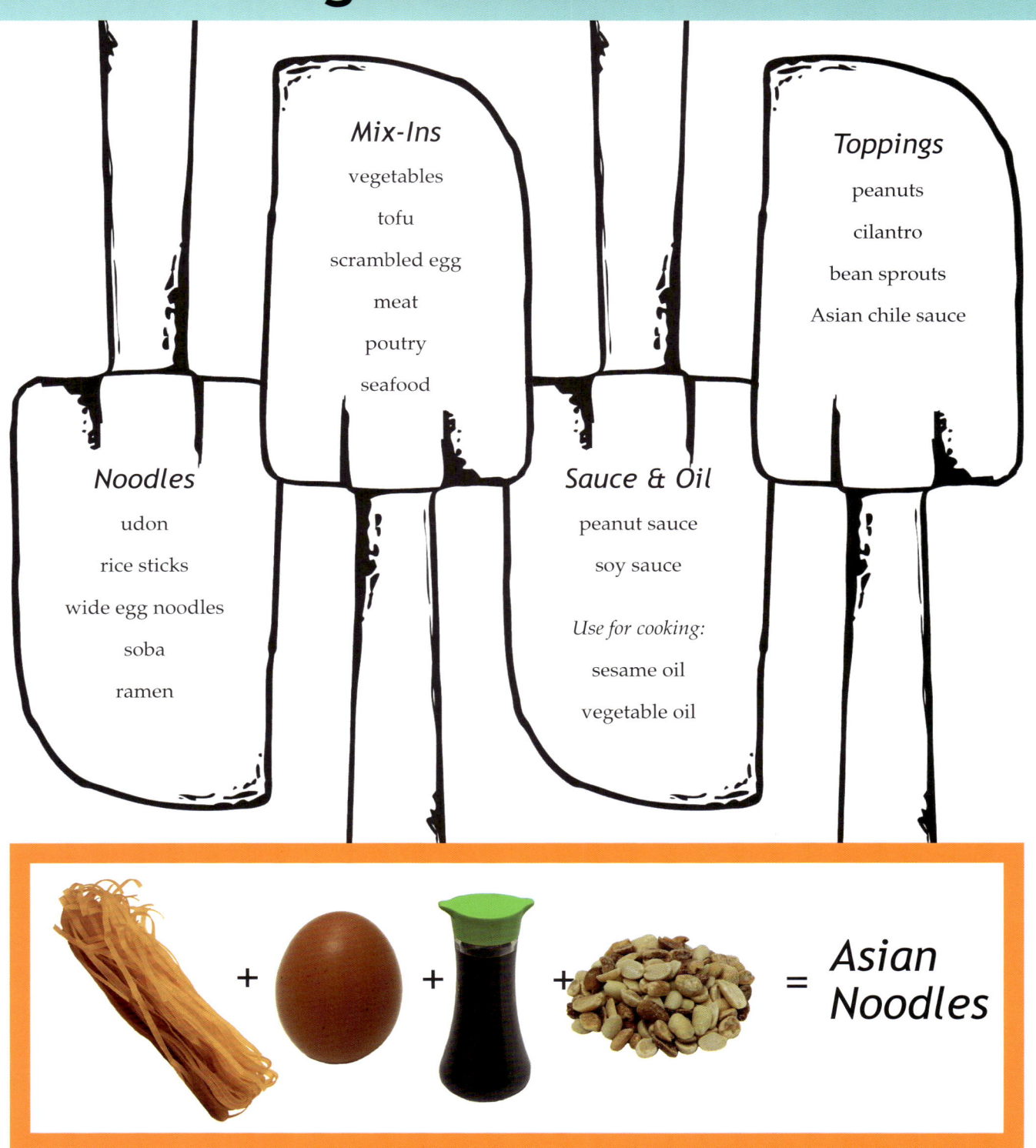

Mix-Ins
vegetables
tofu
scrambled egg
meat
poutry
seafood

Toppings
peanuts
cilantro
bean sprouts
Asian chile sauce

Noodles
udon
rice sticks
wide egg noodles
soba
ramen

Sauce & Oil
peanut sauce
soy sauce

Use for cooking:
sesame oil
vegetable oil

+ + + = **Asian Noodles**

Main Dish ☞ Grain and Noodle Recipes

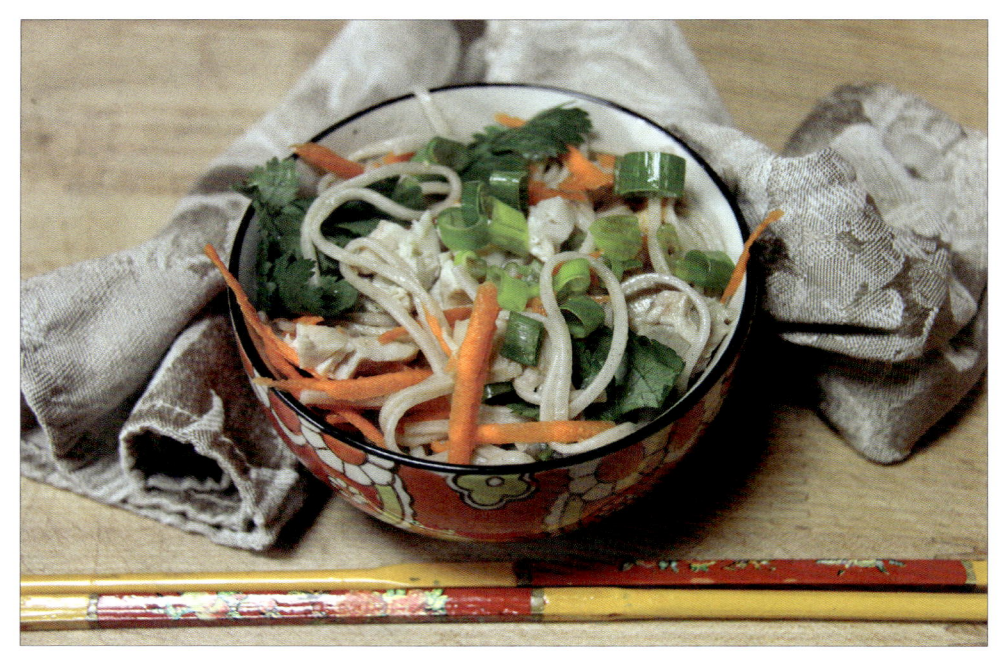

Sesame-Peanut Noodle Salad

4-6 servings

This is a versatile salad that can be made with any kind of Asian noodle.

Salad
- 12 ounces Asian noodles
- 2 cooked chicken breasts, finely sliced, or chopped baked tofu (about 2 cups)
- 1 carrot, grated (about ½ cup)
- 4-6 green onions, sliced (about ⅓ cup)
- ¼ cup dry-roasted peanuts
- 1 tablespoon chopped fresh cilantro (or 1 teaspoon dried)

Dressing
- ½ teaspoon salt
- 1 tablespoon lime juice
- 4 teaspoons vegetable oil (not olive)
- 3 teaspoons sesame oil
- 2 garlic cloves, minced (about 1 tablespoon)

1. Cook noodles (see page 57). Transfer noodles to a large bowl and allow to cool.

2. Prepare the vegetables. Cook the chicken, if necessary, or make Tofu Sticks (see page 145).

3. Add cooked chicken or tofu, carrot, onions, peanuts and cilantro to noodles; toss to combine.

4. Stir dressing ingredients together in a small bowl or shake well in a covered jar. Taste and adjust seasonings. Drizzle over noodle mixture; toss to combine.

Options:

- Save some peanuts and cilantro to sprinkle on individual portions as a garnish.
- Substitute peanut sauce for dressing:

    Combine:
    ¼ cup peanut butter
    2 tablespoons soy sauce
    1 tablespoon brown sugar
    juice of ½ lime

- Substitute 2 cups cooked brown rice for noodles

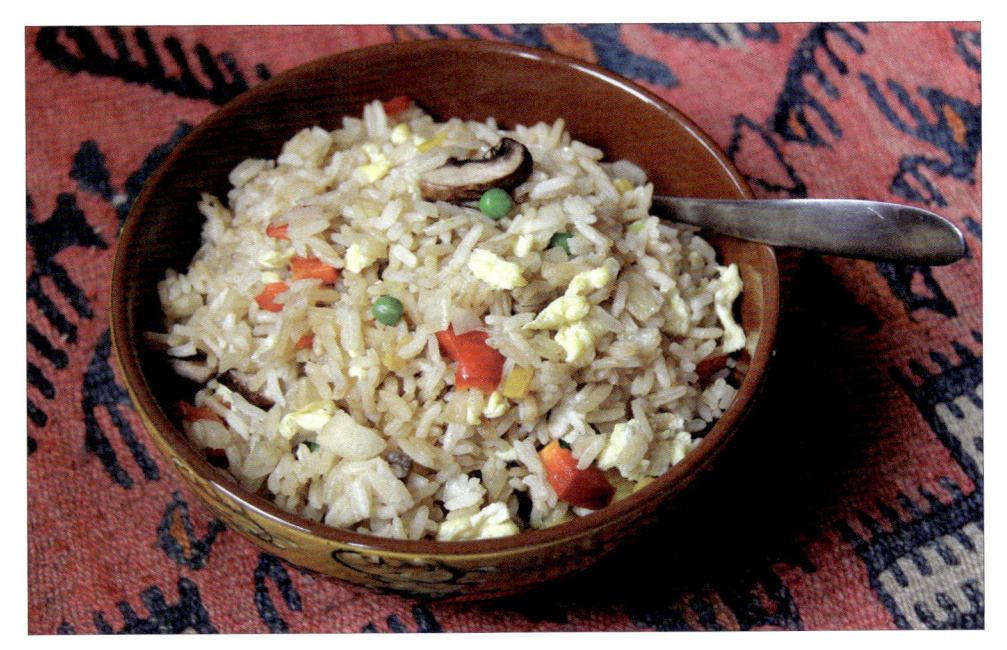

Fried Rice

6 servings

Cut meat and vegetables into small pieces to make a tasty Asian-inspired meal. This is a perfect place to use leftovers.

- 3 tablespoons vegetable or olive oil
- 2 eggs, lightly beaten
- 1 small onion, diced (about ½ cup)
- 4 cups cooked rice (2 cup uncooked, see page 56)
- 2 tablespoons soy or tamari sauce
- ½ cup leftover cooked meat or vegetables, chopped

1. Prepare the vegetables and meats. Cook rice (see page 56). Whisk eggs.
2. Heat 1 tablespoon oil in large frying pan over low heat. Add eggs and scramble (see page 55). Remove cooked eggs and set aside.
3. Add remaining oil, onion and raw vegetables to pan. Sauté about 3 minutes, until onion is softened.
4. Increase heat to medium. Add rice to pan. Stir. Add cooked vegetables and/or meat and stir.
5. Add soy or tamari sauce. Scrape the bottom of the pan every two minutes. Cook for a total of 6 minutes.
6. Chop scrambled egg and add to rice mixture. Mix and remove from heat.

Options:

- At Step 2, chop and cook 2 green onions with the scrambled egg.
- Add optional vegetables—any combination of peas, chopped broccoli, sliced mushrooms, corn, grated carrot, quartered Brussels sprouts.
  - If vegetables are raw, add them at Step 3 after the onion is softened.
  - If vegetables are cooked, add at Step 4.
- At Step 4, add ½ cup of any of the following: chopped ham or tofu, or chopped or finely sliced cooked chicken.
- At Step 5, add ½ teaspoon Asian fish sauce.

Beans and Rice

6 servings

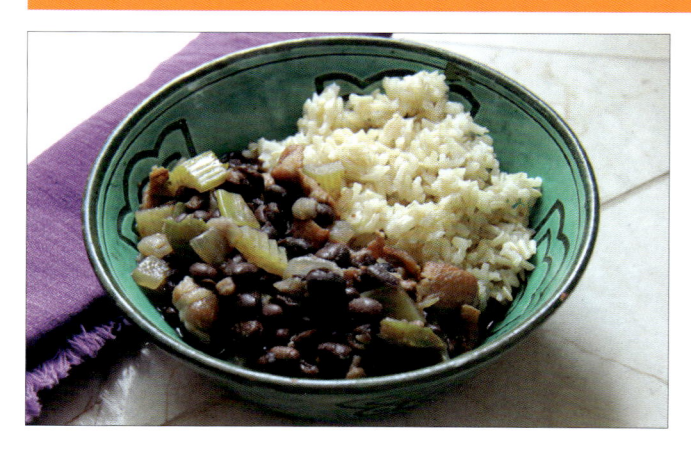

A kid we know refused to eat anything but red beans and rice for one full year. We advocate for a slightly more varied diet, but you really can't go wrong with beans and rice. It's a healthy staple food for much of the world. This version can be made with two different flavor profiles—Mexican or Cajun.

2. Add ½ cup broth to hot pan. Scrape browned bits off bottom of pan. (This process is called *deglazing*).
3. Add remaining broth and drained beans. Add more seasoning to taste and stir.
4. Simmer 15 minutes, uncovered.
5. Mix in tomato paste, and taste and adjust seasonings. Serve with cooked rice.

Options:
- At Step 1, add chopped carrots.
- For a Cajun version, at Step 2, sauté and add 2 sliced Andouille sausages.
- Fry 4 slices of bacon 3-5 minutes. Remove from pan and place on paper towels to drain fat. Let cool. Chop. Drain all but a tablespoon of fat from pan. Add bacon at Step 4.

1	tablespoon vegetable oil or bacon fat
4	cups cooked red, black or kidney beans (2 cups dried, or two 14.5- to 16-ounce cans)
1-2	tablespoons Cajun/Creole or Mexican seasoning (see Spice Mixes, page 193)
1	medium onion, chopped (about 1 cup)
½	bell pepper, seeded and chopped (about ½ cup)
2	celery stalks, chopped (about ½ cup)
3	cups broth, canned or homemade (see page 62)
4	cup cooked rice (2 cups raw, see page 56)
2	tablespoons tomato paste
	Salt to taste

1. Cook rice (see page 56). In oil or bacon drippings, sauté onion, pepper, celery, and 1 tablespoon of seasoning mix. Stir vegetables until brown.

Grains of the World

Grains are grown all over the world. They are human's biggest source of energy.

Ground up into flour, they are used to make bread, noodles and much more.

Different kinds of grains were domesticated in different places, but they have now been spread across the world and adopted into traditional dishes. **Common grains and where they were domesticated:**

- Wheat and barley from the Middle East
- Maize (corn) from North America
- Rice from China
- Oats from Europe

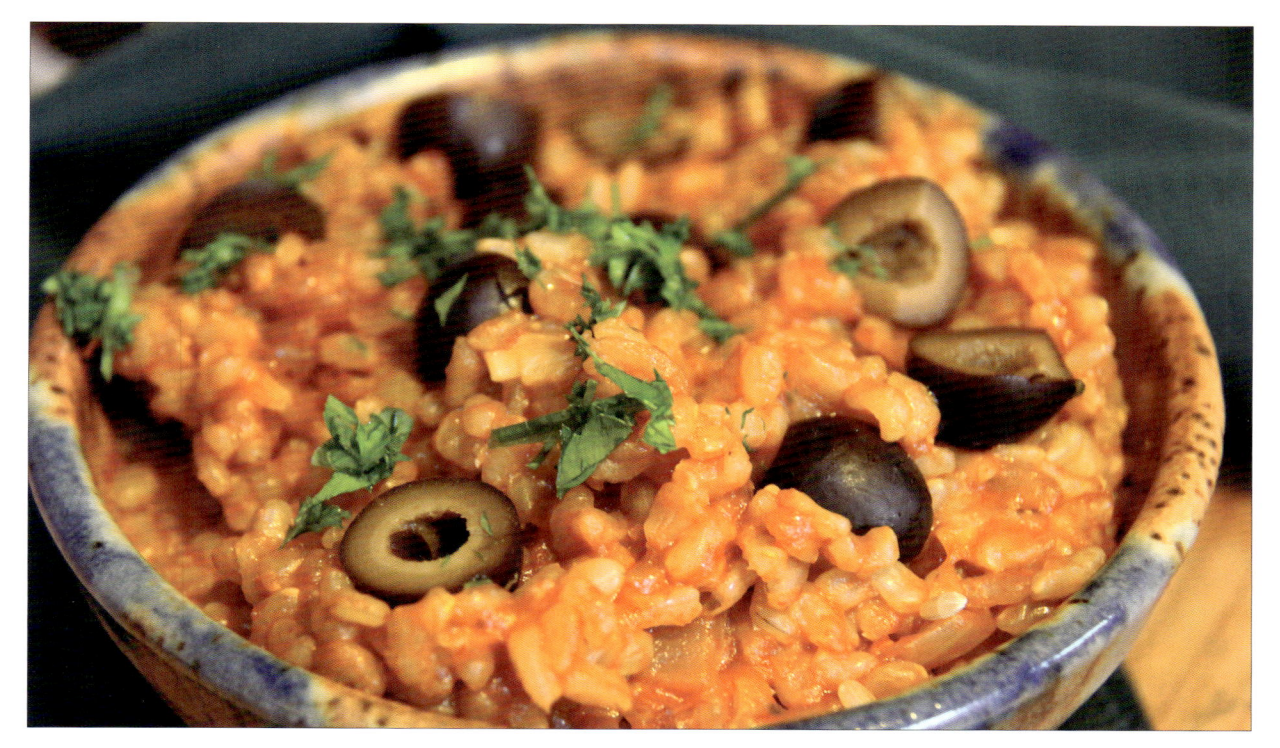

Mexican Rice

6 servings

Mexican rice is a great side dish, a filler for burritos or wraps, or an addition to a frittata, quiche or soup.

- 1 tablespoon vegetable oil
- 1 medium onion, chopped (about 1 cup)
- 1½ cups broth (one 14.5- to 16-ounce can, or homemade, see page 62)
- 1 cup uncooked rice
- 1 small tomato, chopped (about ¾ cup) or (half a 14.5- to 16-ounce can)
- ½ teaspoon chile powder
- ¼ teaspoon salt
- 1 cup corn
- 1 cup peas
- 1 carrot, diced (about ½ cup)

1. Prepare onion and other vegetables.

2. Pour oil into 2-quart pot. Over medium heat, add onion and sauté until soft (about 5 minutes).

3. Add broth, rice, tomatoes, chile powder and salt. Bring to a boil. Reduce heat. Simmer, covered, 25 minutes.

4. Stir in vegetables and let stand for 5 minutes before serving.

Options:

- In Step 3, add 1 tablespoon tomato paste for a darker red, more "tomatoey" rice.
- Garnish with olives.

Main Dish ☞ Grain and Noodle Recipes

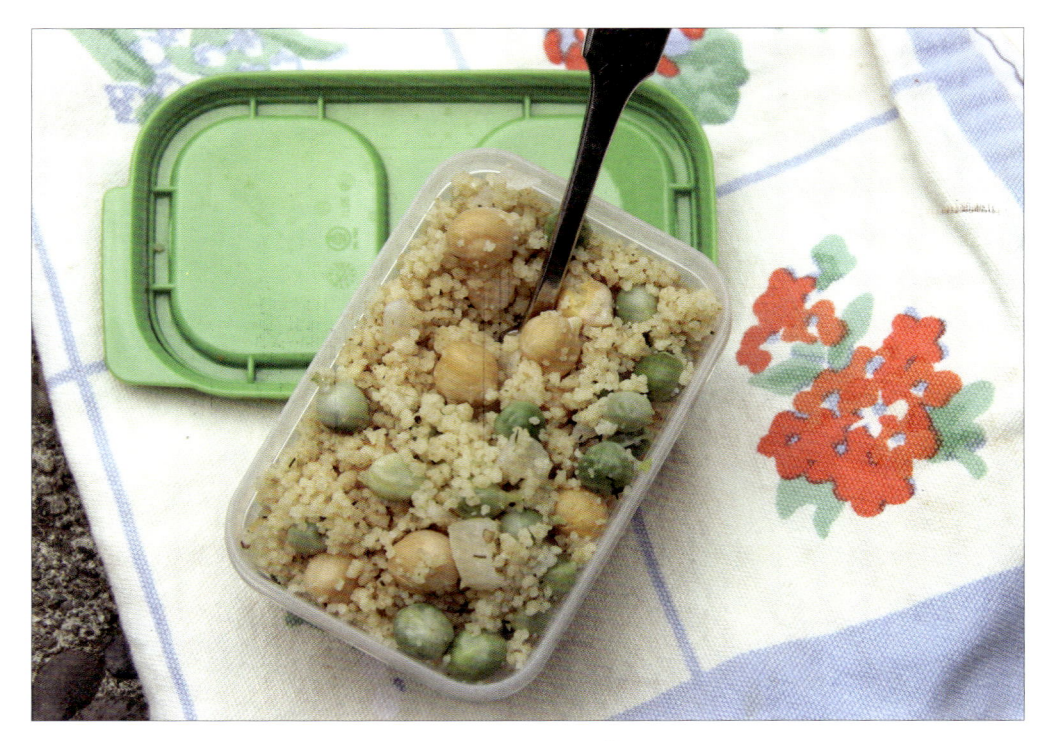

Couscous with Peas

6-8 servings

In a hurry? Then couscous is for you. It cooks in 5 minutes, much faster than other pastas and rice. It's a favorite in North African cuisines. Garbanzo beans will add protein. Make this as a side dish for dinner and use leftovers for lunch.

- 1 tablespoon olive oil
- 1 medium onion, diced (about 1 cup)
- 1 clove garlic, crushed
- 1 cup cooked garbanzo beans (one 14.5- to 16-ounce can)
- 1 cup peas
- 1 tablespoon fresh minced dill (or 1 teaspoon dry)
- 1/8 teaspoon pepper
- 1½ cups vegetable or chicken broth
- 1 cup couscous
- Salt to taste

1. Prepare vegetables.
2. Sauté onion and garlic in a saucepan over medium heat until onion is translucent, about 5 minutes.
3. Stir in peas, garbanzo beans, dill, pepper and broth and bring to a boil.
4. Stir in couscous, return mixture to a boil, and cover.
5. Remove pan from heat and let mixture sit, covered, for 5 minutes, or until the liquid is absorbed. Fluff with a fork. Taste and adjust salt.

Options:
- At Step 3, add peanuts or other vegetables.
- At Step 5, add precooked chopped meats or tofu cubes.

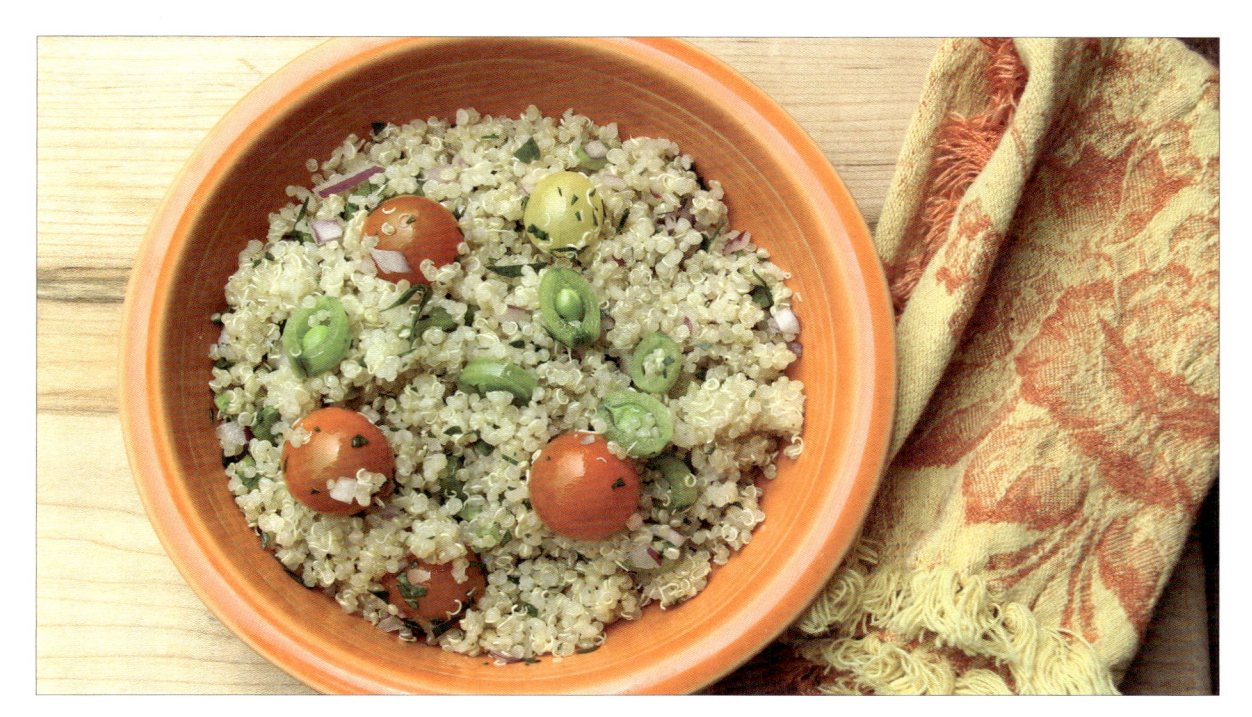

Sugar Snap Peas & Grain Salad

6 servings

Sugar snap peas give a delightful crunch to this salad and little tomatoes add color and sweetness. This salad holds well in the refrigerator for a couple of days.

Salad
- 3 cups cooked pasta, quinoa, or rice
- 2 cups sugar snap peas, cut crosswise
- 1 cup cherry tomatoes, cut in half
- ½ cup fresh parsley, chopped or (2½ tablespoons dried)
- ¼ medium red onion, chopped (about ¼ cup)

Dressing
- 2 tablespoons olive oil
- 2 tablespoons lemon juice
- ¾ teaspoon salt
- ¼ teaspoon pepper

1. Prepare vegetables. Cook pasta (see page 57), quinoa, or rice (see page 56).
2. Mix dressing ingredients together in a small bowl, or shake in a covered jar. Taste and adjust seasonings.
3. Drizzle dressing on salad; mix well.
4. Refrigerate for one hour before serving.

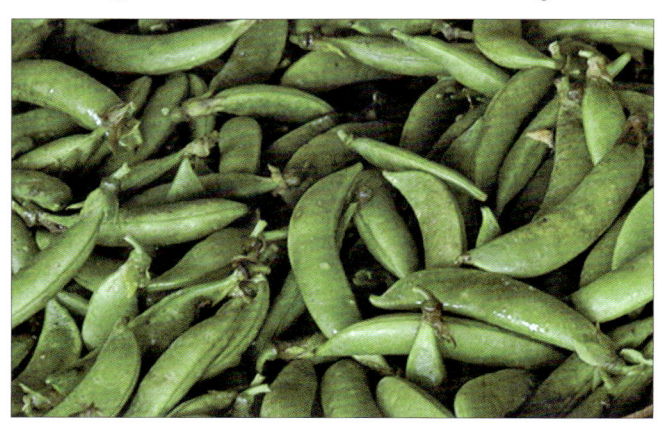

Main Dish ☞ Grain and Noodle Recipes

Quiche/Frittata/Strata Formula

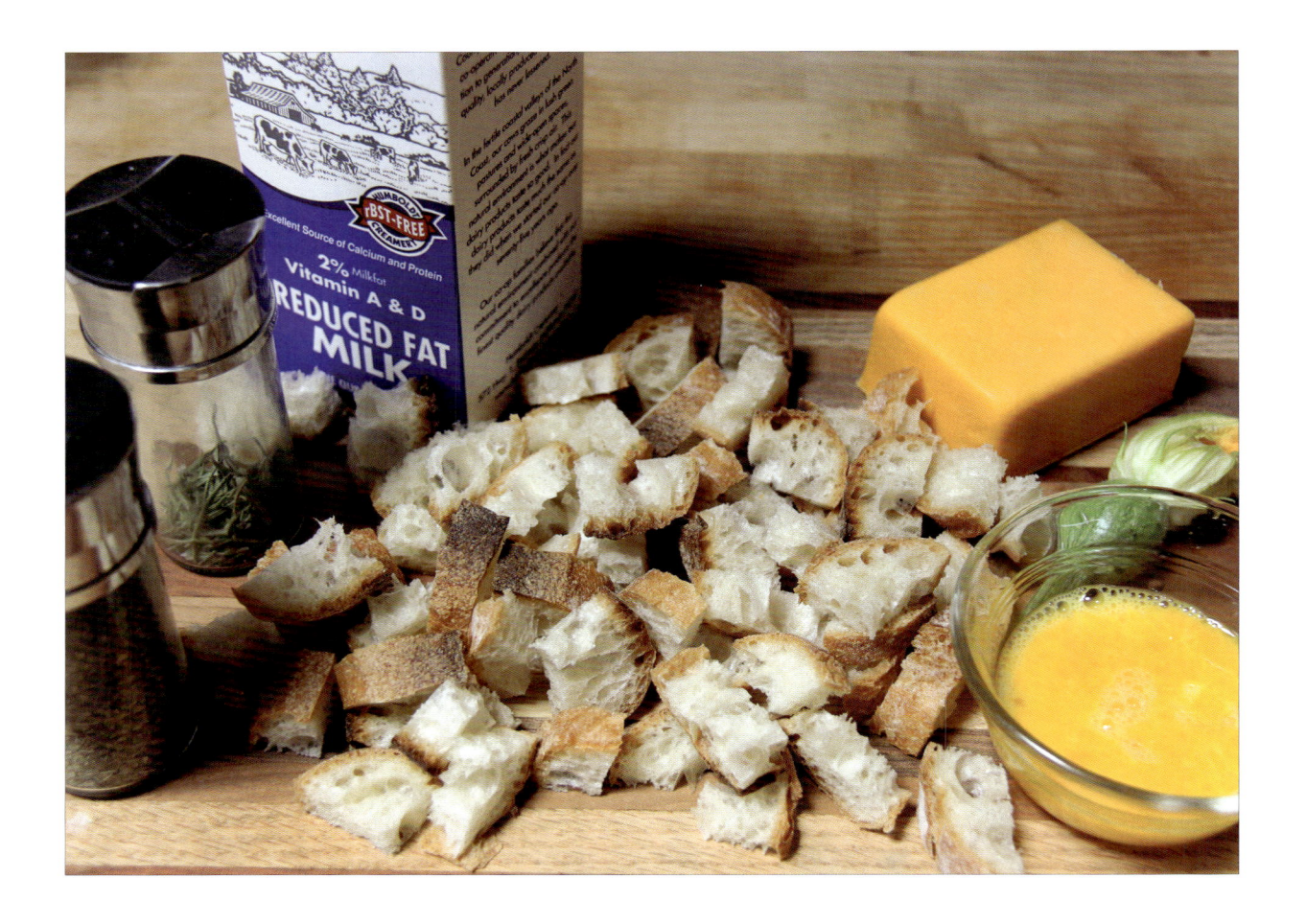

Quiche, Frittata and Strata are all savory egg-custard pies. Quiche has a bottom crust (see page 103), Fritatta has no crust at all (see page 102), and Strata is layered on cubes of bread (see page 104).

1. Choose appropriate pan. Oil lightly.

2. Precook fillings as necessary. Grate cheese.

3. Whisk together eggs and milk. Add seasoning.

4. Layer ingredients in pan in this order: base, fillings and cheese, custard. Top with cheese and bake until custard is firm.

Ingredient Ideas

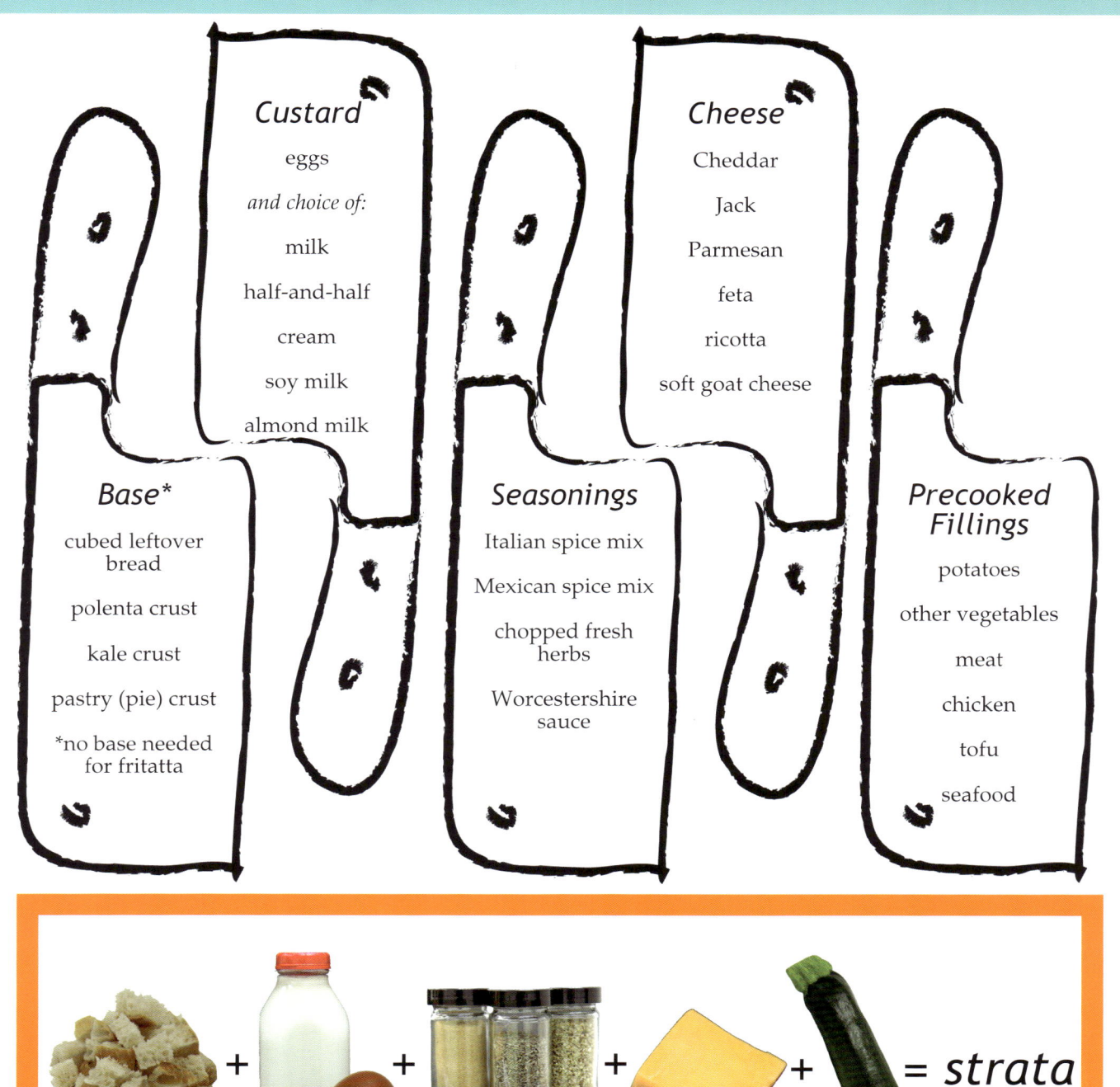

Custard
eggs

and choice of:

milk

half-and-half

cream

soy milk

almond milk

Cheese
Cheddar

Jack

Parmesan

feta

ricotta

soft goat cheese

Base*
cubed leftover bread

polenta crust

kale crust

pastry (pie) crust

*no base needed for frittata

Seasonings
Italian spice mix

Mexican spice mix

chopped fresh herbs

Worcestershire sauce

Precooked Fillings
potatoes

other vegetables

meat

chicken

tofu

seafood

bread + milk & egg + seasonings + cheese + zucchini = *strata*

Main Dish ☞ Egg-Based Recipes 101

Mini Chedder Frittatas

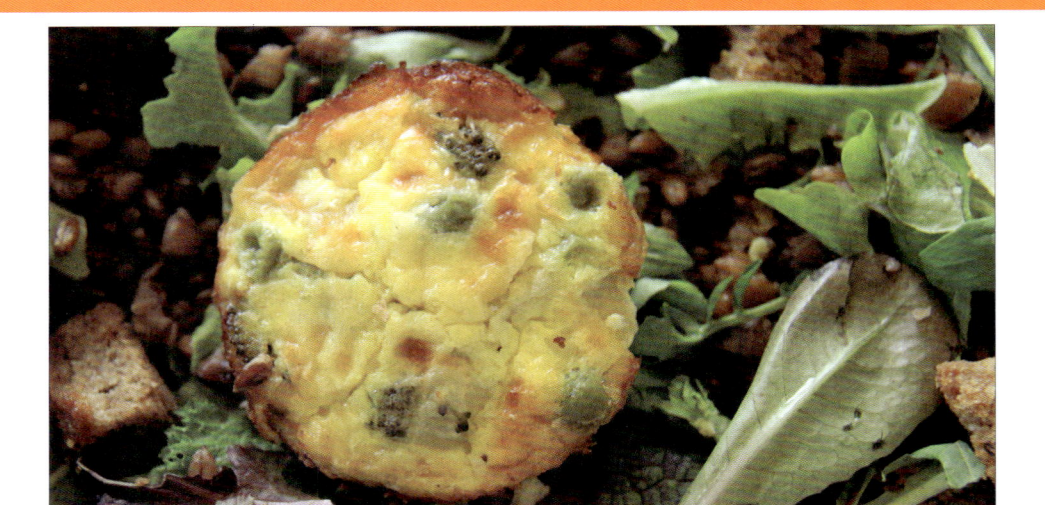

Yield: 12 Frittatas

This is perfect finger food to pack for lunch. It's full of vegetables, with meat as an option.

- 1 tablespoon vegetable oil
- 1 6-inch long zucchini, grated (about 1 cup)
- ½ onion, thinly sliced (about 2 tablespoons)
- 7 large eggs
- ⅔ cup half-and-half or milk
- 1 cup grated Cheddar cheese, divided into two equal portions
- 1 teaspoon chopped fresh thyme leaves (or ¼ teaspoon dried)
- ½ teaspoon salt
- Pepper to taste

Preheat oven to 375°

1. Oil muffin tin. Grate zucchini and cheese.

2. Heat oil in medium frying pan over medium heat. Add zucchini and onions. Cook until soft, 3-5 minutes.

3. Whisk together remaining ingredients in bowl, using half a cup of the cheese.

4. Divide zucchini mixture among 12 muffin cups. Pour egg mixture over zucchini. Top each cup with some of the remaining cheese.

5. Bake 20 minutes, or until centers no longer jiggle. Tops should be puffed and light brown in color.

6. To remove from muffin cups, run knife all the way around frittata.

7. Serve immediately. For lunch, cool and wrap individually. Put in refrigerator if using within two days, or freeze for longer storage.

8. To thaw, remove desired amount from freezer the night before and place in refrigerator.

Options:

- Substitute sautéed green leafy vegetables for the zucchini.
- Substitute a different cheese such as: Jack, Gruyère, Swiss, Cheddar or a mixture of Parmesan and another cheese for the chedder cheese.
- At Step 3, add cooked ham, chicken, or sausage, mushrooms, grilled vegetables.

Corn and Pepper Quiche

Yield: 6-8 slices

This quiche makes an almost complete meal, as it contains protein, vegetables, dairy and grain.

- 1 pie dough for 9- or 10-inch pie crust, homemade (see page 63), or purchased
- 1 tablespoon olive oil
- 2 slices of onion, minced (about 2 tablespoons)
- 1 cup corn, thawed if frozen
- 1 8-ounce jar roasted red peppers, drained and chopped, or 2 oven-roasted red bell peppers, chopped
- 2 tablespoons fresh oregano, marjoram, or thyme (or 2 teaspoons dried)
- 2 beaten eggs, room temperature
- 1 cup milk, room temperature
- 1 cup grated Jack, Swiss, Cheddar or cottage cheese
- 1 teaspoon salt
- ½ teaspoon pepper

Preheat oven to 350°

1. If using purchased pie dough, start on step 2. For homemade, roll out pie dough. Place in pie pan; edges will hang over. Trim off excess dough to the pan's rim. Pinch dough together repeatedly along top of rim to create a fluted edge (see photos below).

2. Prick dough repeatedly with fork on bottom and sides to prevent shrinkage during baking.

3. Prepare onion and corn. Drain and chop peppers, if necessary.

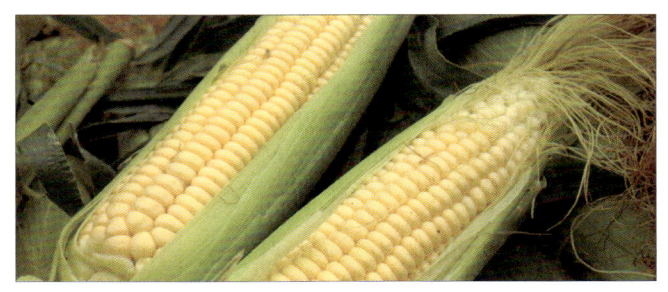

4. Heat oil in a 12-inch frying pan over medium heat. Add onion and corn. Sauté 1-2 minutes. Turn off heat.

5. Pour onion mixture into a bowl. Mix in peppers, spices, eggs, cheese, salt and pepper.

6. Pour into crust.

7. Bake 50-60 minutes, until center no longer jiggles or a knife blade inserted near center comes out clean. Cool 20 minutes before cutting.

Options:

- Substitutions for pie crust:
    - For polenta crust, use cooked polenta (see pages 60-61).
    - For kale crust, oil the pie pan and line with steamed kale leaves.
    - For potato crust, oil the pie pan and line with grated raw potato. Bake at 350° until golden brown before filling.
- Cut into individual portions, wrap airtight and freeze. Thaw in the refrigerator the night before using.

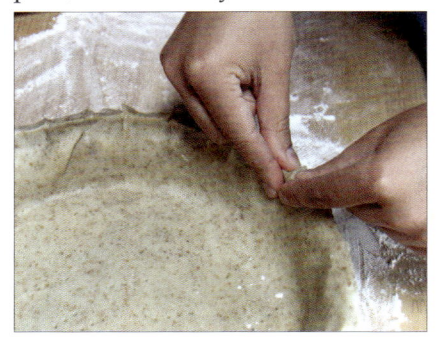

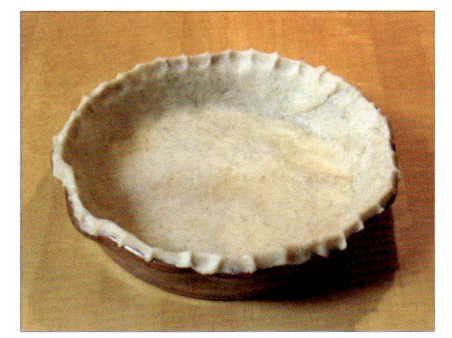

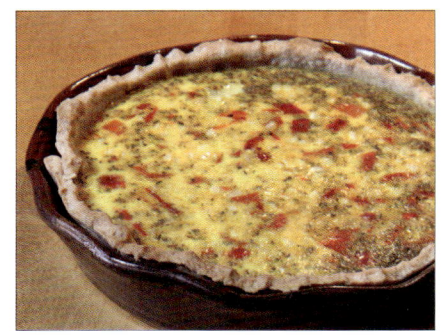

Main Dish ☞ Egg-Based Recipes

Strata with Meat

6-8 servings

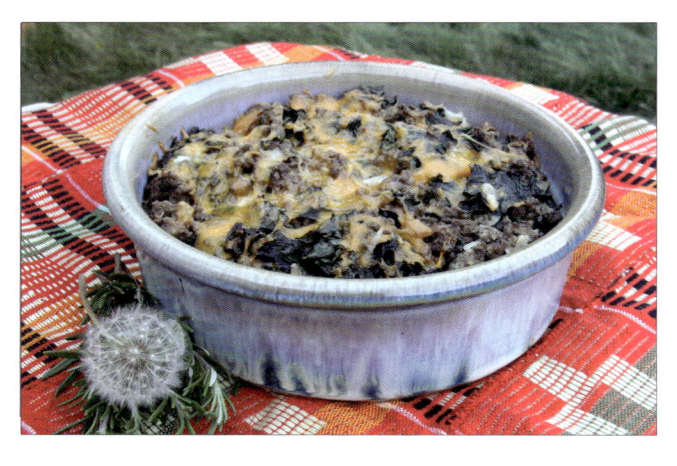

This recipe calls for sausage and greens, but after you've made it the first time, don't be afraid to experiment. You can easily eliminate the meat from this dish to make it vegetarian.

2	cups bread or bagels, cubed
1	tablespoon olive oil
12	ounces any type ground or link sausage meat, chopped
2	garlic cloves, minced (about 1 tablespoon)
1	small onion, chopped (about ½ cup)
6	cups chopped green leafy vegetable such as chard, kale, or spinach
8	eggs, room temperature
2½	cups half-and-half
1½	cups grated cheese (Swiss, Jack, Cheddar, fontina)
¼	teaspoon salt
¼	teaspoon pepper

Preheat oven to 350°

1. Butter a 9 x 13-inch baking dish.

2. Cut bread or bagels into 1-inch cubes; spread in baking dish. (French bread, Italian bread, No-Knead Bread [see page 58] work well.)

3. Remove thick stems from greens (see page 128). Chop garlic, leafy greens, and sausage if necessary. Grate cheese.

4. Heat oil in a large frying pan over medium-high heat. Add onions and garlic. Saute 3-5 minutes. Add meat and cook 4-6 minutes, or until cooked through and no longer pink. Carefully remove meat from pan, using a slotted spoon, and set aside.

5. Add leafy greens to pan. Cook 3-5 minutes, stirring occasionally, until all the leaves are wilted. Turn off heat. Mix meat back in. Distribute mixture over bread cubes in the baking dish.

6. Whisk together eggs, milk, salt and pepper. Pour over ingredients in baking dish.

7. Bake 45-60 minutes, until center no longer jiggles and a knife blade inserted near center comes out clean. The strata should be a light brown. Cool 10-15 minutes before serving.

Options:

- Substitute leftover chicken for sausage.
- Cut into individual portions, wrap airtight and freeze. The night before using, thaw in the refrigerator. Enjoy hot or cold.
- Letting the bread soak in the custard overnight makes this dish even more delicious. Complete Steps 1-6 the night before, cover, refrigerate and bake for brunch the next morning.

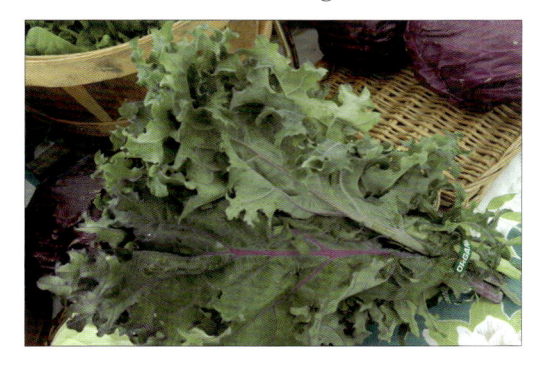

104 Main Dish ☞ Egg-Based Recipes

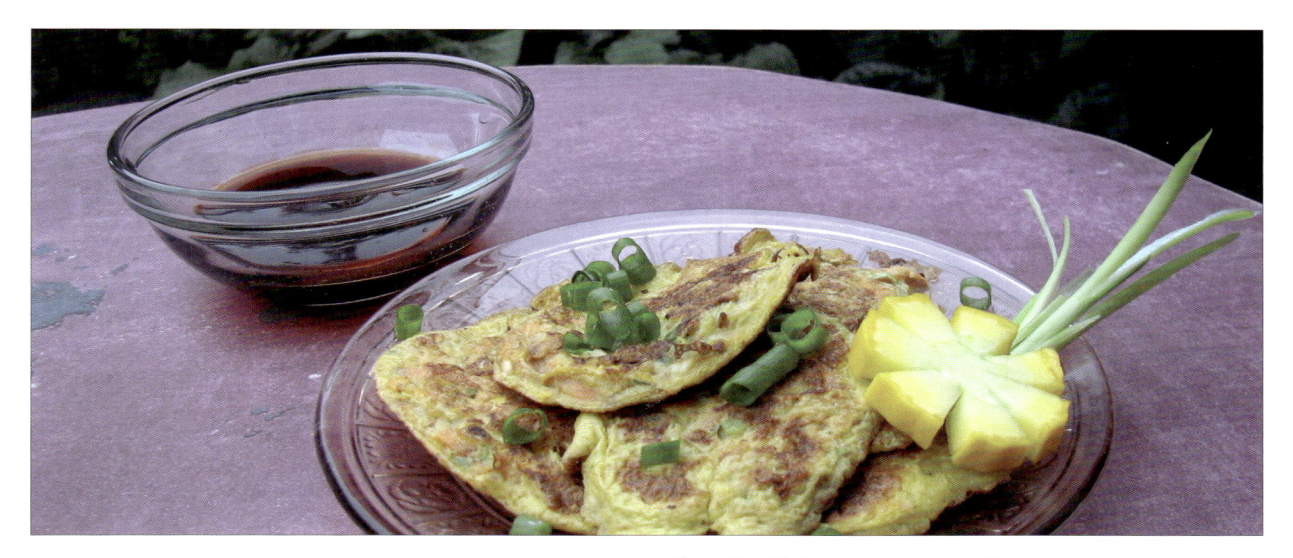

Japanese Griddle Cakes

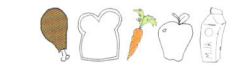

4-6 servings

Japanese vegetable griddle cakes (O-konomi-yaki) make a delicious lunch or breakfast. They are just as tasty cold as they are hot. By using a ladle or smaller spoon, they can be made any size, including bite-size cakes perfect for dipping in soy sauce.

- ½ cup Napa cabbage, finely sliced
- 1-2 green onions, minced
- 2 cups grated vegetables, such as sweet potato, winter squash, zucchini, summer squash, turnips, and/or carrots
- ¼ cup flour
- ½ teaspoon salt
- 4-5 eggs, whisked
- Vegetable or olive oil as needed for frying.

1. Slice the cabbage finely. Mince onion and grate vegetables. Set aside.

2. Whisk eggs in medium bowl. Add all ingredients to eggs and mix well.

3. Heat oil in a frying pan over medium-high heat. Reduce heat to medium.

4. Drop a large spoonful of mixture into a pan. It should begin to sizzle and cook immediately and not spread out. If the egg spreads, increase heat.

5. Using a spatula, flip griddle cakes when the bottom is brown, about 2-3 minutes for a large cake or 1 minute for a smaller one. Add more oil as needed. Griddle cakes should be crunchy on the outside and moist inside.

6. When both sides are brown, remove cakes to a plate and cover to keep them warm.

Option:

- Add chopped mushrooms, ½ cup bean sprouts, bay shrimp, ground or thinly sliced pork.
- Serve with soy sauce, sour cream or yogurt.

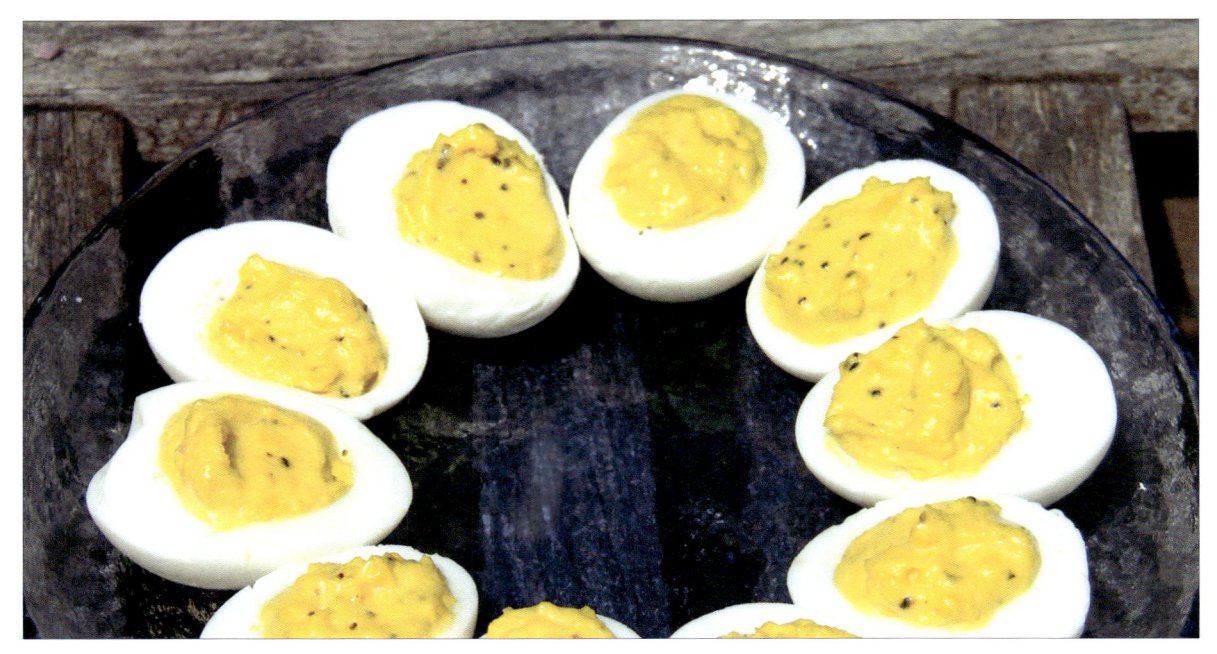

Classic Deviled Eggs

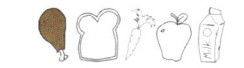

Yield: 12 egg halves

Deviled eggs are a low cost, high quality protein for any lunch.

- 6 hard-cooked eggs
- ¼ cup mayonnaise
- 1 teaspoon prepared mustard (or ½ teaspoon dry mustard)
- ½ teaspoon white vinegar
- ⅛ teaspoon salt
- ¼ teaspoon ground black pepper

1. Hardcook the eggs (see page 55). Cool.

2. Peel eggs and slice in half lengthwise. Carefully remove the egg-yolks with a spoon or gently pop them out of the egg white. Place yolks in a small bowl; mash with a fork. Set halved whites to the side.

3. Add mayonnaise, mustard, vinegar, salt and pepper to the yolks and mix thoroughly.

4. Using a small spoon, fill the empty egg white halves with the yolk mixture. Alternatively, you can fill a plastic bag with the mixture, cut off the tip of one corner of the bag, and squeeze the yolk mixture into the egg white halves.

Options:

- At Step 3, add 2 teaspoons pickle relish to yolk mixture to give a flavor kick.
- Garnish each egg with a sprinkle of paprika.

Perfect Deviled Eggs

To have perfect halves, it's important to peel and slice the hard-cooked eggs carefully.

Tip: Eggs that are more than one week old are easier to peel after cooking.

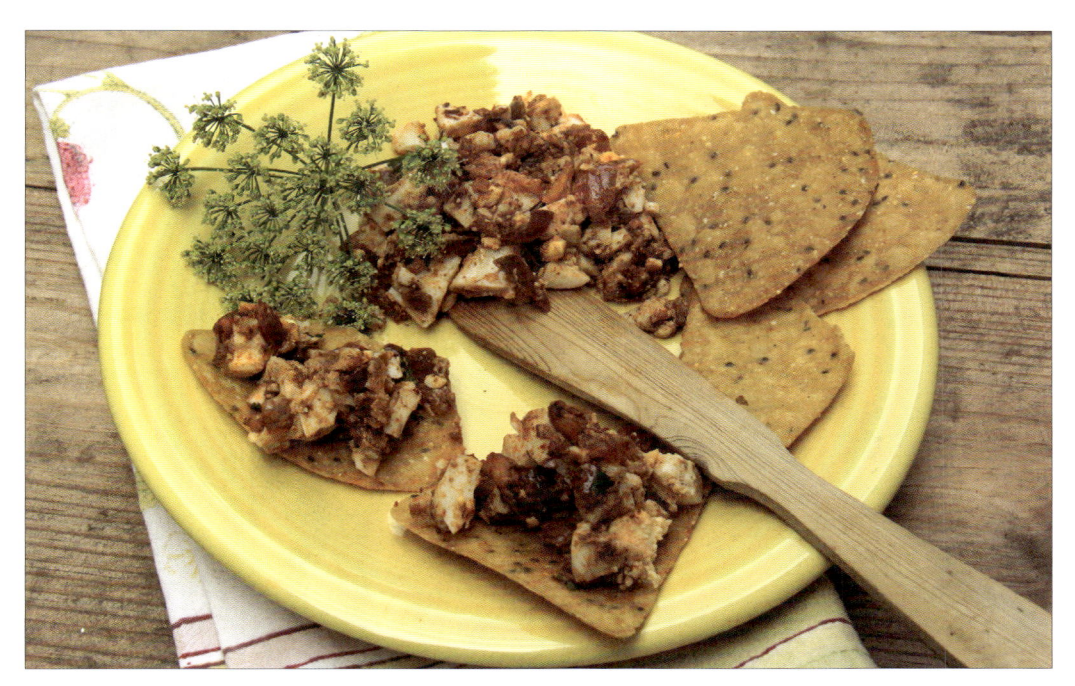

African Egg Salad

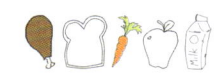

Yield: 2 cups Salad or 10 Deviled Egg halves

Kids' cooking classes prove this to be a very kid-friendly recipe. It makes a flavorful, zippy filling for sandwiches or deviled eggs.

    5   hard-cooked eggs
   ¼   cup olive oil, divided
   ¼   cup unsalted dry-roasted peanuts, chopped
    2   small red onions, finely chopped (about 1½ cups)
    3   garlic cloves, minced
    1   tablespoon paprika
   ½   teaspoon ground ginger
 1½   teaspoons chile powder
    2   tomatoes, chopped
    2   teaspoons chopped fresh cilantro
    1   tablespoon soy sauce
    1   tablespoon lime juice
   ½   teaspoon salt

1. Hardcook the eggs (see page 55). Cool. Peel.

2. Heat 2 tablespoons olive oil in large frying pan. Add peanuts and sauté until lightly brown, about 5 minutes.

3. Stir in onions and garlic and sauté until onions are translucent, about 5 minutes.

4. Add paprika, ginger and chile powder; cook for 2 minutes. Transfer to a bowl to cool.

For Salad:

1. Chop the eggs.

2. Gently combine chopped eggs, tomatoes, soy sauce, lime juice, cilantro, 2 tablespoons olive oil, salt and onion mixture.

For Deviled Eggs:

1. Slice eggs in half lengthwise. Scoop the yolks into the bowl, add all other ingredients, and mix.

2. Fill egg white halves with the mixture.

Main Dish Salad Formula

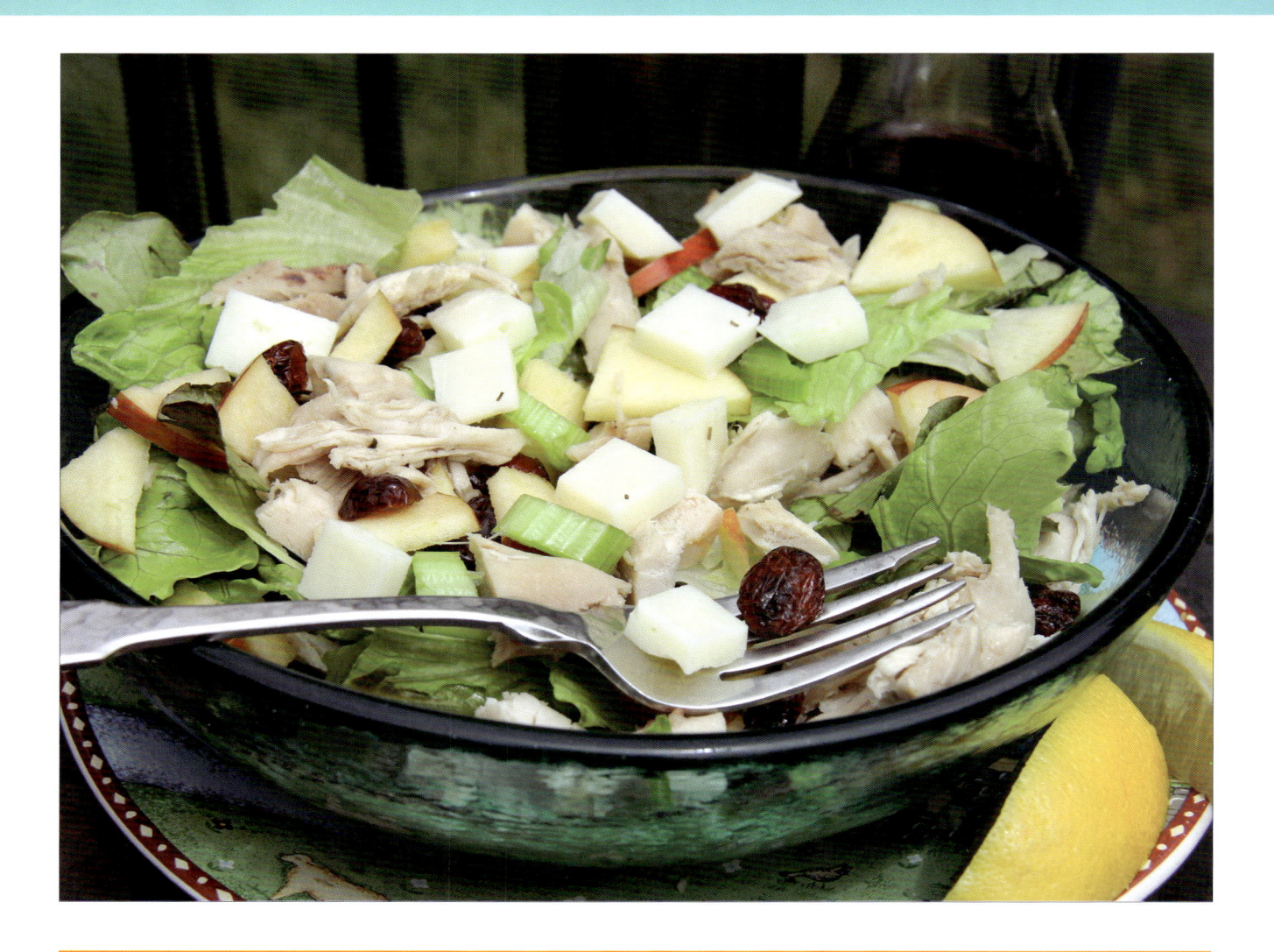

A Main Dish salad is one that has protein in addition to vegetables. Fruit and carbohydrates are optional.

1. Precook all grains, noodles and proteins (meat, egg, beans).

2. Chop fruits, vegetables, and protein items.

3. Toss all ingredients except dressing in a bowl.

4. Stir dressing ingredients together in a small bowl, or shake well in a covered jar. Pour dressing on salad and toss, or serve on the side.

Ingredient Ideas

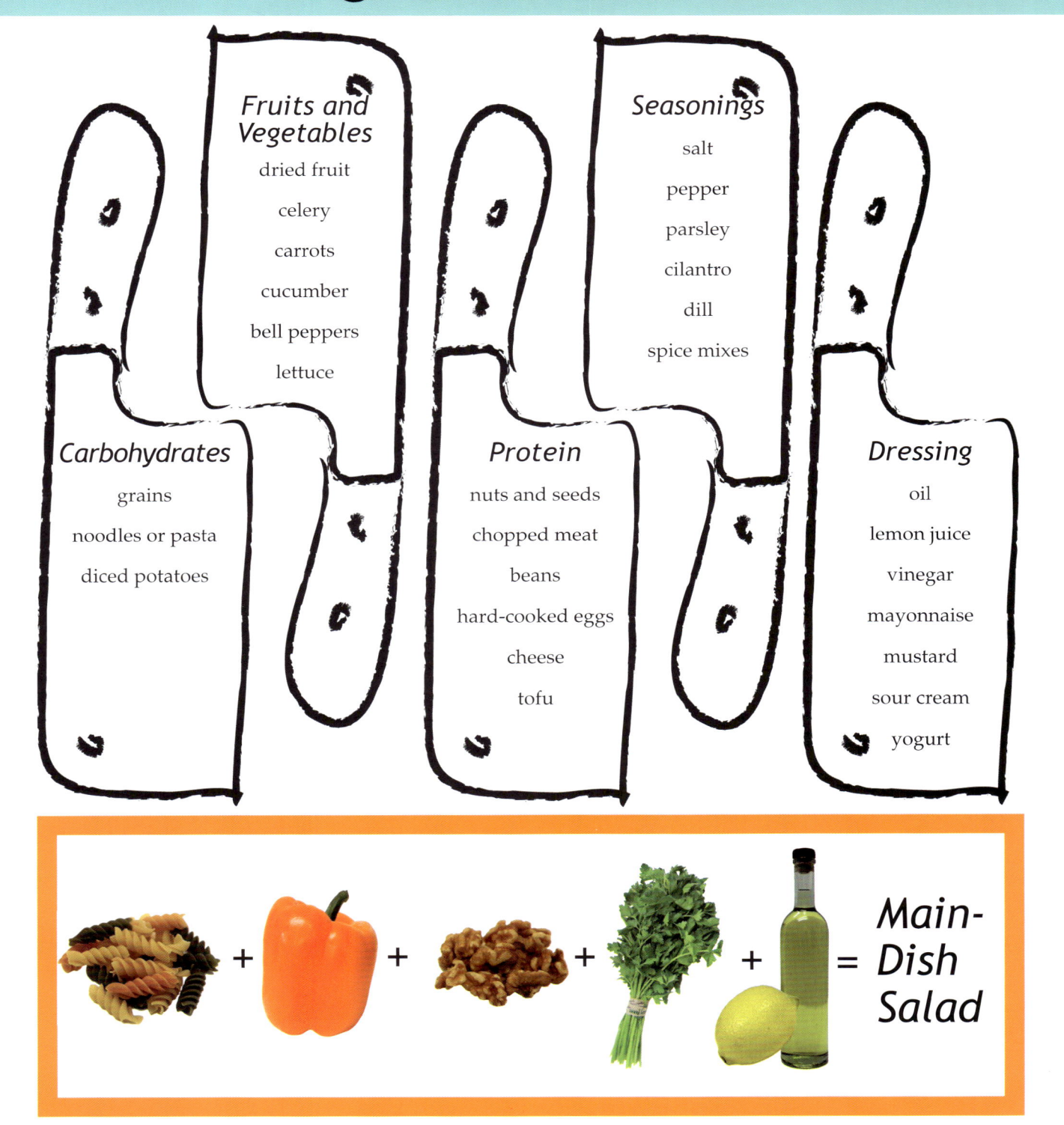

Fruits and Vegetables
- dried fruit
- celery
- carrots
- cucumber
- bell peppers
- lettuce

Seasonings
- salt
- pepper
- parsley
- cilantro
- dill
- spice mixes

Carbohydrates
- grains
- noodles or pasta
- diced potatoes

Protein
- nuts and seeds
- chopped meat
- beans
- hard-cooked eggs
- cheese
- tofu

Dressing
- oil
- lemon juice
- vinegar
- mayonnaise
- mustard
- sour cream
- yogurt

pasta + bell pepper + nuts + parsley + lemon/oil = **Main-Dish Salad**

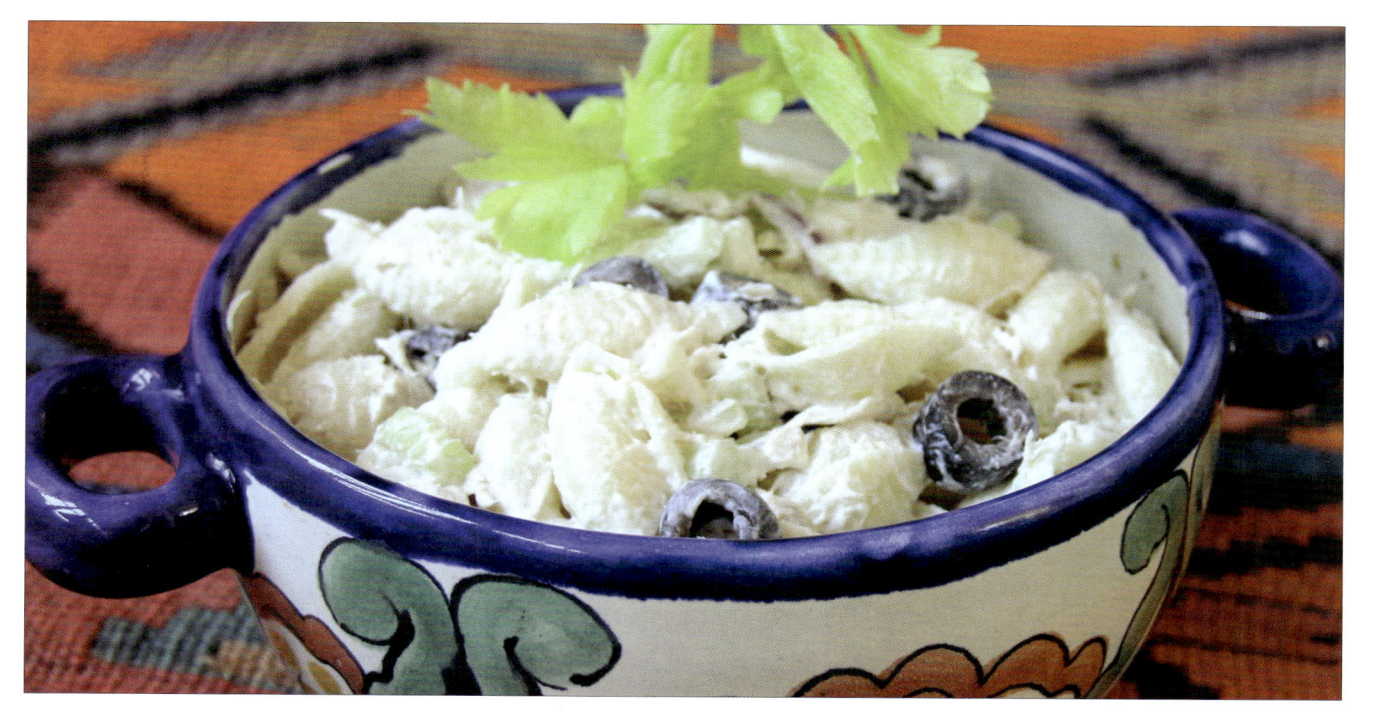

Tuna and Pasta Salad

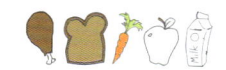

6 servings

Pasta is a simple base for salads. Create innovative recipes with the addition of vegetables, meats, and different dressings. Precook large batches of macaroni to use in other pasta dishes such as Mac and Cheese (see page 90), or other salads.

Salad
- 1½ cups (8 ounces) dry macaroni or other pasta, or 3 cups cooked
- 2 6-7 ounce cans of tuna, well drained
- 1 can (14 ounces) black olives, drained and chopped
- 4 stalks celery, thinly sliced (about 1 cup)
- ½ small red onion, chopped (about ⅓ cup)

Dressing
- 2 tablespoons vinaigrette (see page 161)
- ¼ cup mayonnaise
- Salt and pepper to taste

1. Boil 4 cups of water in a pot. Carefully add dry pasta. Cook until tender, or according to package directions. Drain and set aside.
2. Drain tuna. Chop olives, celery and onion.
3. Combine cooked pasta, tuna, olives, celery and onion in a large bowl. Mix well.

Options:
- Substitute any other small pasta shapes, such as bow ties, shells, rotini, cavatelli, wheels, penne or ziti, for macaroni.
- Substitute low-fat or fat-free mayonnaise or sour cream for regular mayonnaise.
- At Step 3, add chopped sweet pickles, pickle relish or cilantro to taste.

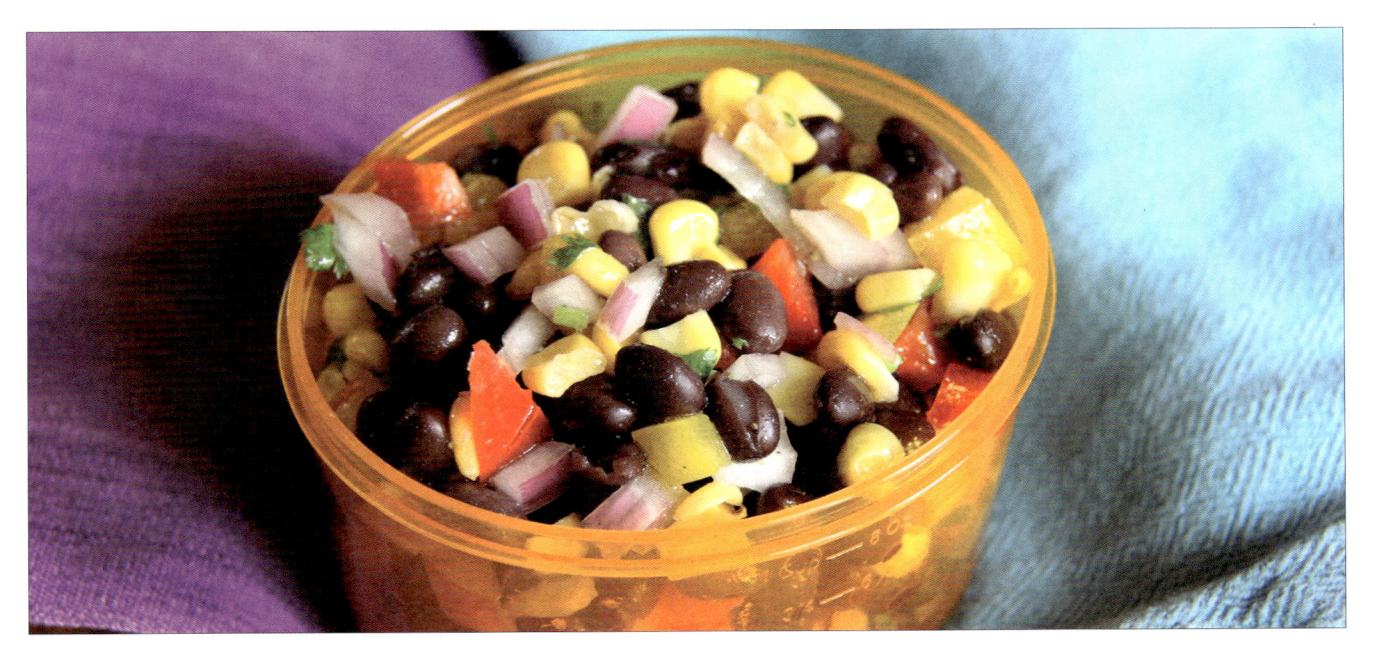

Corn and Black Bean Salad

6 servings

Enjoy this dish as a salad. Mix it with cold cooked rice, or stuff it into a pita pocket. The mixture of corn and beans makes a complete protein. Any oil-and-vinegar dressing works well. Cumin is a nice addition.

Salad
- 1 small red onion, chopped (about ½ cup)
- 2 cups corn, cooked
- 2 cups cooked black beans (1 cup dried or one 14.5 to 16-ounce can)
- 1 bell pepper, seeded and chopped (about 1 cup)
- ½ cup chopped fresh cilantro or parsley

Dressing
- 2 tablespoons vinegar or lemon juice
- ⅓ cup olive oil
- ¼ teaspoon cumin powder
- ¼ teaspoon salt

1. Cook beans (see page 54) if necessary, or drain and rinse canned beans. Wash and prepare vegetables.

2. Stir beans, corn, peppers and cilantro together.

3. Stir dressing ingredients together in a small bowl, or shake well in a covered jar. Taste and adjust seasonings. Pour on salad and toss.

4. Let salad marinate at least one hour before serving.

Options:
- At Step 2, add 2 cups chopped tomatoes.
- At Step 2, add some seeded, minced jalapeño or chile powder to taste, for more heat.
- At Step 3, add ½ teaspoon black pepper, 2 teaspoons Dijon-style mustard and 2 minced garlic cloves to the dressing.
- At Step 3, add ⅛ teaspoon chile powder to dressing.

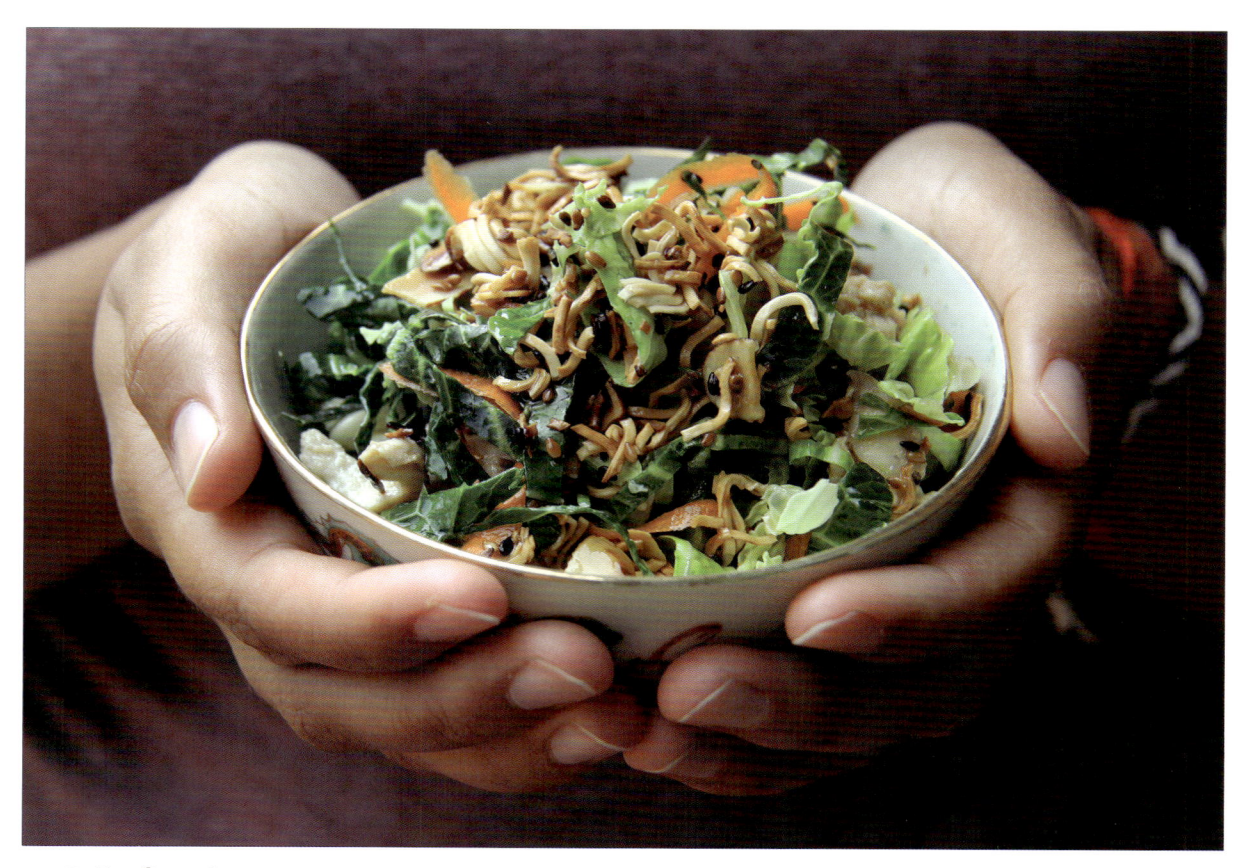

Chicken or Tofu Cabbage Salad

6-8 servings

A taste of Asia in a crunchy nutty salad.

Salad
- 2 chicken breast halves (½ to ¾ pound total) or 1 block of tofu
- 2 tablespoons soy or teriyaki sauce
- 1 tablespoon vegetable oil
- 2 packages ramen noodles (without flavor packet)
- 2 tablespoons sesame seeds
- ⅓ cup sliced or slivered almonds
- 1 small to medium head green cabbage, cored and finely chopped (about 3 cups)
- 4-5 green onions, cut in ½-inch pieces (about ⅓ cup)

Dressing
- ¼ cup vegetable or olive oil
- ¼ cup sesame oil
- ¾ cup rice vinegar
- 1 tablespoon sugar
- 2 teaspoons soy sauce
- ¼ teaspoon salt
- pepper to taste

Preheat oven to 375°
Oil a baking sheet.

For chicken:

1. Rub chicken on both sides with the soy or teriyaki sauce and place on oiled baking sheet.

2. Bake chicken 20 minutes, or until juices run clear when chicken is pierced with a fork. Halfway through baking, turn the chicken over.

3. Remove from oven. Let chicken cool, then cut into bite-size pieces.

For tofu:

1. Cut tofu into ½-inch slices. Rub with soy or teriyaki sauce on both sides and place on oiled baking sheet.

2. Bake 40 minutes or until firm and browned. Halfway through baking, turn the slices over.

3. Remove from oven. Let tofu cool, then cut into bite-size pieces.

For either chicken or tofu:

1. While chicken or tofu bakes, heat the oil in frying pan over medium heat. Break up the ramen noodles and add them to oil, along with the sesame seeds and almonds. Brown lightly, stirring, for a few minutes. Remove fried ingredients and place on paper towels to drain and cool.

2. Wash and cut green onions. Cut cabbage vertically, down through the core. Remove the core, and slice cabbage thinly.

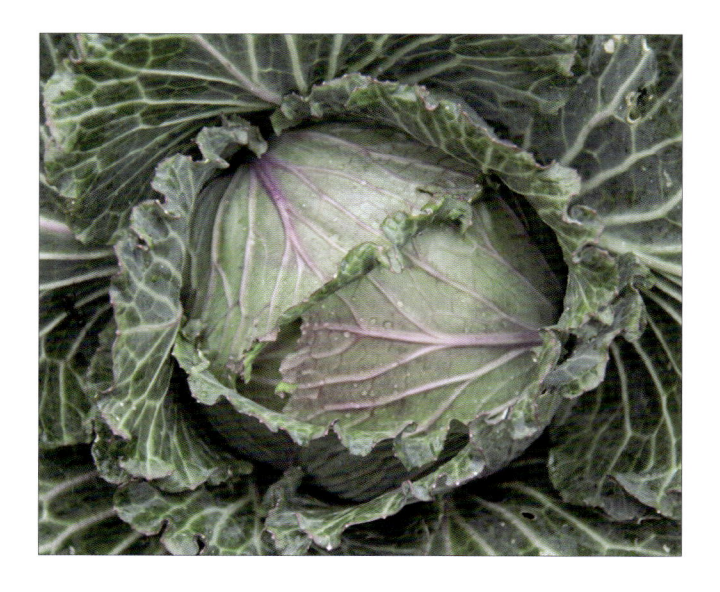

3. Stir dressing ingredients together in a small bowl, or shake well in a covered jar. Taste and adjust seasonings.

4. Place cabbage, green onions, cooled chicken or tofu and noodle mixture in a large bowl. Toss with dressing and serve.

Options:

- Substitute Napa cabbage for cabbage.
- At Step 4, add other chopped vegetables for color: carrots, red or yellow bell peppers, florets of broccoli.
- Save some of the browned ramen noodle mixture to sprinkle over the salad just before serving.

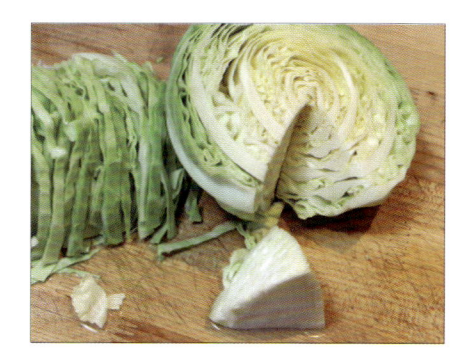

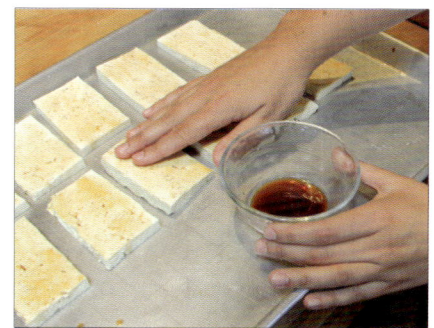

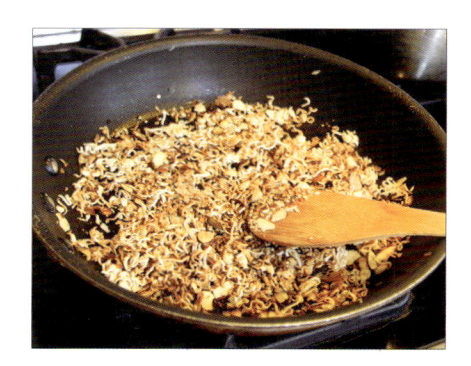

Main Dish ☞ Salad Recipes

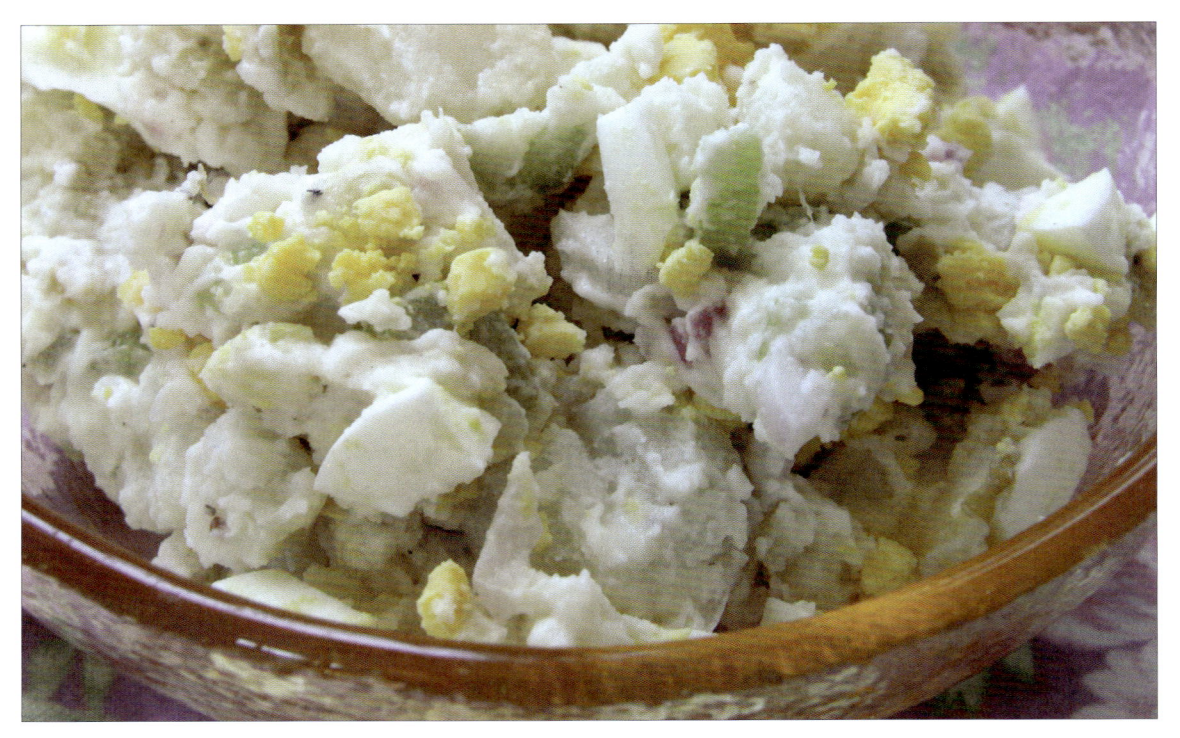

Potato Salad

6-8 servings

Lighten up your potato salad with this version that uses a smaller amount of mayonnaise.

Salad
- 4 large boiling potatoes, peeled or unpeeled
- 2 hard-cooked eggs, peeled and chopped
- 1 teaspoon salt
- 4 celery stalks, chopped (about 1 cup)
- ½ medium red onion, chopped (about ½ cup)

Dressing
- 3 tablespoons vinegar
- ½ teaspoon salt
- ½ cup mayonnaise
- ¼ teaspoon pepper

1. Peel potatoes (if desired), rinse and cut in half.
2. Place potatoes in a 4-quart pot and cover with cold water. Bring to boil, reduce heat and simmer 15-20 minutes, or until a sharp fork easily pierces the potato.
3. While potatoes are cooking, hardcook the eggs (see page 55). Cool, peel and chop.
4. Pour cooked potatoes into a colander. Cool until they can be handled. Cut into 1-inch cubes.
5. Stir the vinegar and salt together in a large bowl until the salt is dissolved.
6. Add the cubed warm potatoes, chopped eggs, celery, onion, mayonnaise and pepper. Mix well and refrigerate.

Options:
- Add pickle relish to taste.
- Add four strips bacon, cooked and chopped.

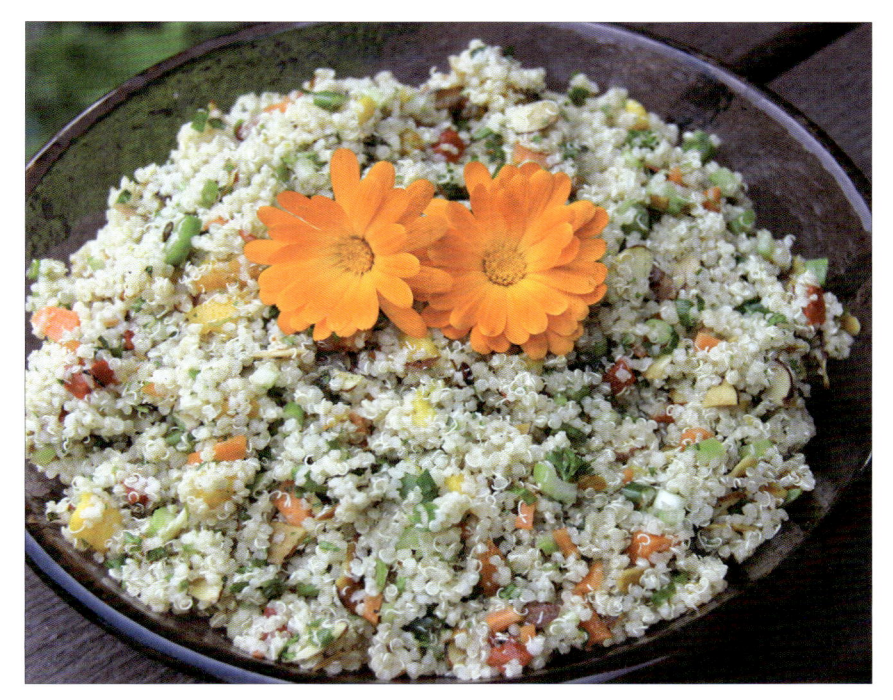

Tabouli

4 servings

This is a classic Mediterranean salad. Bulgur is cracked wheat that has been partially cooked and dried. Quinoa can be substituted. Quinoa, from the Andes Mountains in South America, is not a grain but a seed, and can be substituted for most grains. Quinoa is high in protein as are the garbanzo beans.

Salad
- 2 cups water
- 1 cup bulgur or quinoa
- 1 cucumber, seeded and coarsely chopped (about 1 cup)
- 2 small tomatoes, diced (about ¾ cup) or ¾ cup cherry tomatoes cut in half
- 1 cup cooked garbanzo beans (half a 14.5 to 16-ounce can)

Dressing
- ½ cup minced fresh parsley (or 2½ tablespoons dried)
- 1 clove garlic, peeled and minced
- 1½ teaspoons white vinegar or lemon juice
- 1 tablespoon olive oil
- Salt and pepper to taste

1. Wash and chop vegetables, parsley and garlic.
2. Prepare grain:
   - If using bulgar, boil the water in a small saucepan and add the bulgur. Turn off the heat and cover pot. Bulgar will absorb all the water in about 20 minutes.
   - If using quinoa, rinse and put in a pot with 1 cup of water. Bring water to a boil, reduce heat to medium, and cook 10-15 minutes.
3. Mix cucumber, tomato and grains in a medium bowl.
4. Mix the parsley, garlic, vinegar, oil and salt and pepper together and toss with the grains.

Options:
- At Step 3, add ½ cup chopped red onion
- At Step 3, add 1 small bunch mint, chopped

Soup Formula

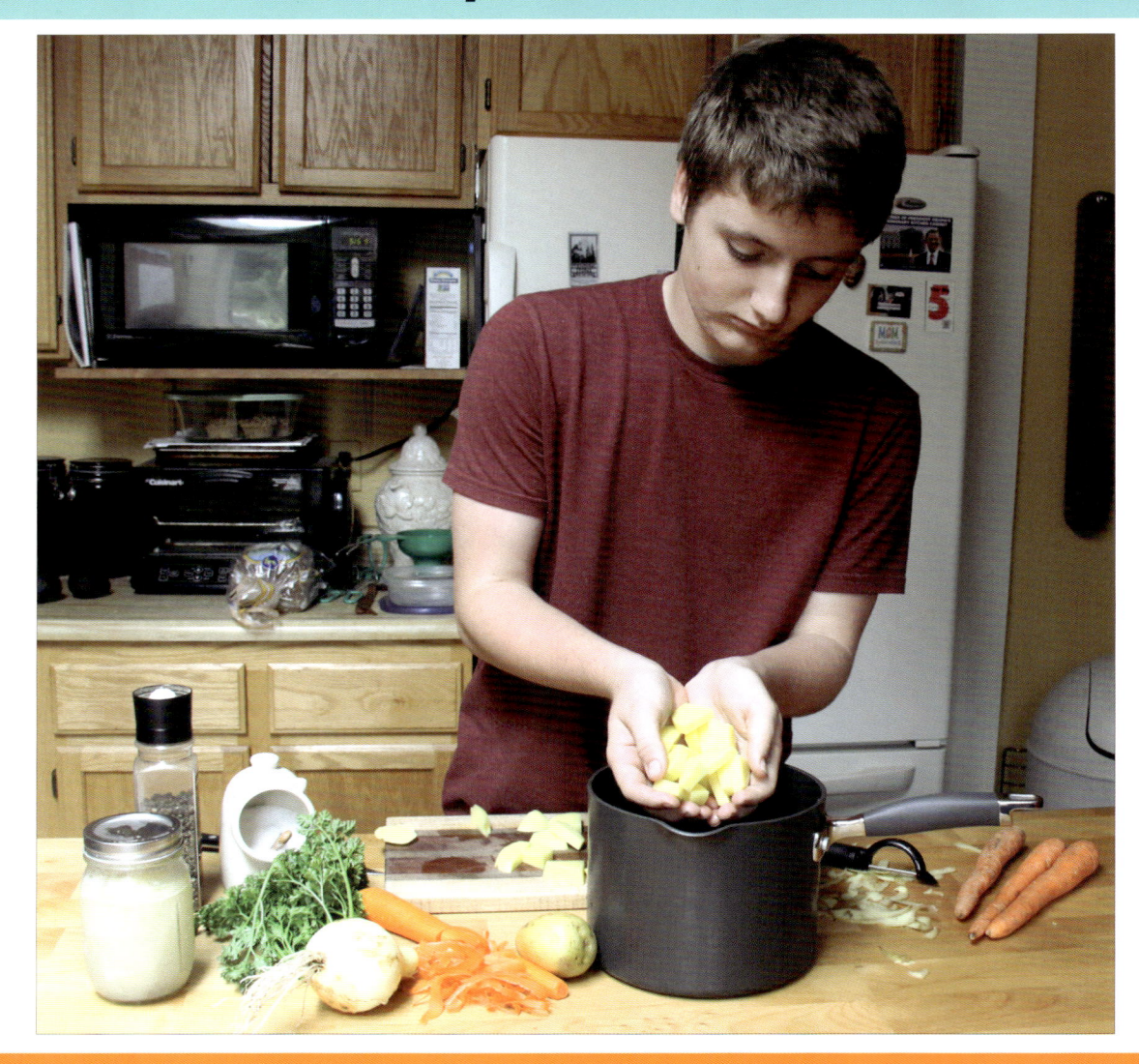

1. Chop and add raw vegetables and/or meat to a large pot.

2. Cover ingredients with broth or water. Bring to a boil. Reduce heat and simmer until meat is cooked and vegetables are soft.

3. Add precooked items, like rice, pasta, or vegetable and meat leftovers.

4. Season with spice mix of choice (see page 193) or your favorite seasonings. Add salt to taste.

5. Simmer for another 5-10 minutes to blend flavors.

Ingredient Ideas

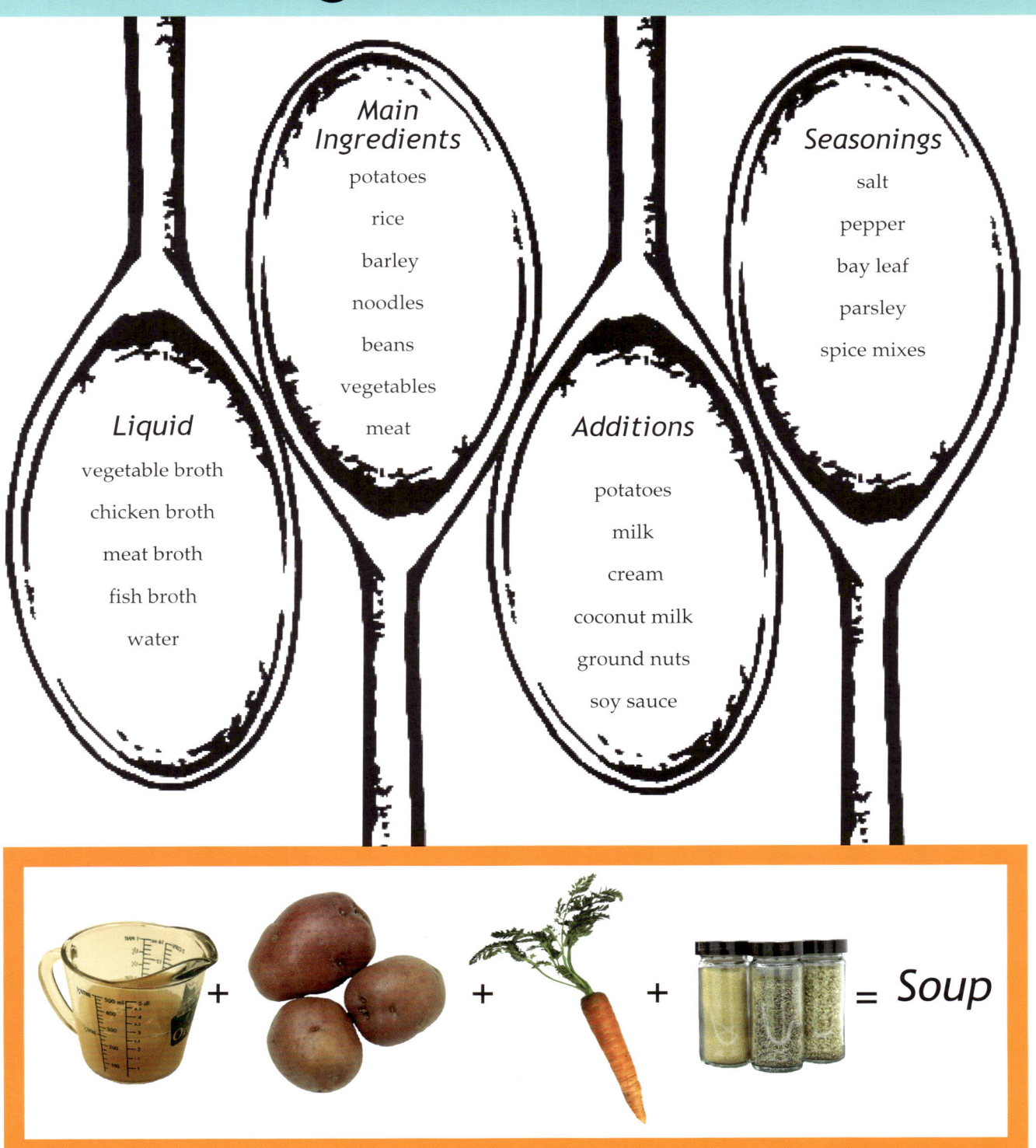

Main Ingredients
- potatoes
- rice
- barley
- noodles
- beans
- vegetables
- meat

Seasonings
- salt
- pepper
- bay leaf
- parsley
- spice mixes

Liquid
- vegetable broth
- chicken broth
- meat broth
- fish broth
- water

Additions
- potatoes
- milk
- cream
- coconut milk
- ground nuts
- soy sauce

+ + + = *Soup*

Main Dish ☞ Soup Recipes

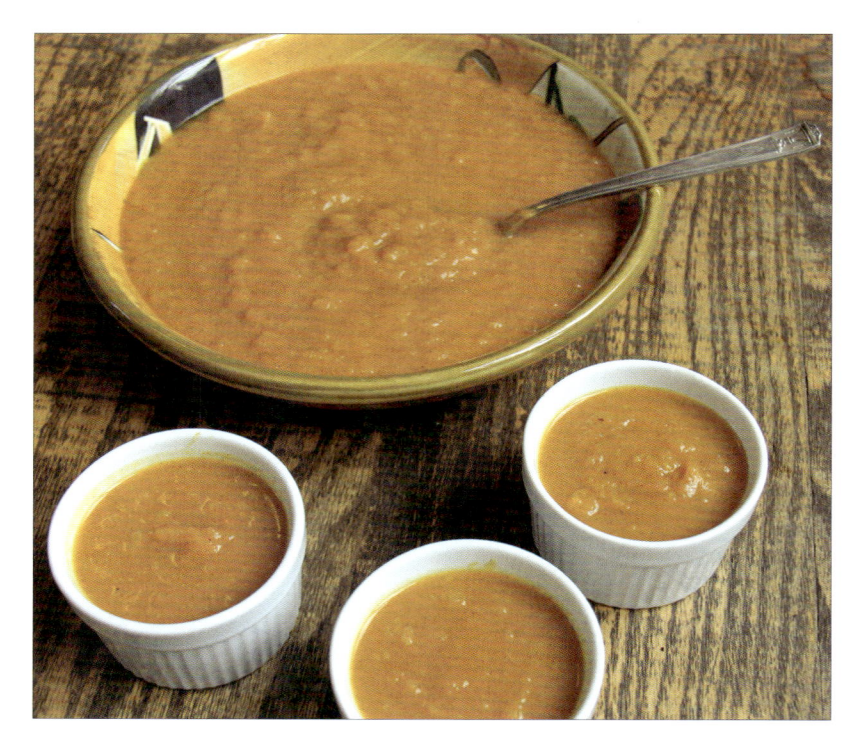

Sweet Squash Soup

4-6 servings

This recipe features one of North America's native vegetables. Winter squash, such as butternut, acorn, Hubbard, or pie pumpkins, work the best. Note: for kids, baking is the safest way to soften the squash and remove the peel.

2	teaspoons vegetable or olive oil
2	medium onions, finely chopped (about 2 cups)
4	cloves garlic, peeled and minced or crushed
½	teaspoon ground cinnamon
⅛	teaspoon nutmeg
1	teaspoon salt
¼	teaspoon pepper
1	2 ½ pound winter squash or pie pumpkin, chopped (about 3 cups), or one 28-ounce can of pumpkin
1	cup applesauce (see page 136)
1	cup apple juice or cider
3	cups vegetable or chicken broth

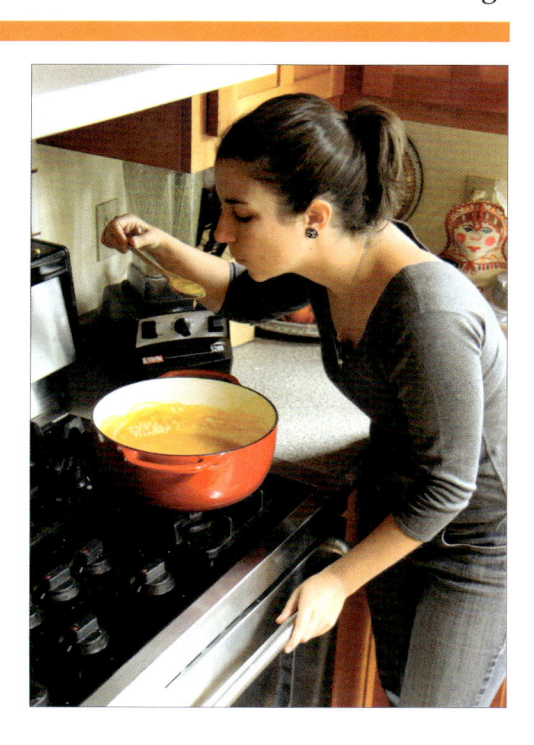

Keeping Soup Warm for School

Use a thermos to keep soup warm. Here's a trick that will make your soup the perfect temperature by the time lunch rolls around:

- In the morning, heat the soup in microwave or on stove.
- Meanwhile, preheat the thermos by filling with boiling water.
- Pour out the boiling water, then pour in the heated soup.
- Stay safe and don't microwave the thermos. Microwave only glass or ceramic.

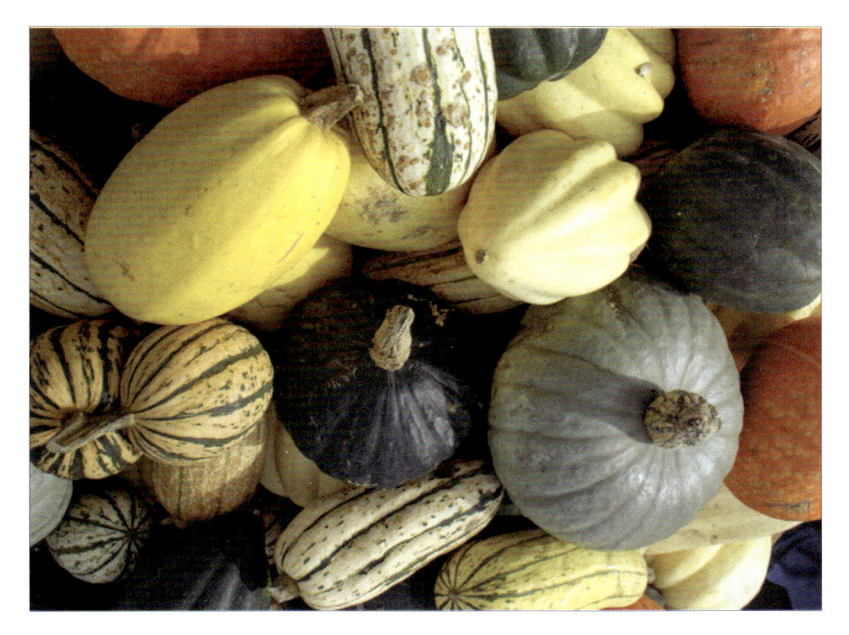

Preparing Winter Squash:

Preheat oven to 350°

1. Oil a rimmed baking sheet. If using fresh squash, cut the ends off. Sit squash on a cut end and cut in half downward (see illustration below). For pumpkin, remove stem, cut in half, and scrape out seeds. Place squash or pumpkin on rimmed baking sheet, cut side down. Pour one cup of water on sheet, cover with foil and place in oven. Cook until a fork pierces the skin easily, about 1 hour. Set aside to cool.

2. When squash is cool, scoop pulp out of peel. Mash the squash.

For Soup:

3. Prepare the onions and garlic.

4. Heat oil over medium heat in a 6- to 8-quart soup pot. Add onions; cook until they begin to brown, about 5 minutes.

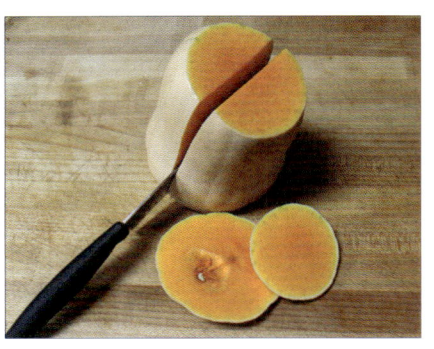

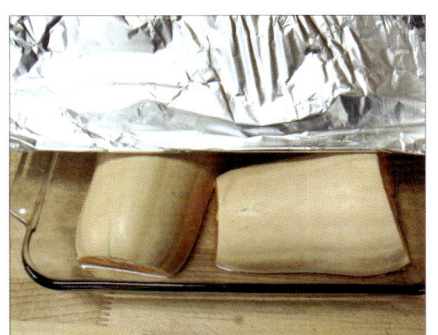

5. Add garlic, cinnamon, nutmeg, salt and pepper to onions and stir until blended, about 30 seconds.

6. Put cooled onion mixture, squash or pumpkin, applesauce, apple juice and broth into a blender, 2-3 cups at a time. Blend or process until smooth.

7. Pour blended mixture back into the pot. Simmer 20 minutes.

Options:

- Substitute 2 leeks for onions. Cut in half lengthwise and rinse thoroughly. Use only the white and light green part.
- Garnish soup with sour cream, fresh parsley or roasted and chopped walnuts.
- Instead of roasting raw squash or pumpkin, cut into several pieces and steam until soft.

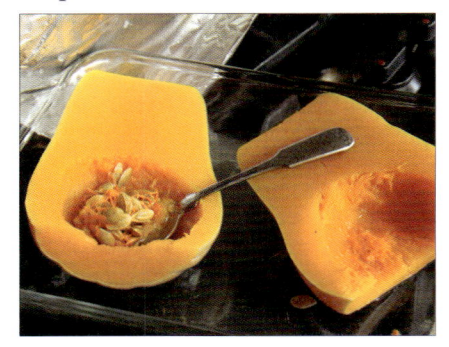

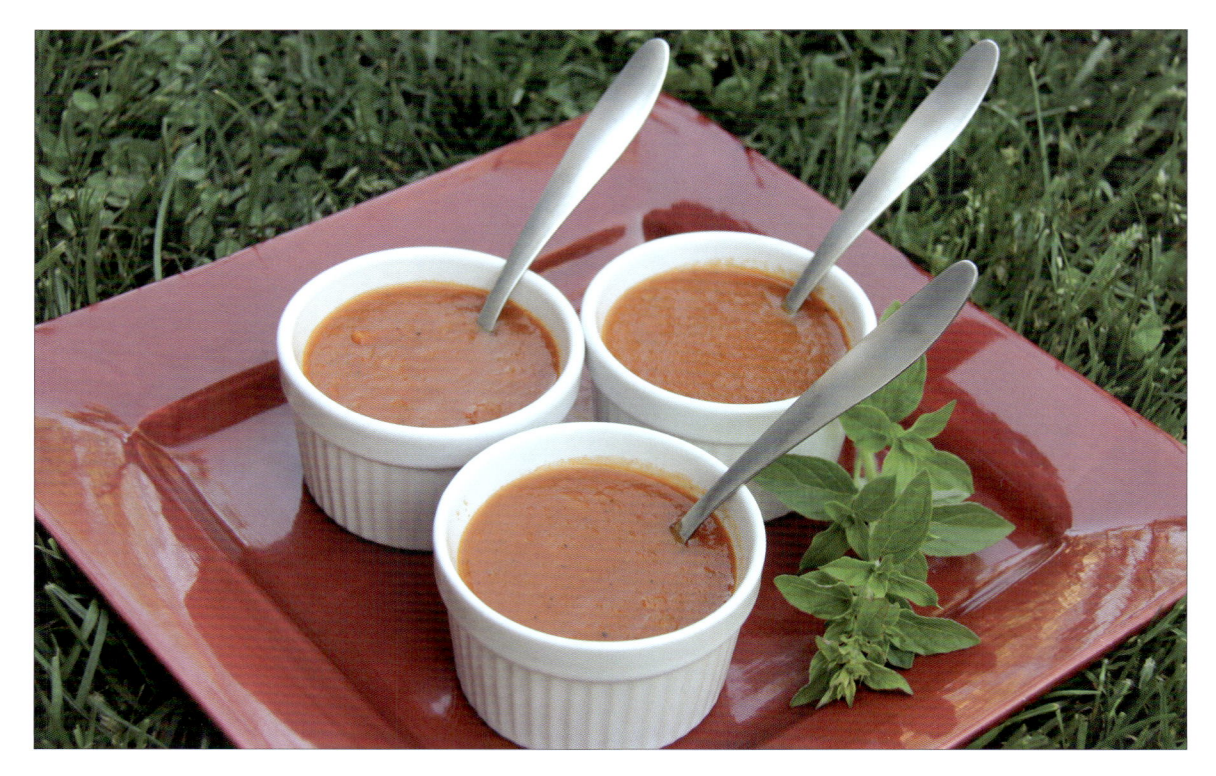

Tomato Soup

6 servings

Warms your heart, warms your tummy! There's nothing like a cupful of this tomato soup in your lunch to brighten your day.

- 4-6 tomatoes, chopped (about 4 cups) or two 14.5- to 16-ounce cans diced tomatoes
- 1 medium onion, chopped (about 1 cup)
- ⅛ teaspoon ground cloves or 2 whole cloves, ground
- 2 bay leaves
- 2 cups vegetable or chicken broth (see page 62)
- 2 tablespoons butter
- 2 tablespoons all-purpose flour
- 1 teaspoon salt
- 2 teaspoons sugar, or to taste
- ¼ teaspoon pepper

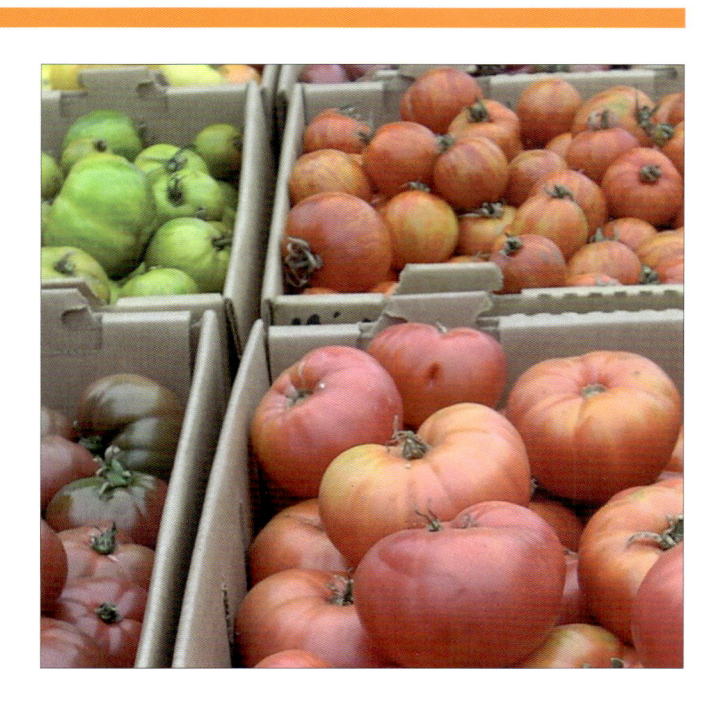

120 Main Dish ☞ Soup Recipes

1. Clean and prepare the vegetables.

2. Combine the tomatoes, onion, cloves, bay leaves and broth in a 4-quart saucepan. Bring to a boil over medium heat. Reduce heat slightly and gently boil for about 20 minutes to blend all of the flavors.

3. Remove from heat and remove the bay leaves. Pour soup into a medium mixing bowl.

4. Leave soup as is, with chunks of tomato, or cool the soup and run it through a blender or food processor for a thicker, smoother texture. Process soup in batches, ½ to ⅓ at a time.

5. In the same saucepan, melt the butter over low heat. Using a whisk, slowly mix in the flour until flour and butter are incorporated, about 2 minutes. The mixture should be smooth. This is called a *roux*.

6. Gradually stir the tomato mixture into the roux so that no lumps form. Season with sugar and salt to taste.

Options:

- For a creamier version, add a can of coconut milk or two cups of milk, cream, half-and-half, soy milk or other nut milk at the end of Step 2. Heat, but do not boil.
- Serve topped with a dollop of sour cream and chopped dill, grated cheese, cooked rice, or crushed crackers.

Thick and Creamy Soups

To make a soup creamier, add:

- milk
- half-and-half
- heavy cream
- soy, almond or nut milks
- coconut milk

Heat on low after adding any of the above. Be careful not to boil the soup after adding a dairy product; the soup could curdle.

To make soup thicker:

- Make a roux described in Step 5 of this recipe and pictured in the photos below.
- Cool soup to lukewarm, then run it through a food processor or blender in small batches until it is smooth.
- Stir in leftover mashed potatoes.

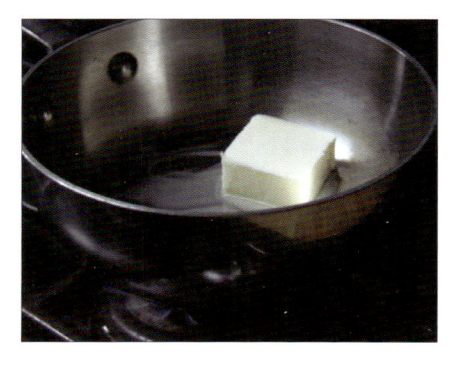

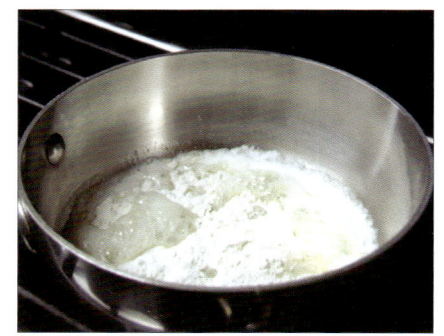

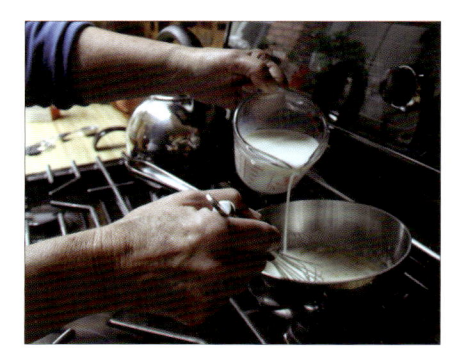

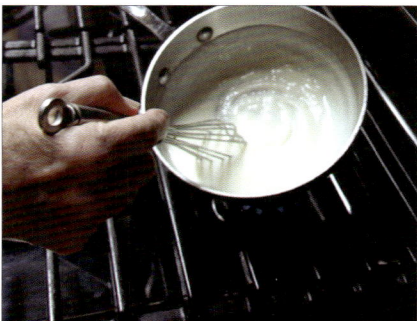

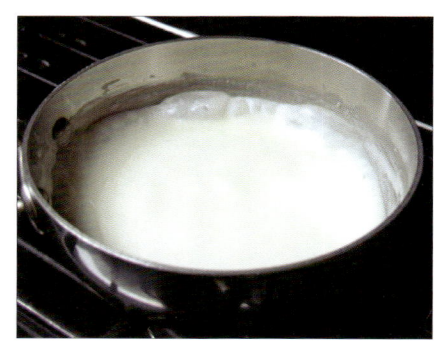

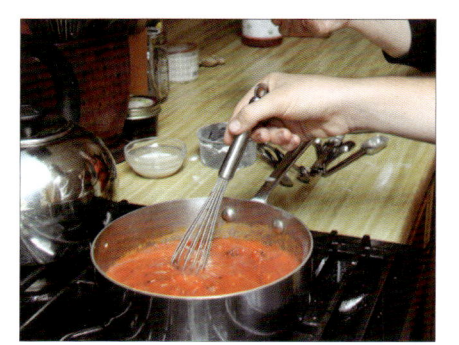

Main Dish ☞ Soup Recipes

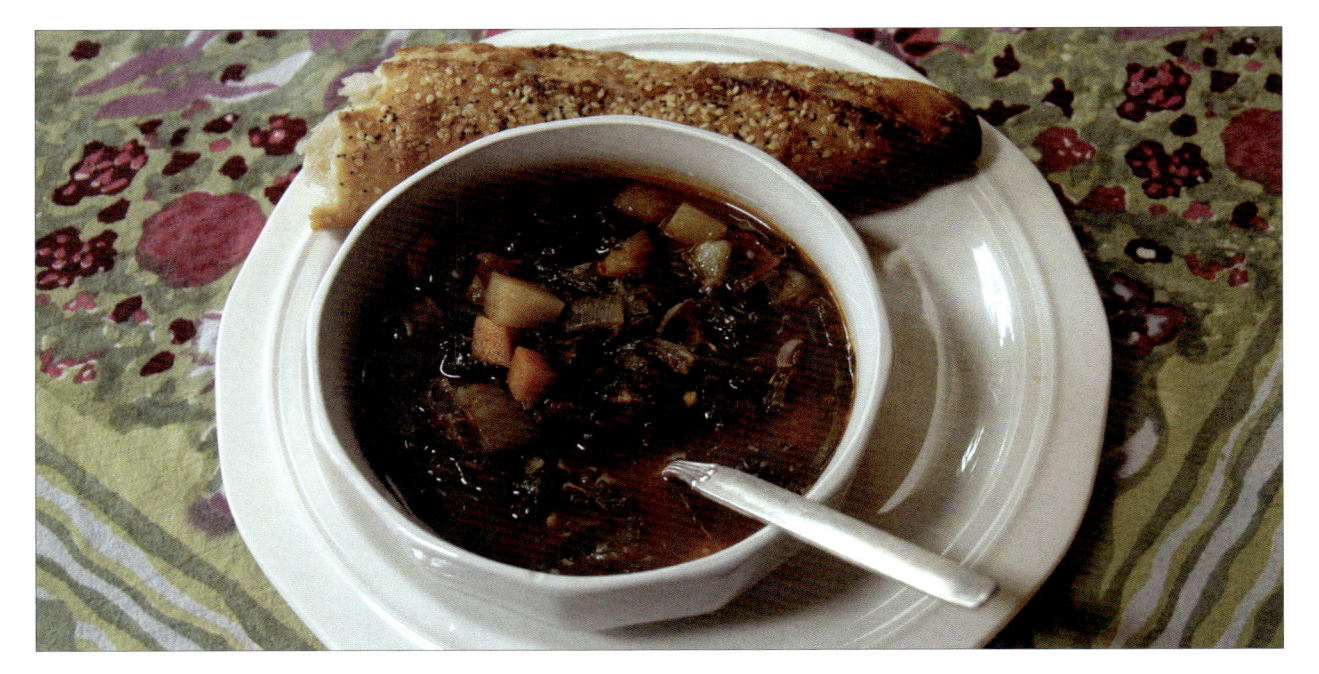

Minestrone Soup

8 servings

Minestrone is an Italian classic. There is no fixed recipe, but most versions include onions, tomatoes, celery, carrots and beans. Like any soup, it tastes better the next day after the flavors have blended.

2	tablespoons vegetable oil
1	large onion, diced (about 2 cups)
4	garlic cloves, minced (about 2 tablespoons)
2	large carrots, diced (about 2 cups)
2	stalks celery, diced (about ½ cup)
2	medium boiling potatoes, diced (about 2 cups)
6	cups broth (see page 62)
½	small green cabbage, sliced finely (about 2 cups)
2-3	medium tomatoes, chopped (about 2 cups), or one 14.5- to 16-ounce can
1	tablespoon salt
2	cups cooked kidney, red, or navy beans and/or black-eyed peas (1 cup dried or one 14.5- to 16-ounce can)

1. In an 8-quart pot, heat the oil and sauté the onion and garlic for 5 minutes or until lightly browned. Add carrots, celery and potatoes. Cook for 10 minutes.

2. Add broth, the rest of the vegetables and salt. Bring to a boil. Reduce heat and simmer 20-30 minutes, or until all vegetables are tender. Stir occasionally.

3. Add cooked beans, pre-cooked ingredients and frozen vegetables. Cook 10-15 minutes, stirring occasionally.

Options:

- At Step 3, add ½ pound fresh or frozen green beans, sliced, or 2 zucchini, diced.
- At Step 3, add 6 cups fresh spinach or one 10-ounce bag frozen spinach.
- Garnish with ½ cup grated Parmesan cheese.

Bean Soup

4-6 servings

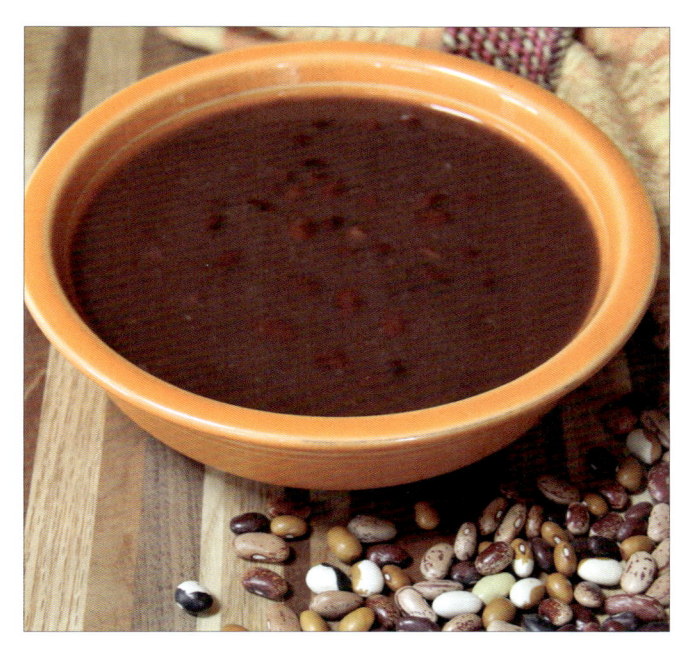

This recipe has two versions. Version one uses canned beans, version two uses dried beans. Black beans are tasty and a good place to start creating a bean soup. Experiment with different types of beans and flavorings.

4	cups cooked beans (2 cups dried beans or two 14.5- to 16-ounce cans beans)
1	medium onion, chopped (about 1 cup)
1	fresh jalapeño chili, seeded and chopped (about 1 tablespoon)
2	teaspoons minced garlic (about 2 cloves)
1	tablespoon chopped fresh oregano (or 1 teaspoon dried)
1	tablespoon chopped fresh thyme (or 1 teaspoon dried)
1½	teaspoons cumin powder
1	teaspoon coriander
3	bay leaves
3	quarts water or broth (see page 62)

For canned or pre-cooked beans:

1. Rinse canned beans well. Prepare the vegetables. (Be aware that the oils in hot peppers can burn you. Wear gloves if you have sensitive skin and don't touch your eyes or face.)

2. Add all ingredients to a 6-quart sauce pan.

3. Bring to a boil, reduce to a simmer, cover and cook 20-30 minutes. Add more liquid, if necessary, to keep the beans from sticking. Adjust seasonings; add salt and pepper as needed.

For dried beans:

See page 54 for cooking directions for beans.

Option:

- To make the soup smoother, puree the beans or the soup in a food processor.

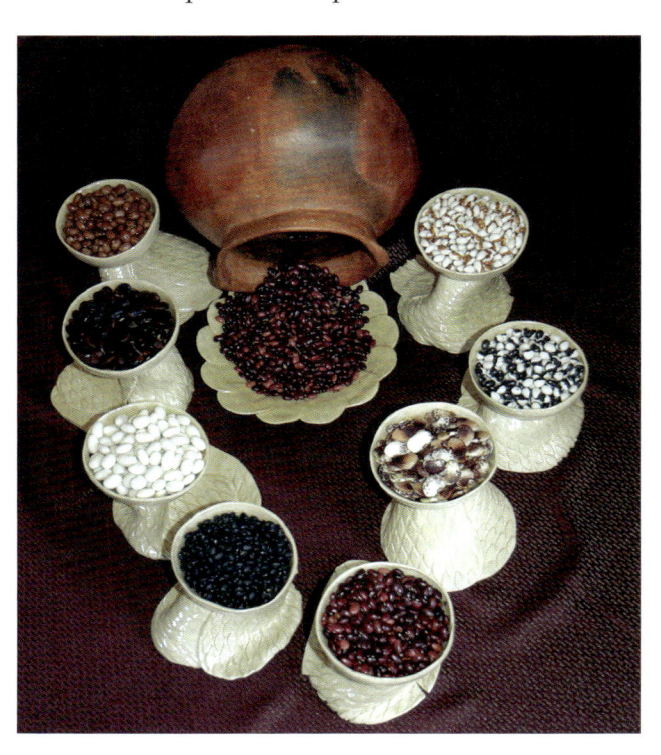

Main Dish ☞ Soup Recipes

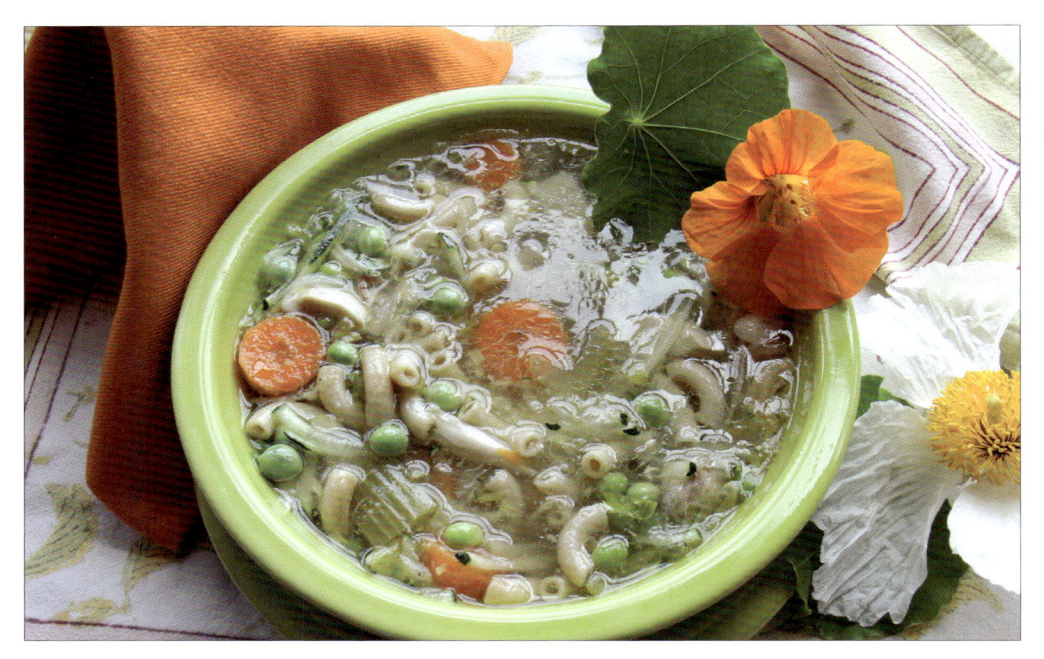

Chicken Noodle Soup

6-8 servings

Whether you're sick or healthy, chicken noodle soup is comforting and delicious.

- 2 tablespoons vegetable or olive oil
- 2 large carrots, peeled and chopped (about 2 cups)
- 4 celery stalks, chopped (about 1 cup)
- 1 medium onion, chopped (about 1 cup)
- 1 clove garlic, minced (about 1 teaspoon)
- 3 pounds of chicken parts (breasts, legs, thighs)
- 1 lemon, cut in half
- 4 cups chicken broth (see page 62)
- 4 cups water
- 2 teaspoons dried thyme
- ¼ cup chopped fresh parsley (about 1½ tablespoons dried)
- 2 bay leaves
- 1 teaspoon salt, or to taste
- 1 teaspoon pepper, or to taste
- 1 cup peas
- 1 cup egg noodles or other small pasta

1. Clean and prepare vegetables.
2. Heat oil in large pot. Add onion, garlic and celery. Cook until tender, about 5 minutes.
3. Add carrots, chicken, lemon, broth, water and seasonings to the pot. Bring to a boil over high heat, reduce heat and simmer, uncovered, for an hour.
4. Remove chicken pieces from liquid with tongs or a slotted spoon. Cool, then remove meat from the bones and break into small pieces. Return meat to pot.
5. Add peas to pot and continue to simmer about 20 minutes.
6. In a separate pot, cook noodles (see page 57), drain, and add to the chicken mixture. Heat through.

Options:

- Cook a whole chicken, use 4 cups of leftover chicken, or use a deli-cooked chicken.
- Save the chicken bones for making broth (see page 62).

Vegetables

Kids are more likely to eat vegetables that are sliced into bite-size portions. Wash and prepare vegetables in big batches. Keep them in the refrigerator for easy snacking and for additions to lunchboxes, with or without a dip or spread. Combine with cottage cheese, nuts (see pages 142 and 143), Hard-cooked eggs (see page 55) or Tofu Sticks (see page 145) for protein to create a Main-Dish item, or serve with a Main Dish that's missing vegetables.

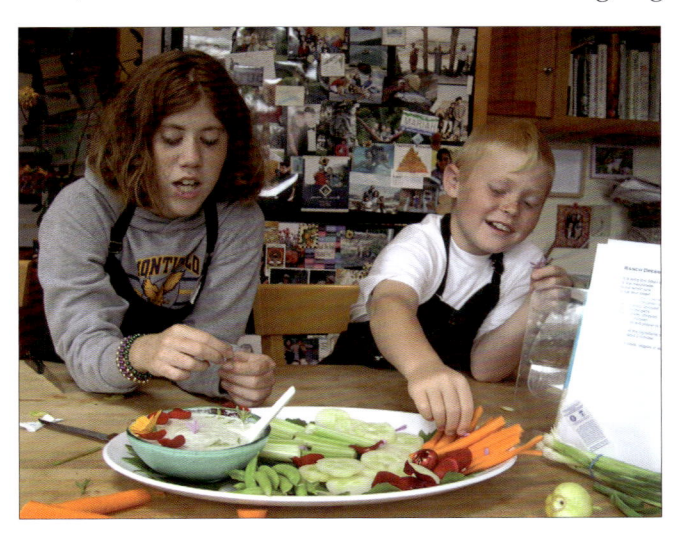

No-Prep
- Bean sprouts
- Cherry tomatoes
- Edamame
- Olives
- Sugar snap peas
- Pickles
- Small or early-picked carrots

Low-Prep
- Bell pepper, sliced long or in rounds
- Broccoli and cauliflower, broken into florets
- Big carrots, sliced into sticks
- Celery, sliced in half or into sticks
- Jicama, sliced into sticks
- Nori snacks—seaweed sheets torn into pieces (see page 81)

Quick Food Carving

Kids! You can do some simple, food carving to make your fruits and vegetables fun to eat...

- **Cucumbers**: Peel away alternate strips of skin until you have a vertically striped cucumber. Slice into rounds.
- **Bell peppers**: Cut in half, scoop out seeds, and use as a bowl for other items.
- **Carrots:** Peel with a hand grater to create lots of ridges. Slice into rounds.

(See page 138 for more food carving ideas.)

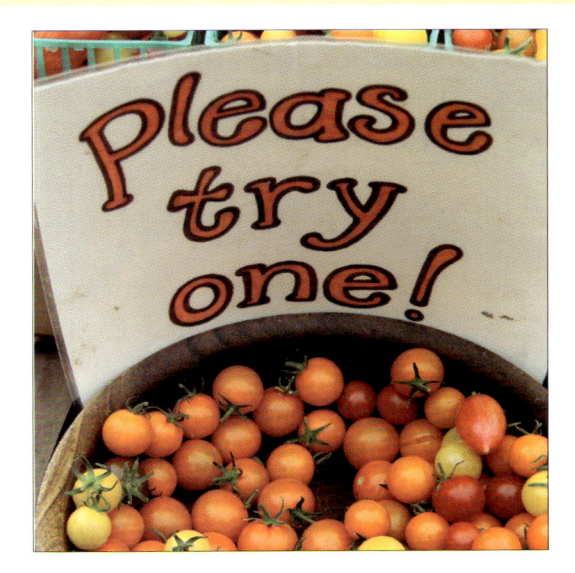

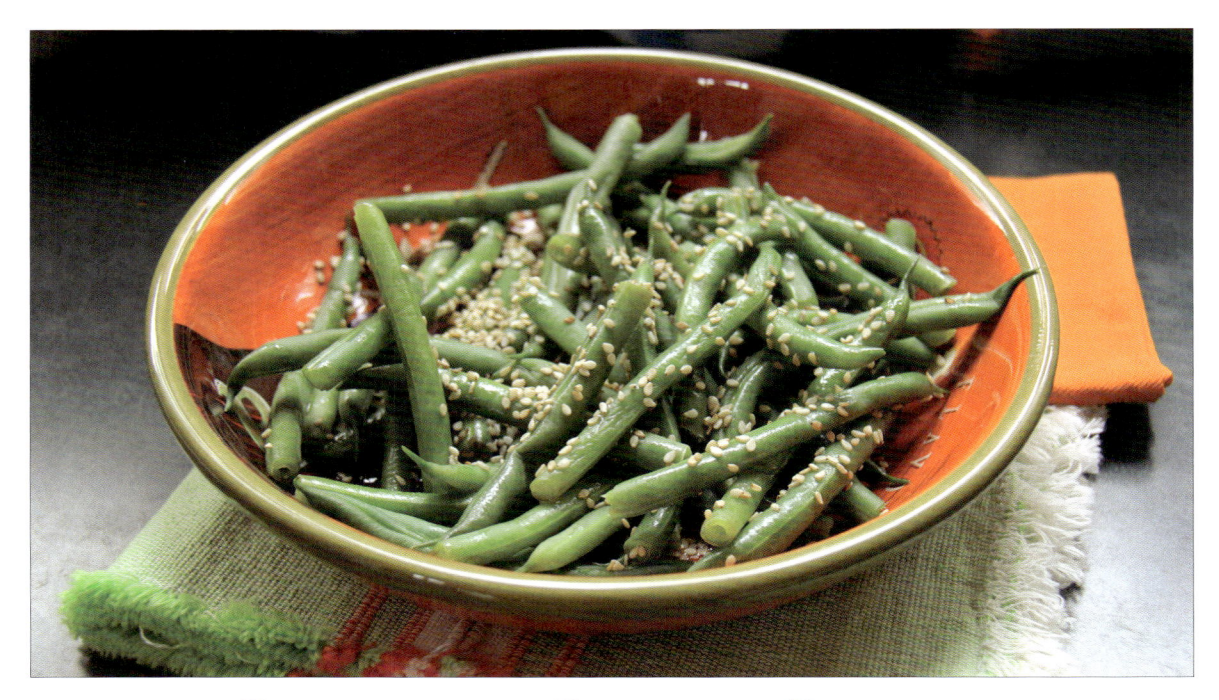

Sesame Green Beans

6-8 servings

These are Asian-inspired green beans. The secret to tasty green beans—keep them crisp by not overcooking them.

- 1 pound green beans, fresh or frozen
- 2 tablespoons rice vinegar
- 2 teaspoons sesame oil
- 2 teaspoons sesame seeds
- Salt and pepper to taste

1. Wash beans. Trim stem end or both ends.
2. If using fresh beans, place 1 inch of water in a pot, place a steamer basket in the pot; place beans in basket. Cover the pot and steam for 5 minutes or until beans are crisp-tender and still bright green. If using frozen beans, steam them lightly.
3. Remove basket from pot, cool beans 10 minutes.
4. Stir vinegar, oil and sesame seeds together in a medium bowl. Add cooled beans and mix well.
5. Season to taste with salt and pepper.

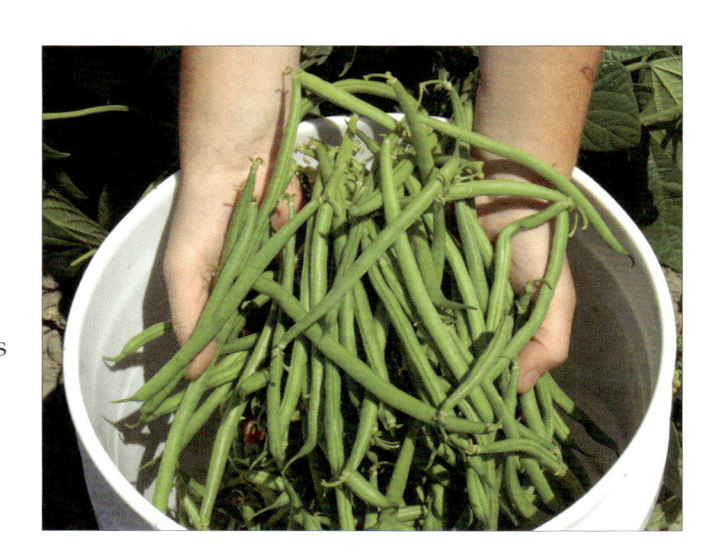

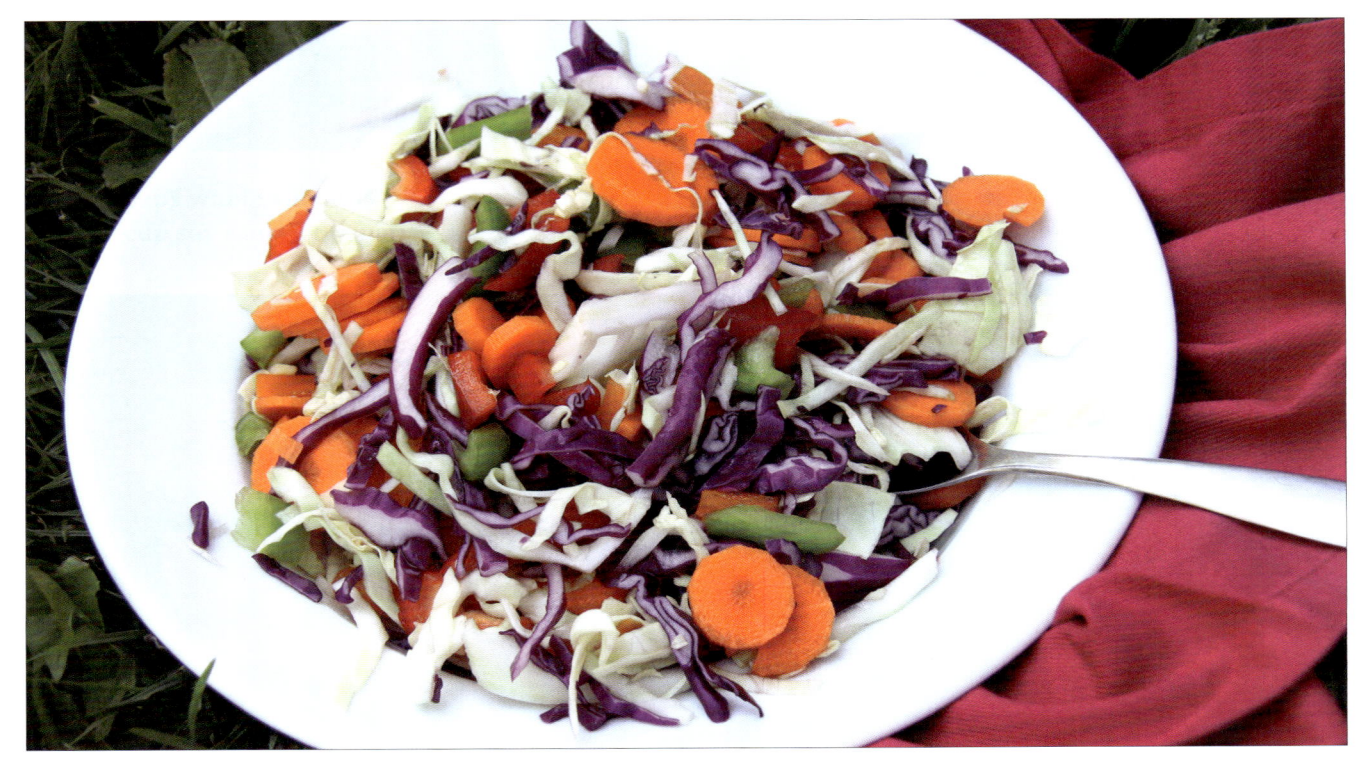

Three-Color Coleslaw

6 servings

This is a colorful cabbage salad that can be expanded and brightened with the suggested options. The salad with its dressing can be refrigerated for a couple of days.

Salad
- 3 cups red or green cabbage, chopped (about half a medium head)
- 3 carrots, peeled and sliced thinly or grated
- 2 bell peppers (one red and one yellow), seeded and chopped (about 2 cups total)
- ¼ teaspoon salt

Dressing
- ¼ cup Vinaigrette (see page 161) or 3 tablespoons olive oil and 1 tablespoon vinegar

1. Wash and chop vegetables.
2. Toss the cabbage, carrots, bell peppers and salt in a large bowl.
3. Drizzle on the dressing. Taste and adjust the amount of dressing.

Options:
- At Step 2:
  - add ¼ cup chopped green onion or green bell pepper.
  - add ½ cup of grated cheese, such as Jack or mozzarella.
  - Add mandarin orange sections or grapes that have been halved, for more sweetness.
  - to add protein, include sliced nuts.
- Just before serving, add dry, broken-up ramen noodles.

Fake Grass Salad

2 servings

The secret to success is to roll the leaves tightly, then slice as thin as a blade of grass.

Salad
- 2 cups thinly sliced collard greens or kale leaves (about half a bunch)
- 1-2 mandarin oranges, peeled and sectioned or ½ can mandarin orange slices, drained
- 2 tablespoons dried cranberries, chopped
- 2 tablespoons toasted almonds or walnuts, slivered or chopped

Dressing
- 1 tablespoon olive oil
- 1 tablespoon vinegar or lemon juice
- Salt and pepper to taste

1. Slice center rib from kale or collard greens. Flatten leaves and stack all together. Roll leaves up tightly. Cut very thin slices off the roll (see photos below).

2. Peel and section fresh orange; drain if canned. Toast nuts if necessary (see page 142). Chop cranberries and nuts.

3. Combine greens, cranberries, orange sections and nuts in a large bowl.

4. Stir dressing ingredients together in a small bowl, or shake well in a covered jar. Taste and adjust seasonings. Drizzle on salad; toss to combine.

Leafy Greens

Dark green vegetables have the greatest concentration of vitamins and minerals of any food. The darker the green, the more powerful the plant!

The nutrients in leafy greens strengthen the eyes, help the blood to clot correctly, reduce inflammation (a contributor to asthma and arthritis), slow down age-related cell degeneration, and more.

Spinach, collard greens, chard and kale are available in many grocery stores, but keep your eyes open for mustard greens, bok choy or pak choy, as well as the greens of turnips, radishes and beets.

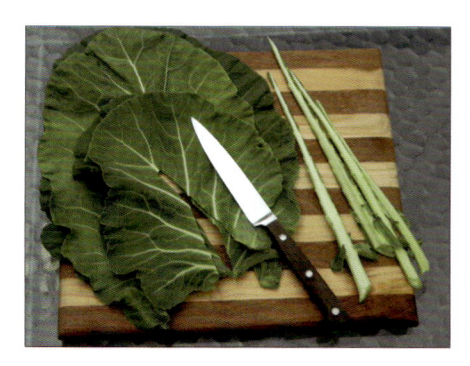

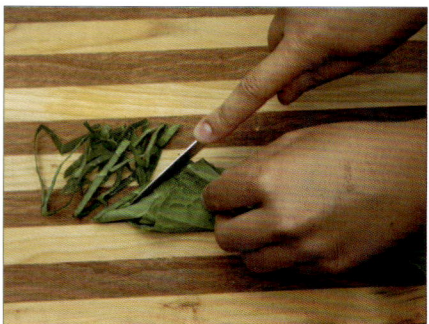

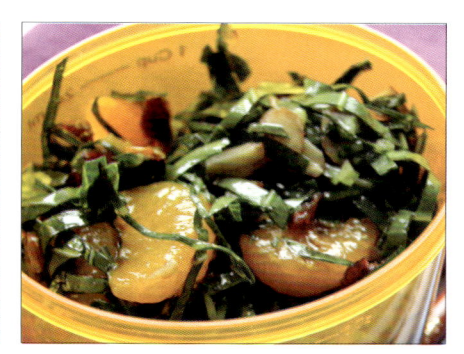

Vegetable Recipes

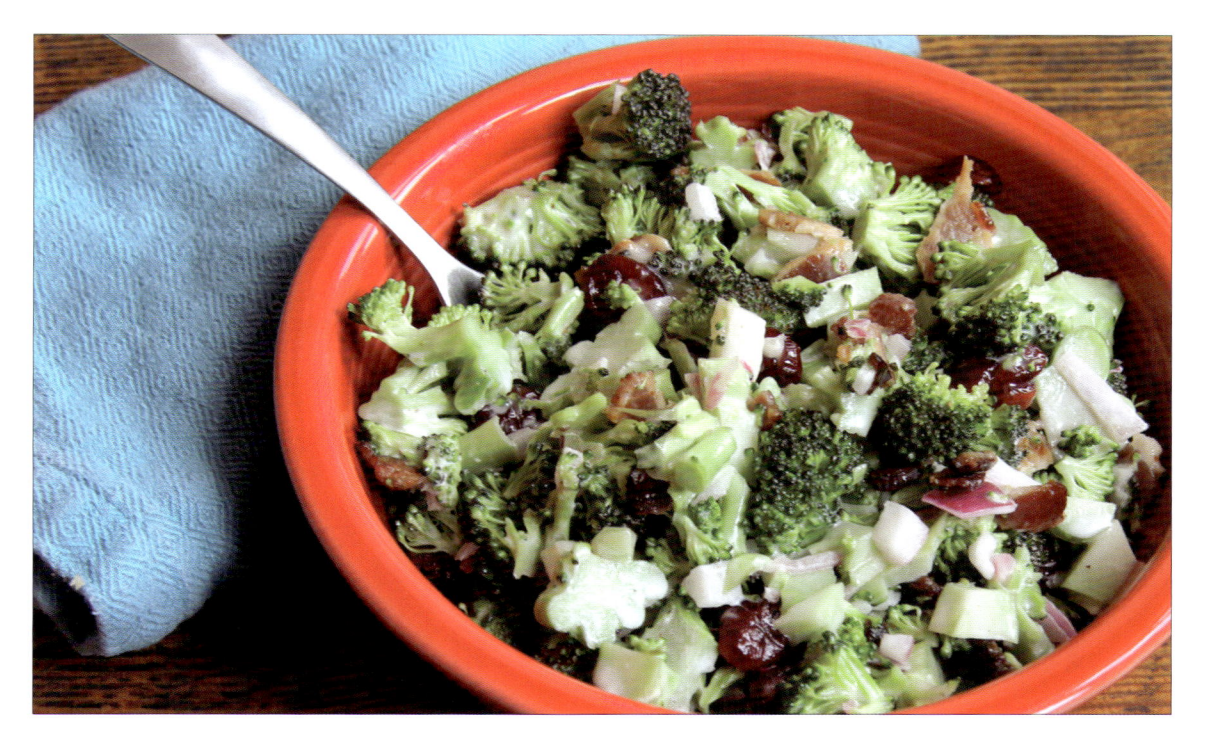

Broccoli & Bacon Salad

4 servings

Here is a salad that will appeal to just about anyone. The sweetness in the dressing really transforms the taste of the broccoli.

Salad
- ¼ pound bacon, either turkey or pork
- 1 bunch broccoli (4-5 cups total)
- ½ cup unsalted sunflower seeds
- ½ cup raisins or dried cranberries

Dressing
- ¾ cup mayonnaise, or use 2 tablespoons mayonnaise and 2 tablespoons plain yogurt
- 3 tablespoons vinegar
- 2 tablespoons sugar

1. Cut bacon into small pieces, then fry until crisp. Remove from pan and place on paper towels to drain fat. Let cool.

2. Wash broccoli and break into florets. Chop stems.

3. Combine all salad ingredients in a medium bowl.

4. Stir dressing ingredients together in a small bowl. Taste and adjust seasonings.

5. Pour dressing over salad and mix well. Cover and refrigerate immediately. Let sit at least one hour.

Options:
- Substitute cauliflower for broccoli, or use half of each.
- Substitute dried cherries for raisins or cranberries.
- At Step 3, add ½ small red onion, chopped.

Vegetable Recipes

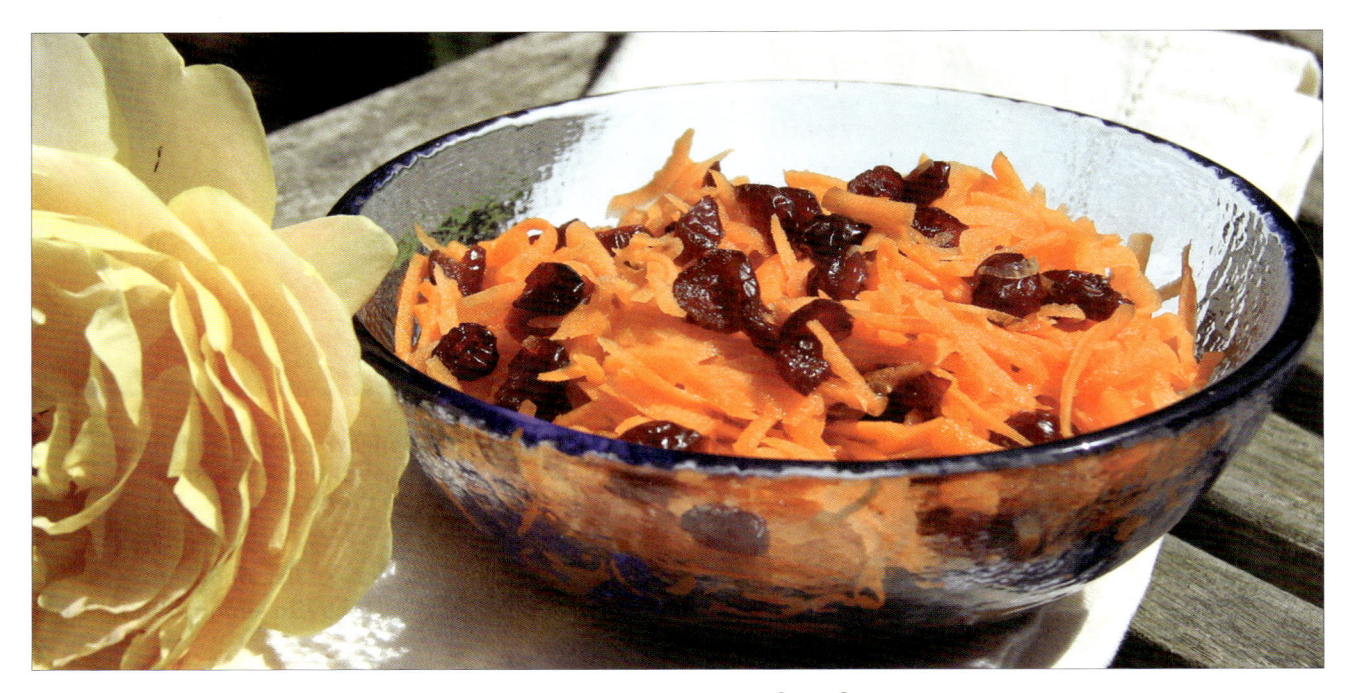

Carrot and Raisin Salad

6 servings

A classic, simple and tasty sweet salad. This is the perfect recipe for beginning cooks to hone their skills.

> 5 large carrots
> 1 cup raisins
> Juice of 1 lemon or small orange

1. Peel and grate carrots. You should have about 5 cups.

2. Combine all ingredients in a medium bowl and stir. Add more lemon or orange juice to taste.

Options:
- For a creamier salad, add ½ cup plain yogurt, mayonnaise, or sour cream.
- Add ½ cup diced celery.
- For protein, toss in ½ cup chopped almonds or walnuts.

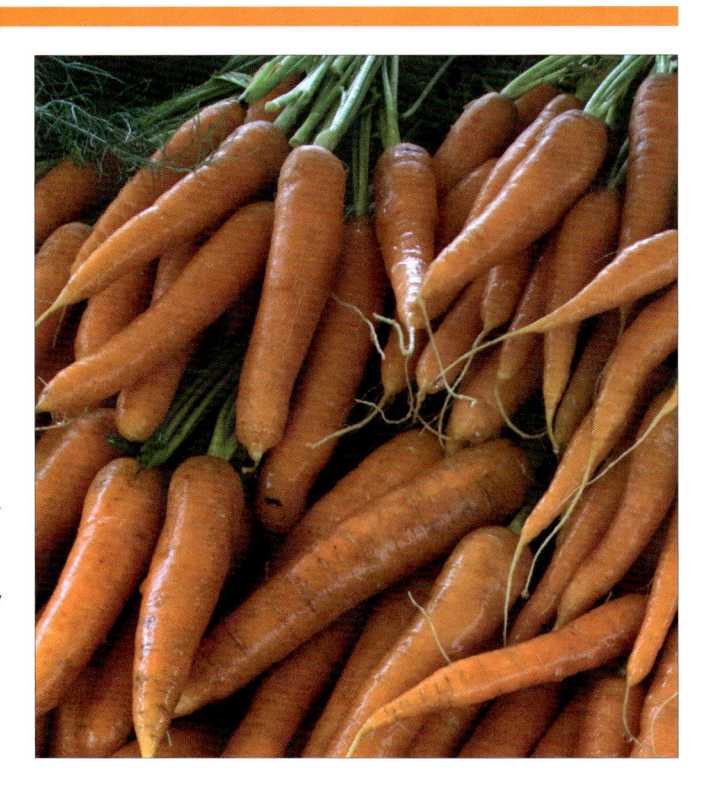

Fruits

Kids are more likely to eat fruits that are sliced into bite-size portions. Wash and prepare fruit in big batches to grab and go throughout the week. Sprinkle cut fruits like apples, pears, and avocados with lemon or pineapple juice to prevent them from becoming brown. Combine cut fruit with cottage cheese, yogurt, nuts.

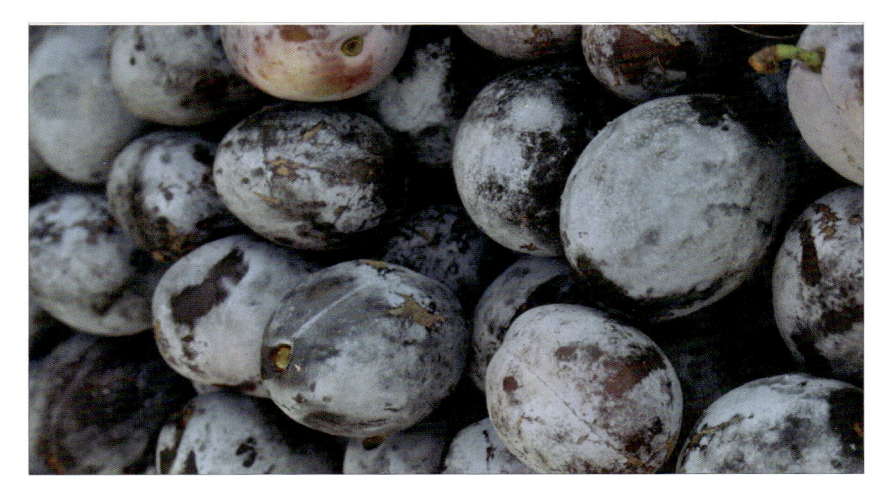

No-Prep

- Apples
- Bananas
- Apricots, peaches, plums
- Oranges, tangerines or mandarin oranges
- Raisins, dried cranberries
- Other dried fruit such as pineapple, mango, figs, dates, apples, apricots, pears
- Blueberries, strawberries, blackberries, raspberries
- Banana chips
- Grapes
- Pears
- Figs
- Kumquats
- Applesauce (see page 136)
- Cherry tomatoes

Low-Prep

- Apple, sliced
- Pear, sliced
- Avocado, sliced or half, packed with spoon
- Orange, sliced into wedges, with rind
- Kiwi, peeled and sliced or half
- Mango, scooped out of rind and sliced
- Melon, cut into chunks or quartered with rind
- Nectarine and peach, sliced
- Papaya, sliced
- Pineapple, canned chunks or fresh, sliced
- Fruit skewered on kebab sticks

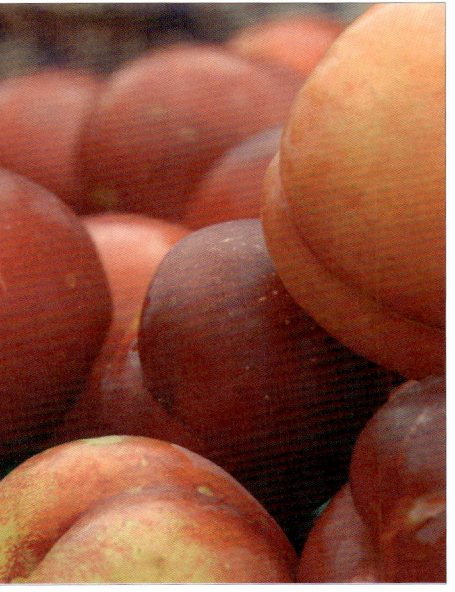

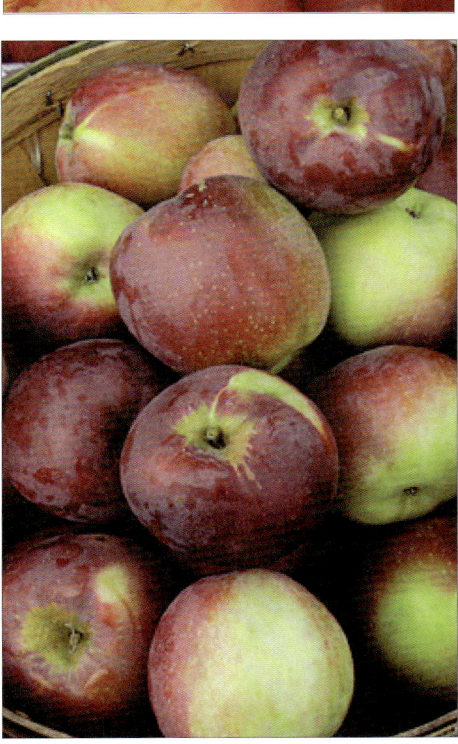

Fruit Recipes 131

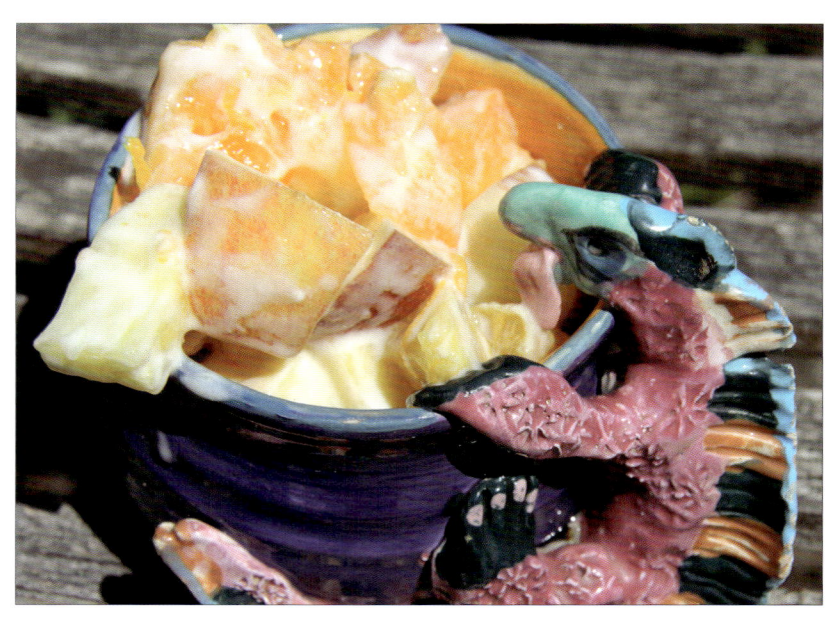

Fruit Salad with Honey & Yogurt

6-8 servings

This salad is perfect for fall or winter.

- 1-2 apples, cored and chopped
- 2 oranges, peeled and sectioned
- 2 kiwis, peeled and chopped
- 2 pears, chopped
- 1 tablespoon warmed honey
- 1 cup plain yogurt
- ¼ cup slivered almonds, toasted

1. Wash and chop the fruit. Combine fruit in a large bowl.
2. Warm honey to thin liquid consistency. (On a stove top, place glass container of honey in a small pot containing 2 inches of water. Simmer until honey thins. In a microwave, heat in a glass container until honey thins. Microwaves vary in time and power, but start with 5 seconds.)
3. Combine yogurt and honey in a small bowl. Stir into the fruit mixture; toss gently to combine.
4. Sprinkle with almonds.

Seasonality

Buying seasonally keeps salads interesting, new, flavorful—and lower cost.

A summer green or vegetable salad is a whole different creature from a winter one. During the summer, tomatoes, cucumbers, peppers, and peas make salads sweet, bright, and colorful. Summer fruit salads include peaches, strawberries and melons.

Winter green salads are nutritious and hardy. They can include leafy greens such as spinach, kale and mustard greens, as well as root vegetables such as carrots and beets. Mix in a variety of citrus fruit. The key is to be creative.

See Chapter 3, page 29, for more about In-Season Food.

Options:
- Substitute maple syrup for honey.
- Add tropical fruits like banana, pineapple, mango or flaked coconut.

Fruit Smoothie

Yield: 2 cups

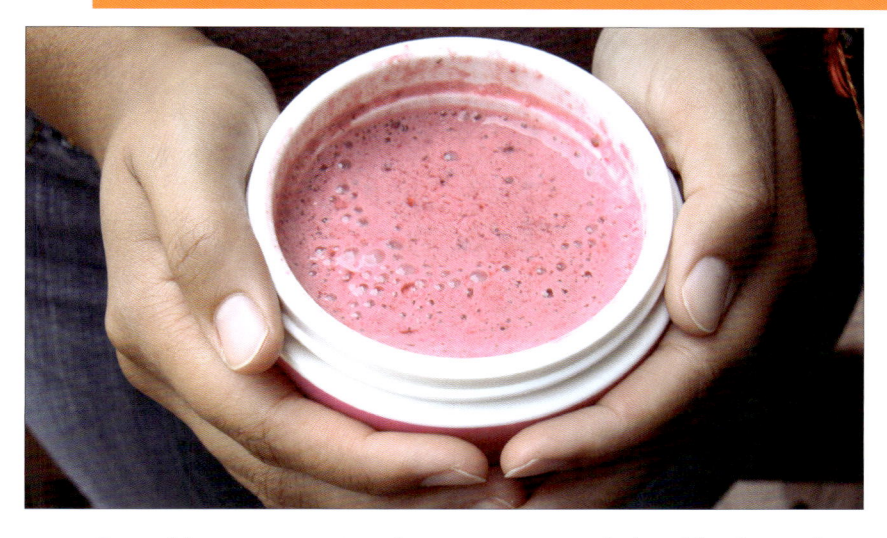

Cost Comparison: Plain Yogurt

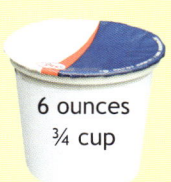

6 ounces
¾ cup

21.5¢ per ounce
$1.73 per cup

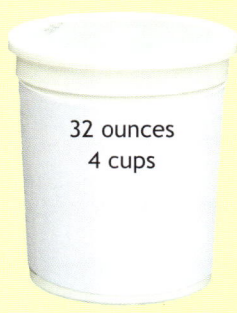

32 ounces
4 cups

8.5¢ per ounce
67¢ per cup

Prices vary. Estimate based on nationwide chain grocery store generic brands, 2012.

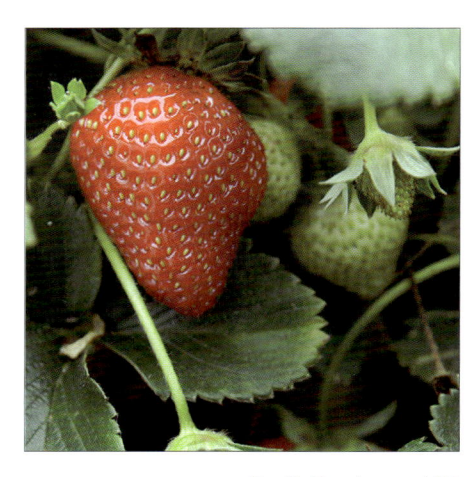

Smoothies are a sweet and creamy treat made in a blender and are full of fruit, calcium, vitamins and minerals. Experiment with different combinations of fruit.

- ½ cup favorite fruit, fresh or frozen (peaches, bananas, blueberries, blackberries, raspberries, strawberries, mangos)
- 1 cup plain yogurt
- 1 cup milk or other liquids (See Options, below)
- 4-5 ice cubes

1. If using fresh fruit, peel, chop into small pieces and place in blender. If using frozen fruit, pour it straight into the blender.
2. Put yogurt and milk into blender with fruit. Puree until smooth. Test to see if it is sweet and creamy enough (see Options, below).
3. To keep smoothies cold until lunch, pour into insulated thermos.

Options:

- Substititue calcium-added orange juice, 100% fruit juices, soy milk, nut milk or coconut water for milk.
- Test first, then add 1 tablespoon honey or sugar if desired.
- Add a banana or more yogurt to make smoothie creamier.
- Add peanut butter for more protein (goes best with banana).

Fruit Recipes

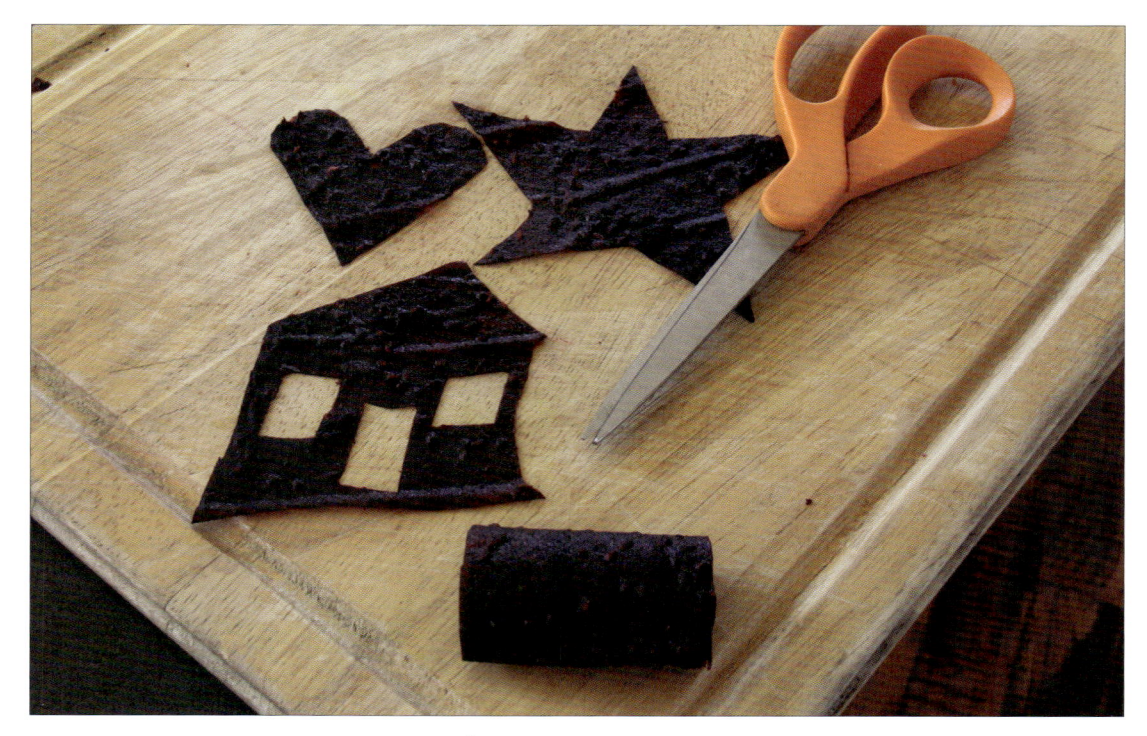

Fruit Leather

8 servings

Capture the flavors of summer in easy-to-make fruit leather. When fruit is abundant and inexpensive, make a large batch to carry you through the winter. Depending upon how sweet the fruit is, you may not need to add extra sugar or honey.

- 4 cups fresh fruit (any combination you like)
- ¼ cup water
- 1-3 tablespoons honey or sugar (optional)
- 1-3 teaspoons lemon juice

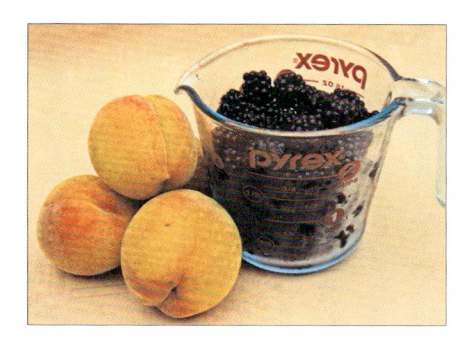

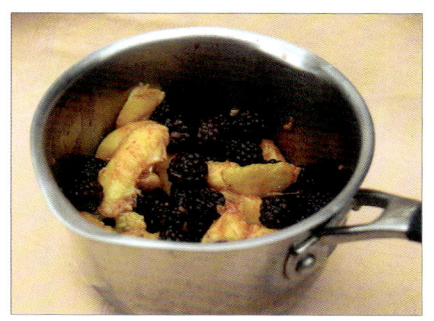

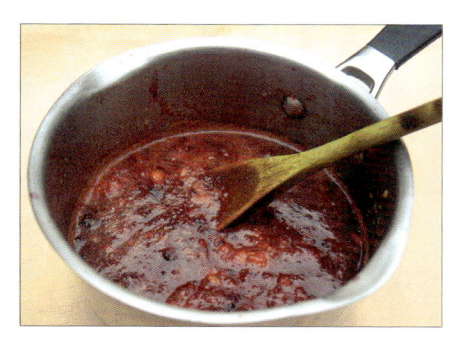

1. Wash the fruit. For stone fruit (apricots, peaches, plums), remove the pits. For apples and pears, remove cores and stems. De-stem grapes. For berries with tougher seeds, such as blackberries, cook separately and strain out the seeds.

2. Place fruit in a large saucepan and add water. Bring to a simmer, cover, and let cook over low heat 10-15 minutes, or until fruit is cooked through. Uncover and stir.

3. Taste the fruit. If sugar is needed, add a tablespoon at a time, to taste. Add lemon juice, 1 teaspoon at a time, to make the leather a little tangy.

4. Continue to simmer and stir until any added sugar is completely dissolved and the fruit mixture has thickened—10 or more minutes.

5. Cool the mixture and puree in a blender until very smooth, or use a potato masher and mash as much as you can—the leather will end up a little lumpier, but it will still taste great.

6. Dehydrate the puree, using one of the methods described in "How to Dehydrate." Pour puree into a rimmed baking sheet or tray that will fit into your dehydrator. Spread evenly to about ⅛- to ¼-inch thick. Tipping the baking sheet will allow the puree to spread.

7. Bake at 120°-150° (135°-145° is ideal) for 5-8 hours. The fruit leather is ready when it's no longer sticky, and has a smooth surface. Start checking after 4 hours, as it's very easy for it to get too dry and burn.

8. Cut the leather into 8 equal pieces and peel them from the baking sheet. Place each portion on a piece of plastic wrap and roll up tightly.

9. Store in an airtight container in the refrigerator or freezer.

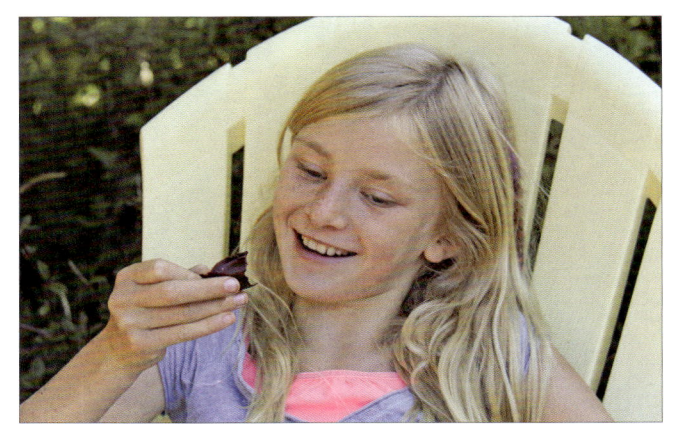

Option:

- After Step 5, add spices, such as cinnamon, nutmeg or ginger.

How to Dehydrate:

- Dry in the sun: On a hot day you can put the fruit on the tray, make a tent from cheesecloth to keep the bugs off, and leave the tray in the sun all day.

- Make the solar dehydrator described in Chapter 6 (page 174) and use it to dry the leather. Temperatures in the dryer will probably reach from 125°-150° and leather may be ready in about 6-8 hours.

- Dry in a food dehydrator: If you have control of the temperature, dehydrate at 135°-145°. Drying time will vary, but 5-8 hours is a good estimate. Trays for some dehydrators may not need oiling. Check the owner's manual.

- Dry in an oven: Set temperature to 125°-150° (135°-145° is ideal). Drying time will vary, but 5-8 hours is a good estimate. **Warning:** Above these temperatures, it's very easy to burn the leather.

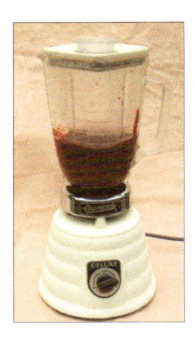

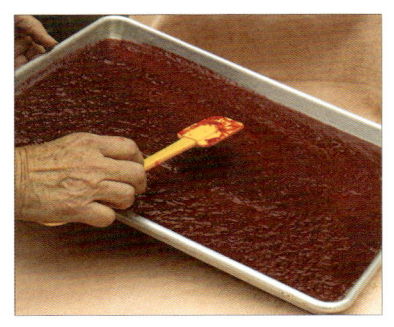

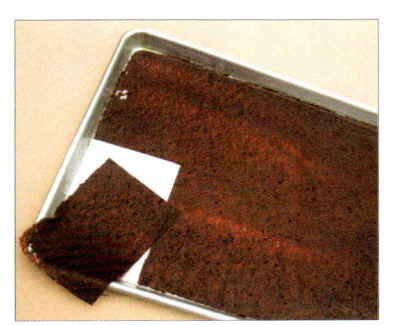

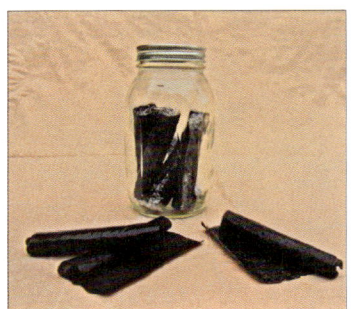

Fruit Recipes 135

Applesauce

Yield: 1 quart

Applesauce is delightful all by itself or with the addition of a bit of cinnamon or nutmeg. Try it warmed for breakfast or for a simple dessert. All apples can be made into applesauce, but the following varieties work best: Pippin, Rhode Island Greening, McIntosh, Elstar, Cortland, Fuji, Gala, Gravenstein. Apples that are no longer crisp work well for applesauce.

    6   medium apples
¼-½   cup water

1. Wash, peel, quarter and core the apples.
2. Put water and apples in a 4- to 6-quart saucepan and bring to a boil over medium heat—you'll hear the water sizzling in the bottom of the pan. Immediately lower the heat to a simmer and partially cover the pan.
3. Cook until apples are very tender, 15-25 minutes. Stir often to prevent burning.
4. Remove pan from heat. Add sugar or spices, to your liking. Cool to room temperature.
5. Place applesauce in a tightly lidded container and refrigerate. It will keep for up to two weeks. It can also be frozen in serving-size containers.

Canning

When apples are in season, they are plentiful and cheap. You can preserve them for the coming months by freezing or canning large batches of applesauce.

To get started canning, visit the National Center for Home Food Preservation, USDA publications, online at *http://nchfp.uga.edu/publications/publications_usda.html*

Two excellent books for canning recipes are the *Ball Blue Book* and *So Easy to Preserve*. The latter book is available from the Cooperative Extension at The University of Georgia.

Options:
- At Step 4, add nutmeg and/or cinnamon to taste.
- At Step 4, add brown or white sugar, or honey, to taste.
- For smoother applesauce, put it through a blender or food processor after cooling.
- Cook with half an unpeeled lemon. Remove lemon before serving or storing.

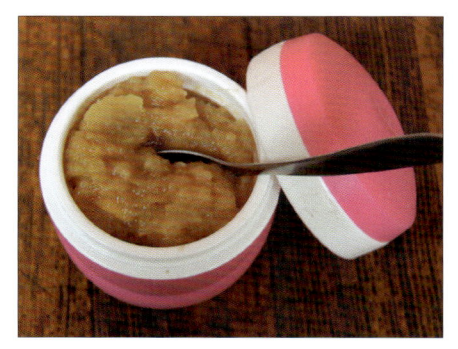

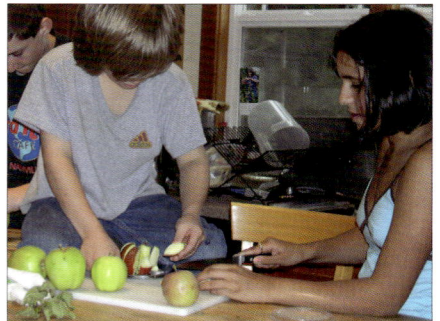

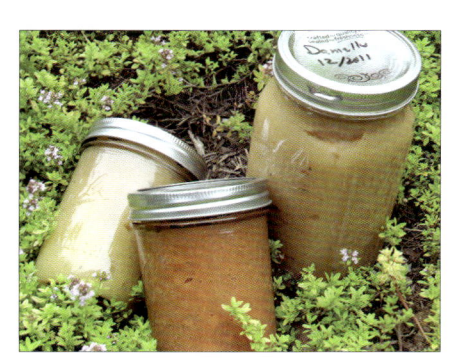

Dehydrating Fruit

Drying food (dehydrating) is an ancient method of preservation. It concentrates fruit sugars, making the fruit very sweet and a great replacement for processed sugary snacks. Dehydration is one method to save money. Buy fruit in season when it is less expensive and dry it for enjoyment all year.

Use an oven with a low setting (125°-150°; 135°-145° is ideal) or a dehydrator. Make your own solar dehydrator (see page 174). Use a cookie sheet for drying in the oven. Use a cooling rack in the solar dehydrator or the dehydration trays that come with the dehydrator. (See page 135, "How to Dehydrate".)

Drying time varies with temperature and thickness of the fruit. The range is generally 4-12 hours. Start checking after 4 hours.

Fruit is completely dehydrated when no moisture comes out when it's squeezed, or when no condensation forms if it's sealed in a bag or jar while still warm.

Store fruit in air-tight bags or jars. Keep in a cool, dry place, away from direct light. Dried fruit can last up to a year because mold and bacteria can't grow without moisture.

Easy-to-dehydrate fruit choices:
- apples
- pears
- peaches
- plums
- strawberries

To remove peach skin before dehydrating, cut a small "X" in the skin at the bottom. Place peaches in boiling water for 30 seconds, then into ice cold water. Remove the skin using your fingers.

Dehydrating Peaches and Plums

1. Wash and cut peaches or plums in half. Remove pit and slice halves into ¼-inch-thick slices.

2. To prevent browning, dip fruit in a solution of ¼ cup lemon, lime or pineapple juice and 1 cup water, or use ascorbic acid (follow directions on package).

3. Dry fruit in an oven or dehydrator.

Dehydrating Strawberries

1. Wash and cut leafy crown from strawberries.

2. Slice ¼ inch thick. Place the berries in a single layer on a baking sheet or the dehydrator tray.

3. Dry fruit in an oven or dehydrator.

Dehydrating Apples and Pears

Firm, crisp apples work best and any variety of semi-ripe pear is suitable.

1. Wash and slice the fruit into ¼- to ½-inch-thick slices.

2. To prevent browning, dip fruit in a solution of ¼ cup lemon, lime or pineapple juice and 1 cup water, or use ascorbic acid (follow directions on package). Place fruit in a single layer on a baking sheet or the dehydrator tray.

3. Dry fruit in an oven or dehydrator.

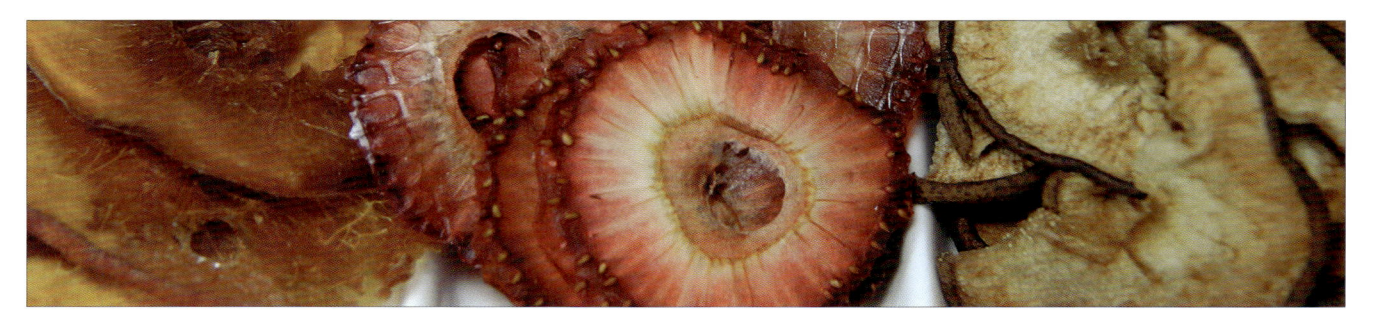

Carving Fruits & Vegetables

Enjoy the fun of vegetable carving all through the year. Carving is a fun after-school or birthday party activity. Kids love to use their creations as centerpieces.

Vegetable carving began in the Far East, most particularly in Japan and Thailand. Carving fruits and vegetables is about the concept that the more beautiful food looks, the more delicious it is to eat. Students in both countries are taught food carving from an early age.

Create imaginative shapes, silly critters or fantasy creations with a few fruits, vegetables and cutting tools. Kids can carve fruits and vegetables safely when they follow some basic knife rules and tips. Use a sharp paring knife rather than a dinner knife; it requires less pressure and is safer to use.

Included are some suggested vegetables and fruits to choose for carving. Remember, the sky's the limit, so be creative and use any vegetable or fruit to turn into an edible masterpiece.

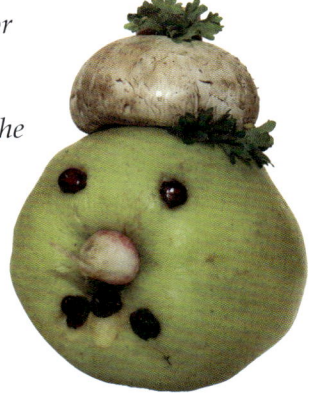

Tools
- paring knife
- vegetable peeler
- toothpicks or skewers
- metal cookie cutters
- forks

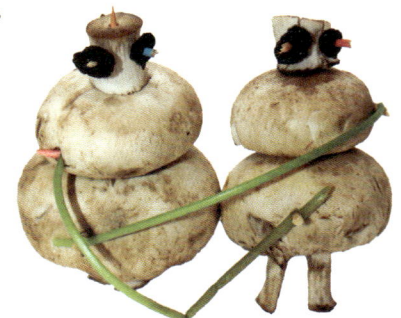

Carving Ideas

broccoli	trees
cauliflower	clouds, huge flowers
potatoes	strong base
bell peppers	a bowl, boat, or funny face
cucumbers	boat or car (sliced in half, seeds scooped out)
cabbage	strong base when halved
pineapple	boats, wings, sun or moon
melons	heads or bowls (sliced in half, seeds scooped out)
olives and raisins	eyes, noses, ears, car wheels, buttons
strawberries	flower centers, wings or hearts (when cut in half)
blueberries	heads, eyes

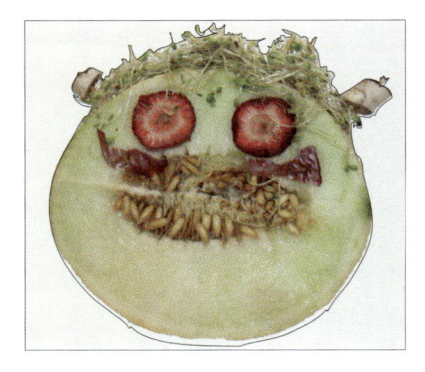

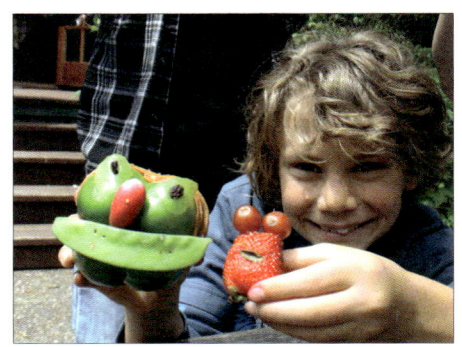

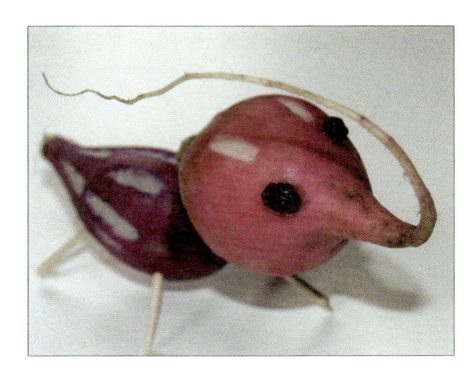

138 Food Carving Fruits and Vegetables

General Food Carving

1. Read Knife Safety (see page 43). Show younger children how to hold a knife and cut away from their bodies. Adults should supervise carving.

2. Spread newspaper or a tablecloth under all the tools and food. This will make clean up much easier.

3. For creations that might tip over, cut off one rounded end of the fruit or vegetable. This flat base will keep a round item steady on the table.

4. Add smaller pieces to the base, connecting them with toothpicks and skewers.

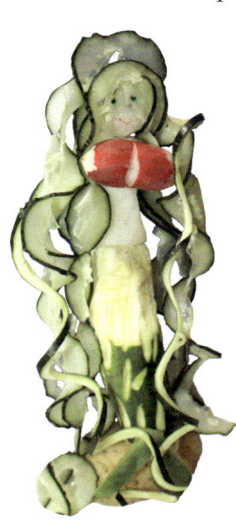

5. Use a peeler to expose different colored layers of fruit or vegetable, as seen in the radish flower photos at the bottom of the page.

6. For cucumbers, peel alternate stripes; run the tines of a fork down the sides of the cucumber just where the skin has been peeled away. Slice into rounds. Try a cucumber, sliced in half lengthwise; scoop out the seeds and use the shells to hold other, smaller, diced or chopped vegetables.

Radish Flower Bouquet

For Flowers:

1. Use a vegetable peeler to peel away some of the skin, revealing the white part of the radish. Be careful to leave the peeled part still attached to the radish—this takes some practice! Repeat around the whole radish to create a flower.

2. Put your finished radishes into a bowl of water from 1 hour to overnight and the little flaps you've cut will open up.

For Green Onion Stems:

3. Cut off the white end. Cut sections the same length as a toothpick.

4. Lay a section flat on the table and make an ⅛-inch-long slit from one end. Turn and repeat.

5. Put a toothpick inside the onion tube. The end you cut the incisions in will be at the top of the toothpick. Now stick a radish on top of the green onion and the onion piece will be the stem of the flower.

6. Stick the other end of the toothpick into the larger vegetable that you're using for a base.

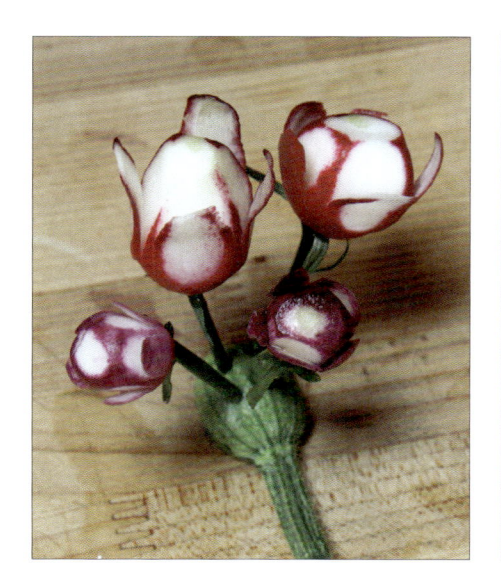

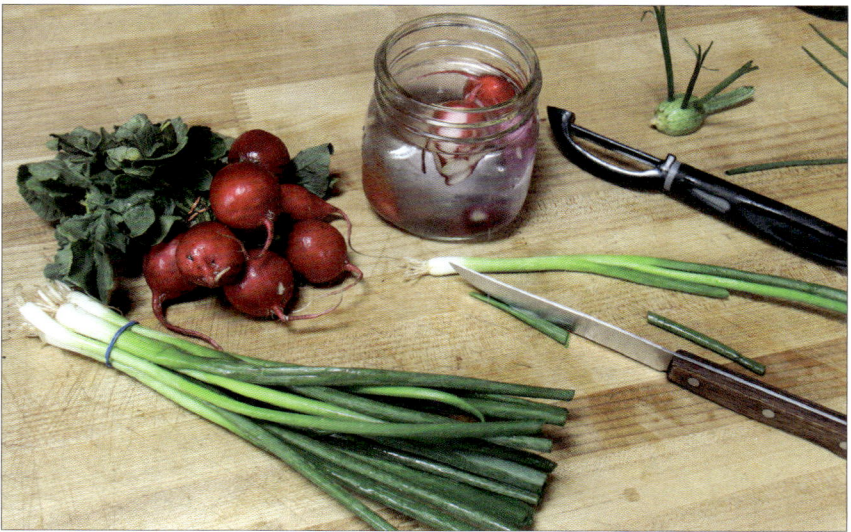

Drinks

Drinks are an easy part of the lunch and one that can make a big difference in the health of a child. Sugary drinks are the single biggest source of additonal sugar. These extra calories lead to weight gain, which can increase the risk of health problems such as type 2 diabetes and heart disease.

No-Prep
- Water
- Milk
- Soy, rice, almond milk
- 100% fruit juice (best diluted 1:1 with water)

Low-Prep
- Unsweetened iced tea
- Water with a squeeze of juice
- Flavored waters (see below)

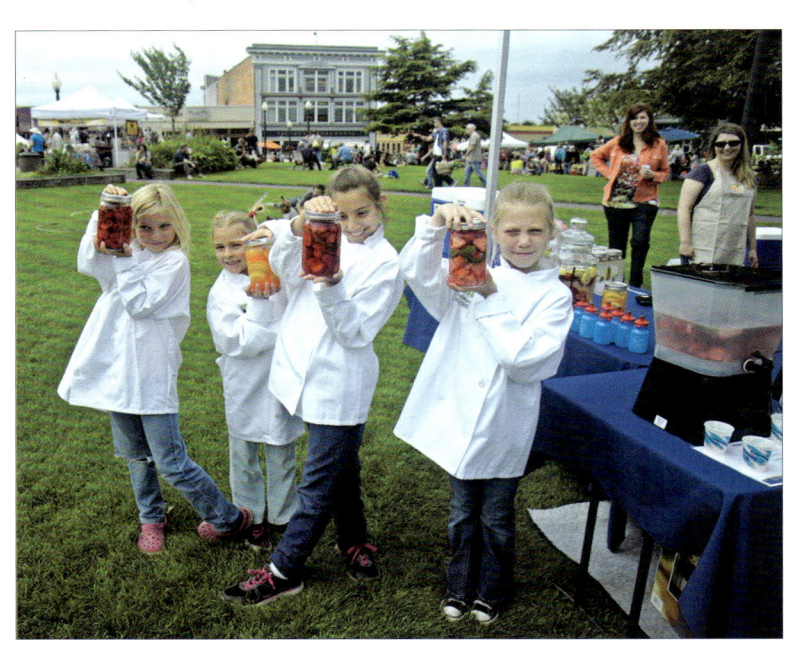

Kid-Created Flavored Waters

Try these delicious flavored water combinations created by the Culinary Allstar kids in Humboldt County, California:

- **Anthony's Tasty H_2O**: orange, carrot, lemon
- **Berry Minty**: strawberries, raspberries, lime, mint
- **Red Dream Drink**: watermelon, strawberries, basil

Flavored Water

Water can be flavored with sweet fruits and vegetables and delicious herbs—no extra sugar needed! Use fruits such as raspberries, strawberries, watermelon, cantaloupe, peaches, oranges, lemons, or limes. Use vegetables such as carrots or cucumbers. Use herbs such as basil or mint.

1. Slice, thickly chop, or grate larger ingredients. Use whole herb leaves.
2. Fill a 1-quart glass jar or bowl with 2 cups of ingredients.
3. Pour very hot water over ingredients until jar is filled, or pour two cups of very hot water over ingredients in the bowl. Place a lid on the jar or cover the bowl with a plate.
4. Cool to room temperature. Add cold water until you have ½ gallon (about 4 more cups of water.) Chill for at least two hours.
5. Pour flavored water through strainer or colander to remove fruit or vegetables.
6. Use an insulated thermos to take drink to school.

Treats and Snacks

Treats and snacks are lunch items to be eaten occasionally. High-protein snacks can be combined with fruits and vegetables to create a balanced lunch that has all the MyPlate components. Other grain-based snacks can provide a boost of energy for active kids.

Eat sparingly and enjoy to the fullest.

No-Prep
- Walnuts
- Almonds
- Cashews
- Peanuts
- Pistachios
- Pretzels
- Pumpkin seeds (pepitas)
- Sunflower seeds
- Soy nuts
- Raisins
- Dried fruit

Low-Prep
- Sliced fruit
- Sliced vegetables
- Sliced cheese

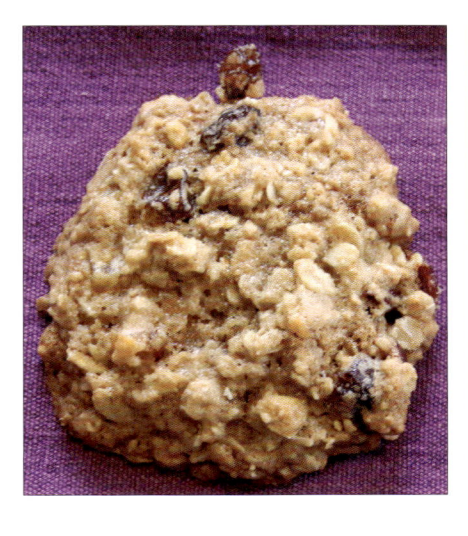

Bulk Snack Bins

Bulk bins are generally the cheapest way to buy some foods (see page 16). Many stores have bins specifically for snacks. If you make your own snack mix, you know exactly what is going into it.

Check out the bin labels for ingredients of items that are not whole foods (see Food Labels, page 190). As you choose, be aware of the extra sodium or salt that is added to your diet through snack items.

Make your own trail mixes. Aim for less of the sweet or sugar-coated items and more whole items such as dried fruits or nuts.

Choose a variety of nuts, seeds such as sunflower or pumpkin, and dried fruit.

Remember not to snack from the bulk bins. Please always use the tongs or spoons provided, for health and safety reasons.

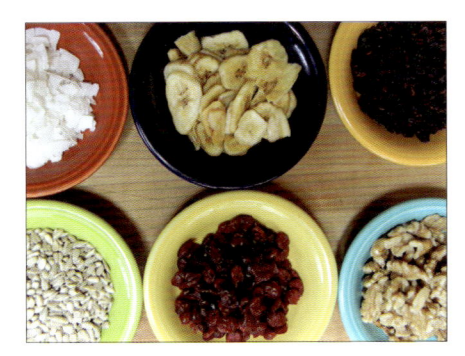

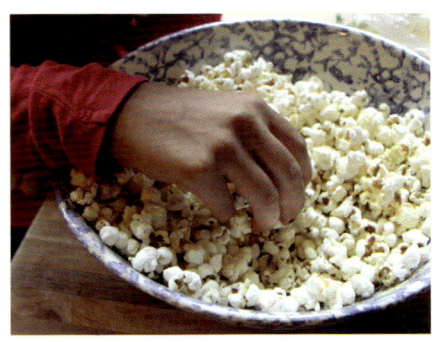

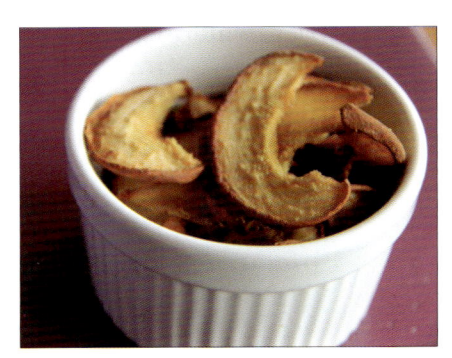

Treat and Snack Recipes

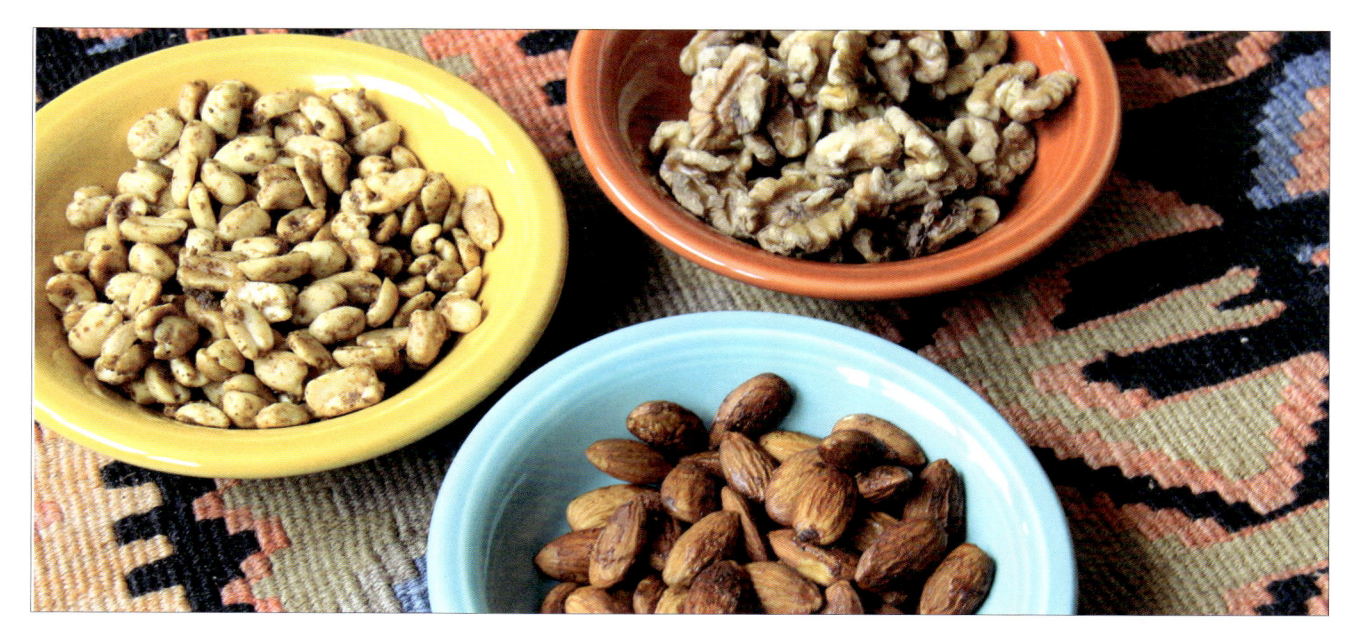

Go Nuts!

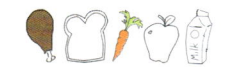

Yield: 2 cups of nuts

Nuts, an easy-to-prepare snack, are high in unsaturated fat (that's a good kind of fat). They are high in protein; and they lack cholesterol. Toasting intensifies the flavor and makes them crispy. You can add a variety of flavorings to plain nuts. Always cool nuts completely before storing in an airtight container so they will stay crisp. Nuts store best in the refrigerator for up to 3 months, or longer in the freezer.

Fast Roasted Nuts

Check these nuts frequently—it's very easy to burn them at this temperature.

almonds, peanuts, walnuts, hazlenuts, pine nuts, cashews

Preheat oven to 325°

1. Place nuts on a rimmed baking sheet.
2. Roast 10-15 minutes. Stir every 5 minutes.
3. Remove, cool and store in airtight containers.

Crunchy Walnuts or Pecans

Soaking before roasting makes these nuts easier to digest and releases some of their nutrients.

2 cups walnut or pecan halves
1 teaspoon salt
2 cups water

1. Mix salt and water together and add the nuts. Let sit 3-4 hours.
2. Drain.

Preheat oven to lowest setting (200° maximum)

3. Spread nuts on a rimmed baking sheet.
4. Roast 6-8 hours. Stir occasionally.
5. Remove, cool and store in airtight container.

142 Treat and Snack Recipes

Tamari Almonds

Tamari is a type of soy sauce with a different flavor. Gluten-free tamari is also available.

- 2 cups whole almonds
- ¼ cup soy sauce or tamari

Preheat oven to 250°

1. Place almonds and tamari in bowl and mix until almonds are well coated.
2. Spread almonds on a rimmed baking sheet.
3. Roast almonds about 45 minutes. Stir a few times during roasting.
4. Remove, cool and store in airtight container.

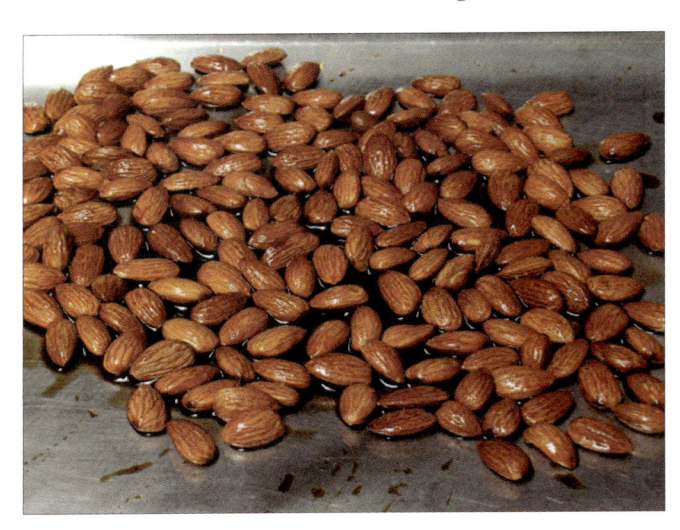

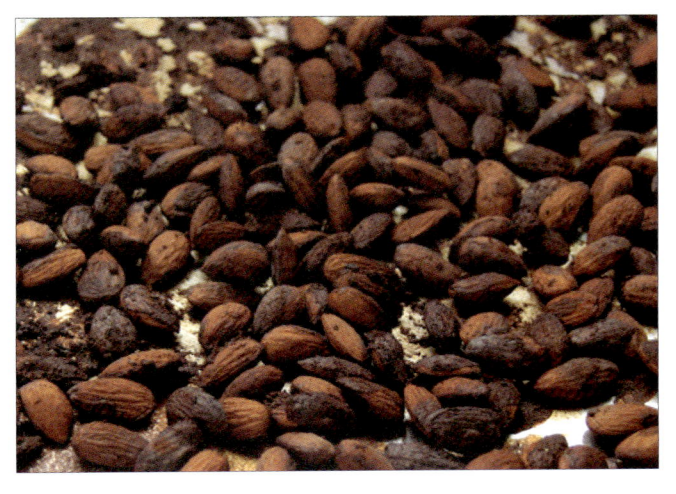

BBQ Peanuts or Pecans

You'll be licking your fingers as you make this. Sprinkle some on top of rice or in salads for a tasty, crunchy extra.

- 3 tablespoons melted butter
- 2 tablespoons Worcestershire sauce
- 1 tablespoon ketchup
- ¼ teaspoon hot pepper sauce
- ½ teaspoon chile powder
- ½ teaspoon salt
- 2 cups raw peanuts or pecan halves

Preheat oven to 200°

1. Lightly oil a rimmed baking sheet.
2. In a medium-sized bowl, combine everything and mix well. Place on the baking sheet in a single layer.
3. Bake 45 minutes or until browned. Stir every 10 minutes.
4. Remove nuts from oven and spread on a brown paper bag or a paper towel to absorb extra oil.
5. Cool and store in airtight container.

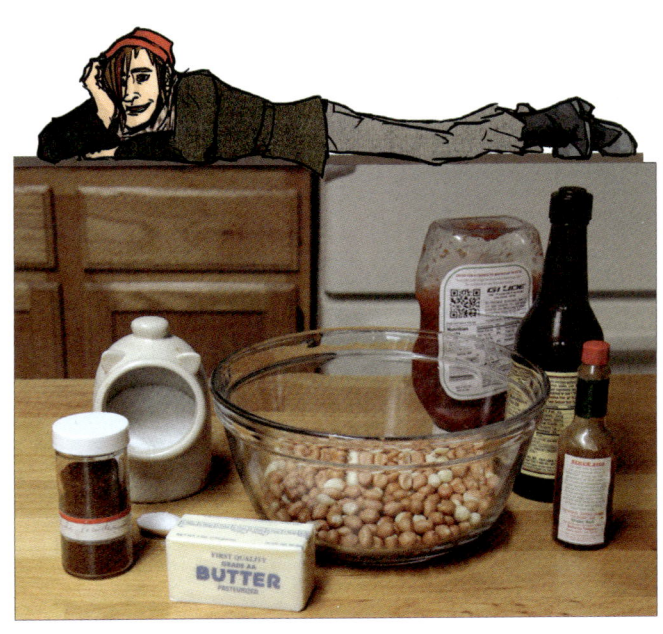

Popcorn

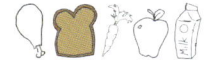

Yield: 10 cups

Popcorn is simple to make. It's also a nutritious whole grain. The grains are called kernels. They're available in bulk food bins. This recipe makes twice as much as purchased microwavable popcorn bags and is much cheaper. Store popped corn in an airtight container up to 2 days for an easy-to-grab snack.

- ½ cup popcorn kernels
- 1 teaspoon vegetable oil
- ½ teaspoon salt, or to taste

In a Microwave:

1. Mix the kernels and oil in a bowl. Place in a brown paper bag and sprinkle with salt. Fold the top of the bag over twice.

2. Cook in the microwave at full power 2½ to 3 minutes, or until you hear a 2-second pause between pops. Open the bag carefully to avoid steam burns. Pour popped corn into a container and seal securely to keep fresh.

On the Stove top:

1. Mix oil and kernels in a 5-quart lidded saucepan.

2. Cover pan and heat on high until popping begins. Using a potholder in each hand, hold the lid securely closed, then pick up the pot and shake it. Replace on heat and repeat every 10-20 seconds until you hear a 2-second pause between pops. Remove from heat.

3. Leave lid on until all popping stops (around 30 seconds), and tilt lid away from you to open.

Options:

- Stir in extra toppings, like melted butter, garlic salt, Parmesan cheese, and/or 1 tablespoon nutritional yeast (available at natural food stores).

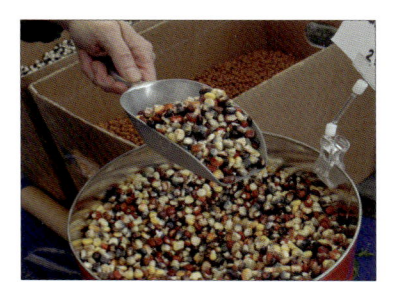

Home-popped vs. Purchased Microwave Popcorn Bags

Be aware: Studies show that the plastic that lines the inside of purchased microwave popcorn bags, as well as some artificial butter flavorings, release cancer-causing chemicals when heated.

When you pop popcorn on the stove or in your own bag in the microwave, you avoid unnecessary danger, save money, and get to choose the toppings. Find kernels in the popcorn aisle or bulk foods section of a grocery store.

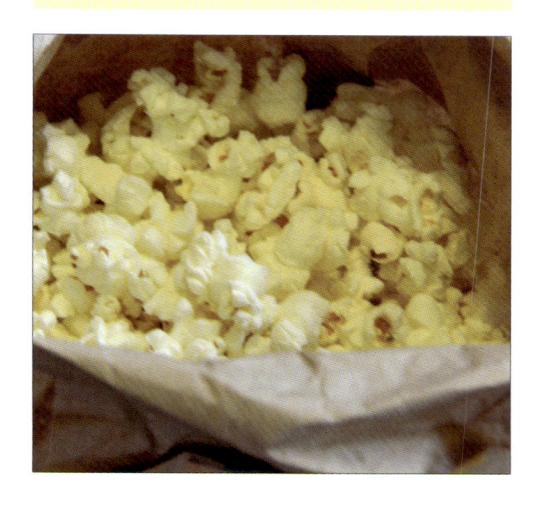

Tofu Sticks

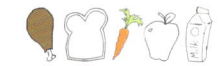

Yield: 32 Sticks

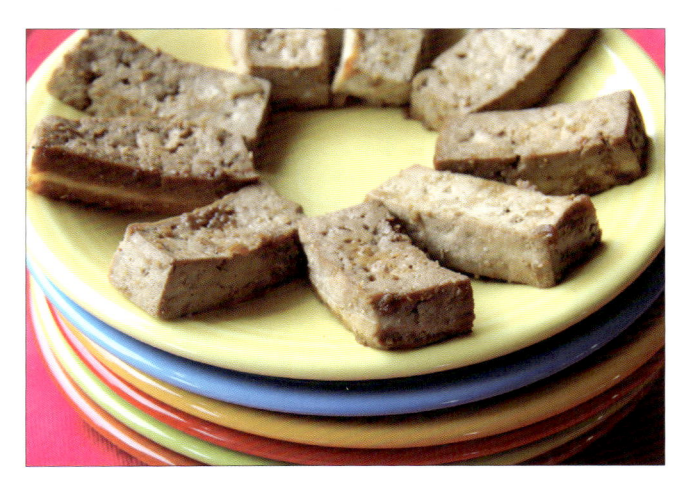

Kids adore these snacks. This recipe transforms tofu into something enticingly delicious.

1½ tablespoons dry mustard powder
1½ tablespoons finely grated onion
1½ cups water
½ cup honey
½ tablespoon finely chopped garlic
1 cup soy sauce or tamari sauce
2 blocks extra-firm tofu (about 2 pounds)

1. Grate onion and garlic.
2. Mix all ingredients except tofu in a medium-sized bowl. This is the marinade. Set aside.
3. Drain the tofu and cut into 1 x 4-inch strips.
4. Oil a sheet pan and pour in enough of the marinade to just cover the pan.
5. Lay the tofu sticks next to each other over the marinade, with the sides of the tofu not touching.
6. Pour the remaining marinade over the entire pan of tofu sticks, cover, and let sit in the refrigerator for at least 1 hour or overnight.

Preheat oven to 300°

7. Bake in preheated oven 45 minutes. Turn the sticks over and bake another 15 minutes, until all the liquid is absorbed and the sticks are browned. Remove from oven and allow to cool.
8. Store in the refrigerator in a lidded container.

Tofu is an excellent source of protein. It is also high in iron and calcium or magnesium. Your body uses it the same way it uses animal protein, but tofu is lower in fat. It can be used in hundreds of different recipes because it absorbs the flavors in which it is cooked.

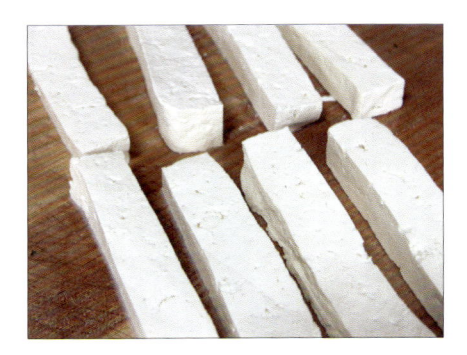

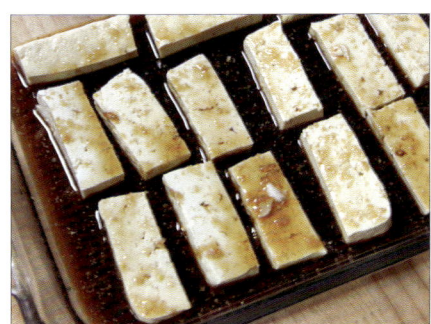

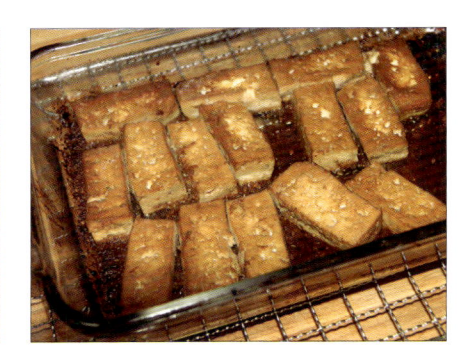

Treat and Snack Recipes

Kale Chips

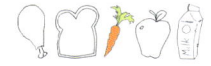

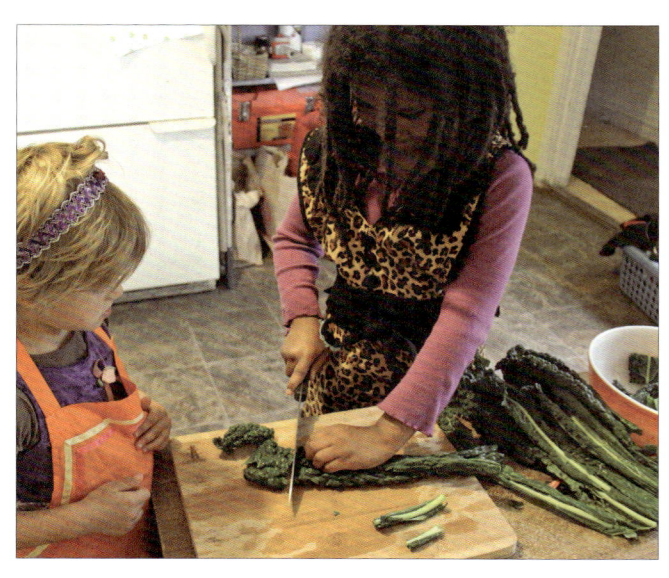

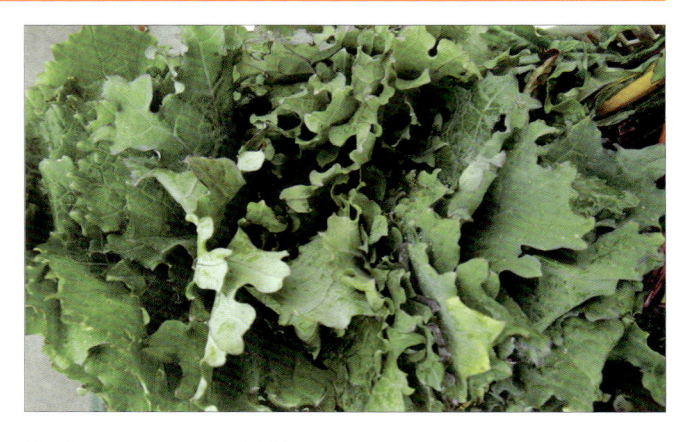

Yield: 8-10 cups

Kale chips are the best-ever vegetable snack. Your friends will be crowding around to have a taste. Believe us—we've seen it happen.

- 2 bunches of kale, washed, dried, and stems removed (See Fake Grass Salad, page 128, for photo of removing stems.)
- 1 lemon, juiced
- 1 tablespoon salt
- 1-2 tablespoons olive oil

Preheat oven to 250°

1. Stack the prepared kale leaves. Cut across the whole stack, making 2- to 3-inch-wide strips. Place strips in a large bowl.

2. Mix lemon juice, salt and oil in a small bowl or jar. Add this to the kale and thoroughly but gently mix to coat the kale. Leave the kale in the oil mixture 30 minutes.

3. Place kale on a baking sheet and bake in the oven 20 minutes or until it is totally crisp. Remove from the oven and cool.

Options:

- The kale can also be dehydrated. It comes out a beautiful deep green color. Dehydrate 3 hours or until absolutely dry.
- Substitute tamari sauce for salt.

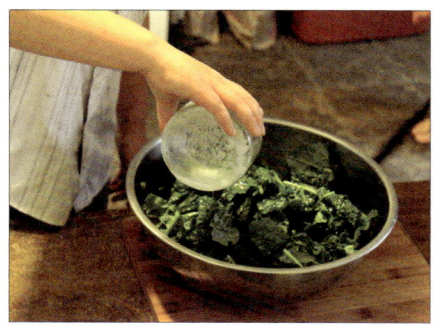

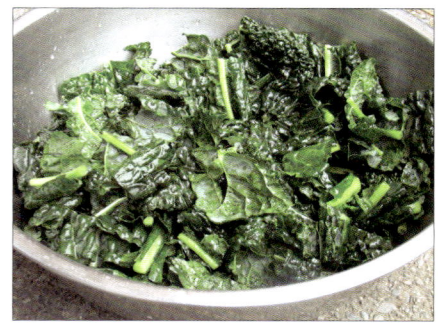

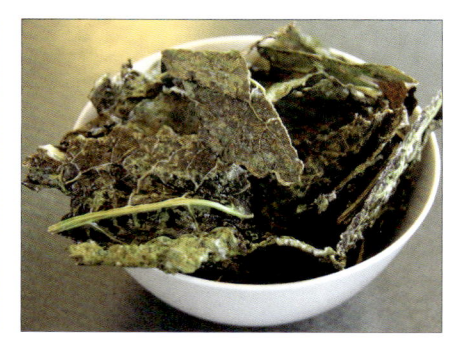

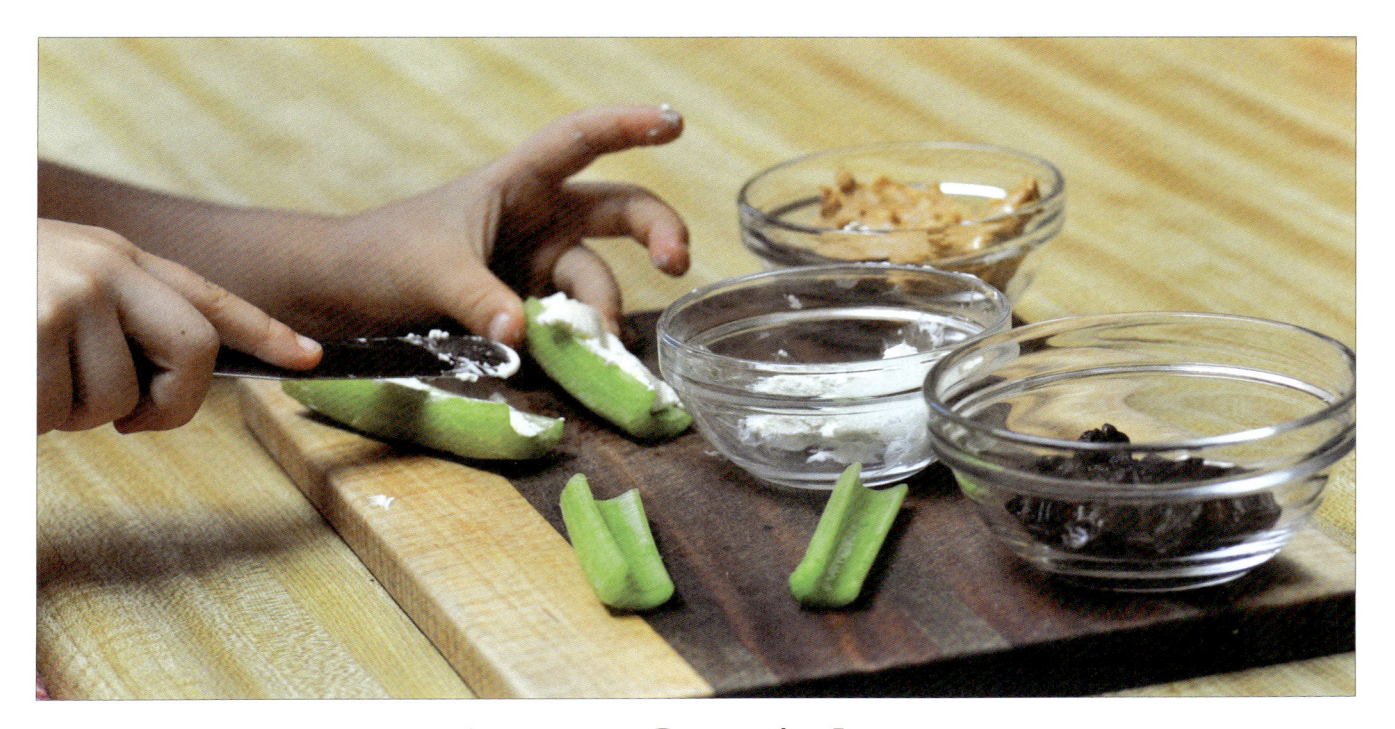

Ants On A Log

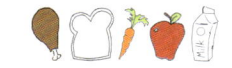

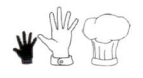

Yield: 15 Logs

Even very young kids can create this delightfully simple snack.

 5   celery stalks
 ½   cup peanut butter
 ¼   cup raisins

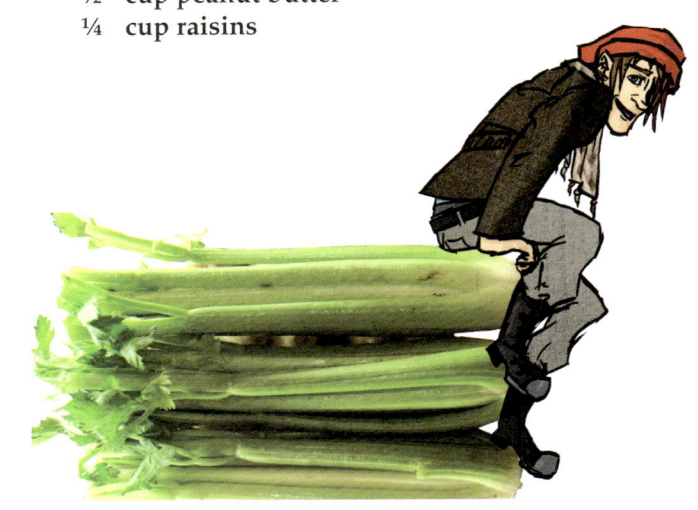

1. Wash the celery stalks, dry and cut into thirds.
2. Spread peanut butter in the U-shaped part of the celery, from one end to the other.
3. Press the raisins ("ants") into peanut butter.

Options:

- Substitute cream cheese, or another type of nut butter (cashew, almond, sunflower seed) for the peanut butter.
- Substitute dried currants, cranberries or blueberries for raisins.
- Ants On An Apple: Use apple slices instead of celery.

Treat and Snack Recipes

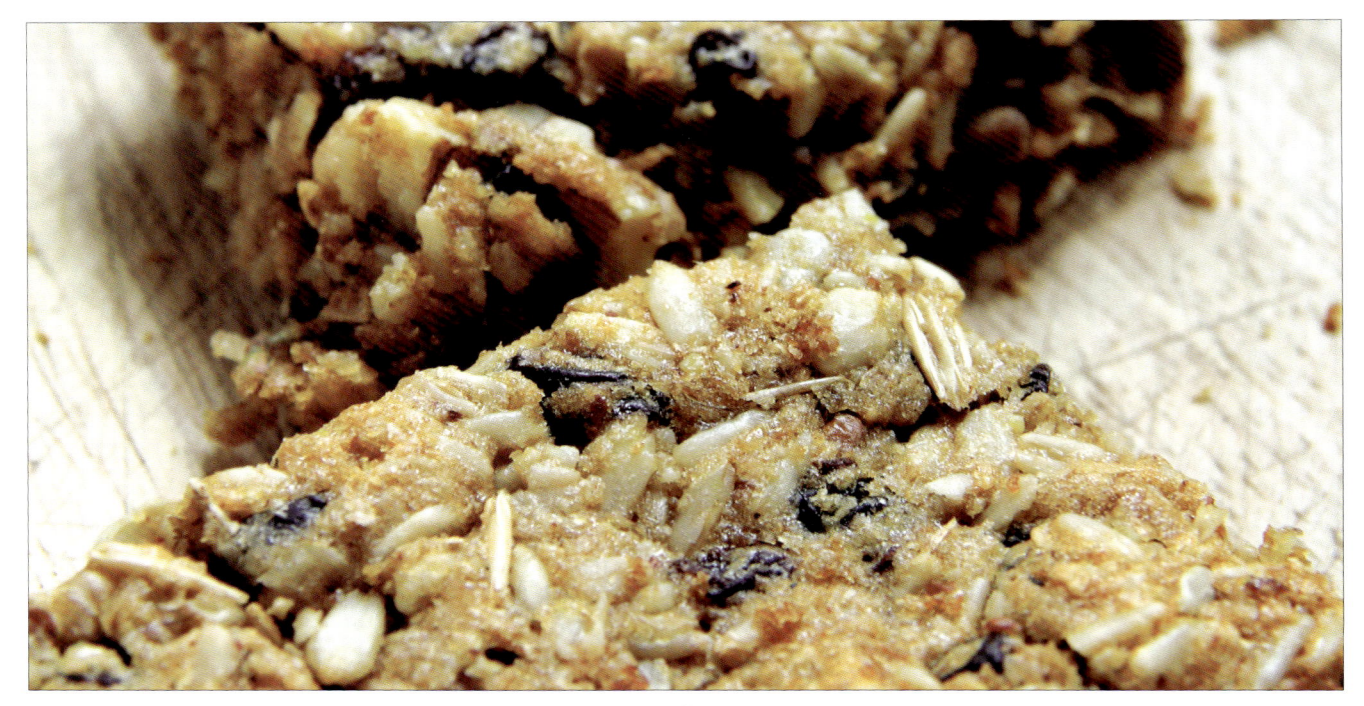

Granola Bars

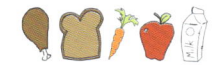

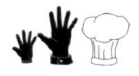

Yield: 20-24 Bars

Young student chefs think these bars are awesome. Delightful any time of day, the bars are especially tasty still warm, just ten minutes out of the oven.

3	cups old-fashioned rolled oats
1½	cup all-purpose flour (gluten-free flour can be substituted)
⅓	cup brown sugar, packed
⅔	cup butter, melted
1	teaspoon baking soda
½	teaspoon salt
1	teaspoon vanilla extract
1	cup raisins or currants
1	cup walnuts, almonds or peanuts, chopped
1	teaspoon ground cinnamon (optional)
½	cup honey, warmed

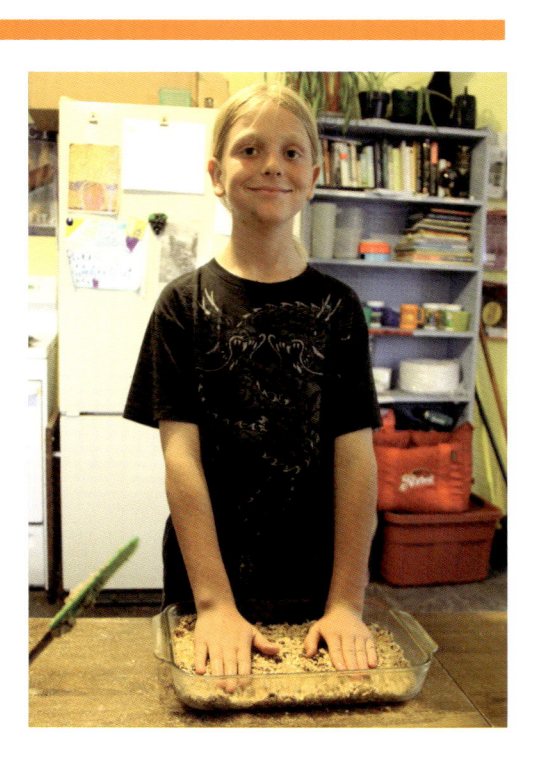

Preheat oven to 325°

1. Grease and flour a 9 x 13-inch baking pan.

2. In a bowl combine the oats, flour, sugar, baking soda, salt, raisins and toasted nuts.

3. Melt the butter and honey together in a small saucepan or in a glass container in the microwave. (Microwaves vary in time and power, but start with 15 seconds.)

4. Add the vanilla to the honey mixture.

5. Pour the honey mixture over the dry ingredients and mix well.

6. Lightly press mixture into the prepared pan. Bake 18 to 22 minutes, or until golden brown.

7. Cool 10 minutes before cutting into bars. Allow bars to cool completely in pan before removing.

Options:

- At Step 4, add 2 tablespoons flaxseed meal that has first been dissolved in 6 tablespoons water. Flaxseed meal is high in omega-3 fatty acids, fiber and phytochemicals. It can be found at natural food stores.
- For a vegan bar, substitute coconut oil for the butter.
- Substitute ½ cup sunflower seeds for ½ cup of the nuts.

Granola Cereal

Homemade granola cereal is a great alternative to processed, high-sugar, purchased cereals.

Yield: 5-6 cups

4½	cups old-fashioned rolled oats
1	cup chopped nuts
1	teaspoon ground cinnamon
⅓	cup brown sugar, packed
2	tablespoons oil
2	tablespoons honey
1	teaspoon vanilla extract
1	cup dried fruit

Preheat oven to 300°

1. Oil a rimmed baking sheet.

2. Combine oats and nuts in a medium bowl.

3. Heat cinnamon, sugar, oil, vanilla and honey in a pan. Add to oats and nuts and stir well.

4. Pour onto baking sheet and spread evenly.

5. Bake 1 hour. Stir every 20 minutes. Remove and cool.

6. Mix in dried fruit when cooled. Stores well up to one month in an airtight container.

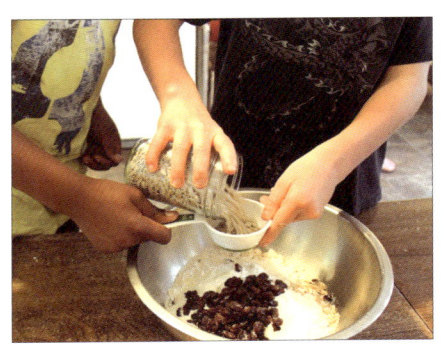

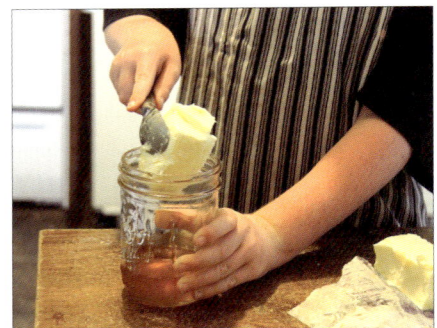

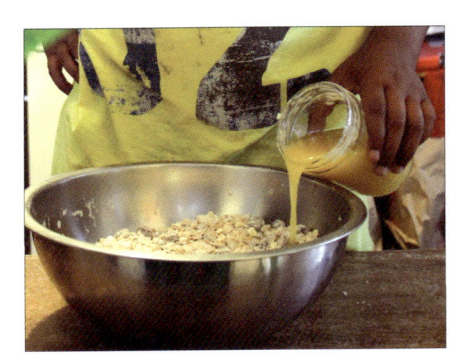

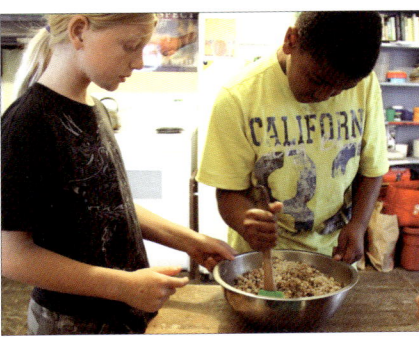

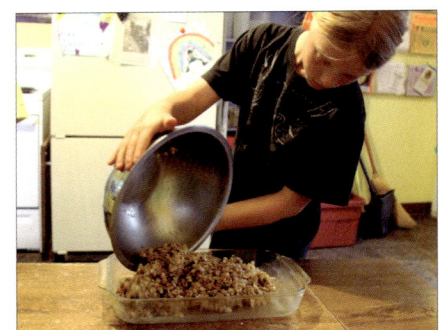

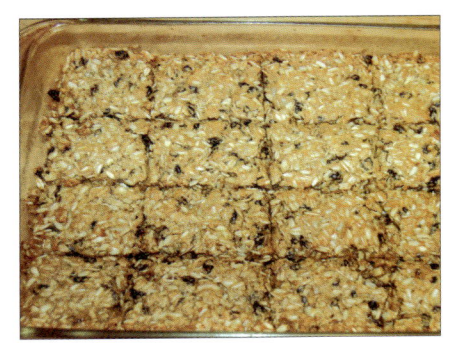

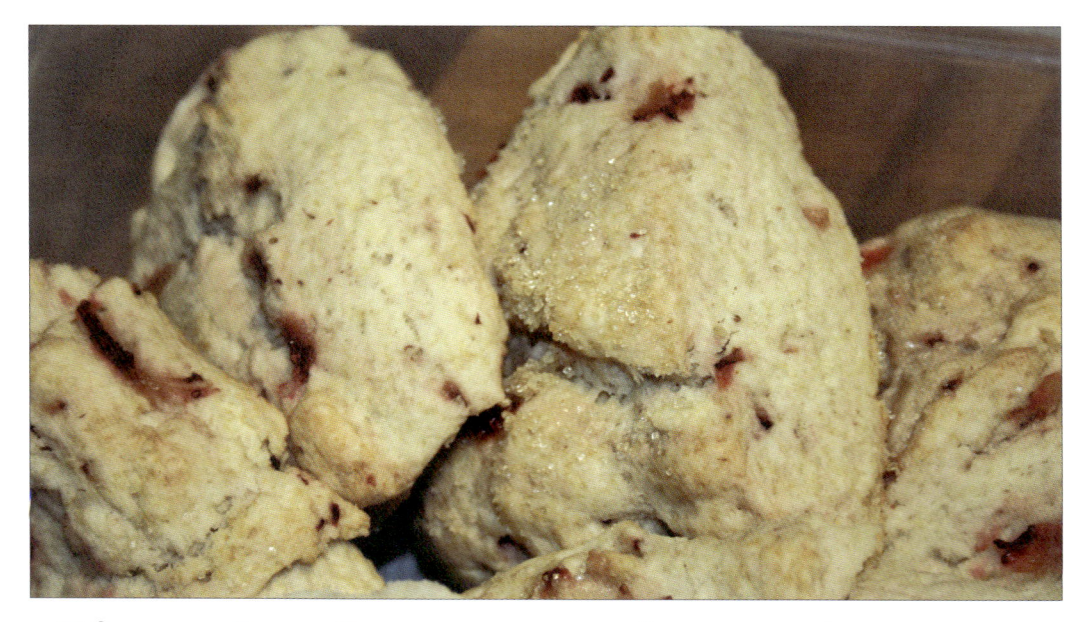

Simply Scrumptious Scones

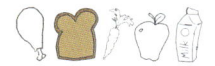

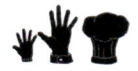

Yield: 6 Scones

This versatile recipe adapts to the addition of any of the following: dried fruit, nuts, flours or herbs. If you want a more savory scone, reduce the sugar to 2 tablespoons.

- 2½ cups all-purpose flour
- 1 tablespoon baking powder
- ½ teaspoon salt
- ⅓ cup sugar
- 8 tablespoons well-chilled butter
- 1 cup milk

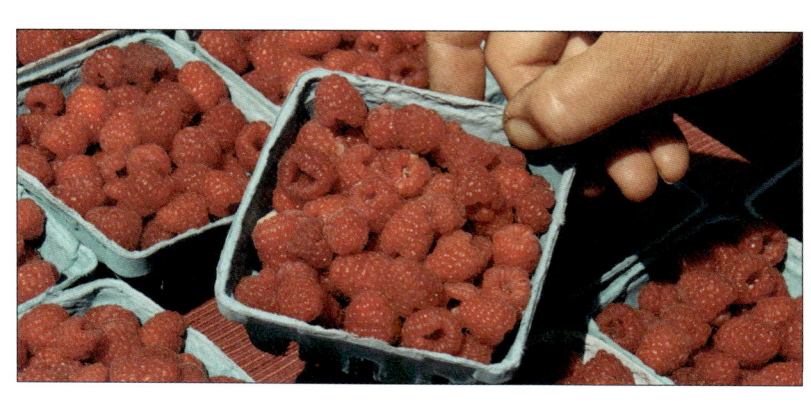

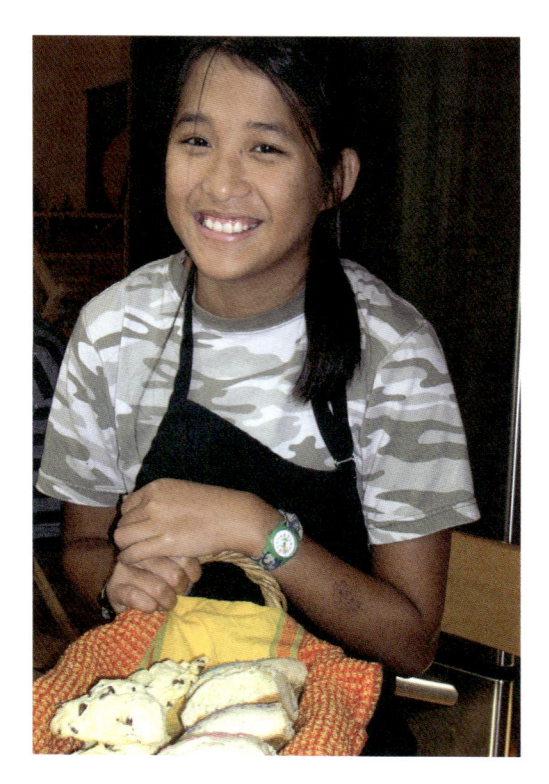

Preheat oven to 375°

1. Mix all of the dry ingredients in large bowl or food processor.

2. If hand mixing, grate the chilled butter into the dry mixture. Mix until you have a texture that resembles cornmeal. If using the food processor, cut the stick of butter into 8 pieces by hand, then drop one section at a time into the processor while mixing. When mixed, place ingredients in a separate bowl.

3. Add the milk slowly to the dry ingredients. Stir to incorporate. Go slowly. If you don't need that much liquid, don't use it. If mixture still seems too dry, add milk, a teaspoon at a time, until a soft dough forms.

4. Turn dough out onto a floured surface and knead 10 times. Shape into a ball (see kneading photos, below).

5. Flatten the ball into a 6-inch circle, cut it in half, then cut each half into 3 or 4 triangles.

6. Place triangles 2 inches apart on an ungreased baking sheet.

7. Bake 15-20 minutes or until slightly brown on top.

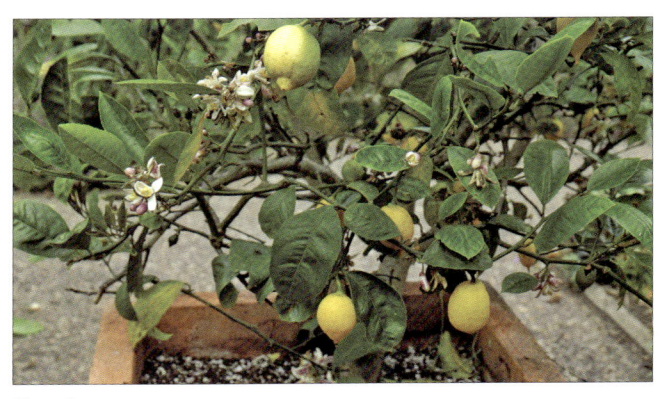

Options:

- Whole wheat scones: Replace 1 cup white flour with ¾ cup whole wheat flour.
- Lavender scones: At Step 3, combine 1 tablespoon lavender flowers with the milk.
- Lemon scones: At Step 1, add 1 tablespoon grated lemon peel to mixture. At Step 6, mix 2 teaspoons fresh lemon juice with 2 tablespoons sugar and sprinkle some on top of each scone before baking.
- Parmesan cheese scones: At Step 1, add ½ cup grated Parmesan cheese to mixture. At Step 6, top scones with an additional sprinkle of cheese before baking.

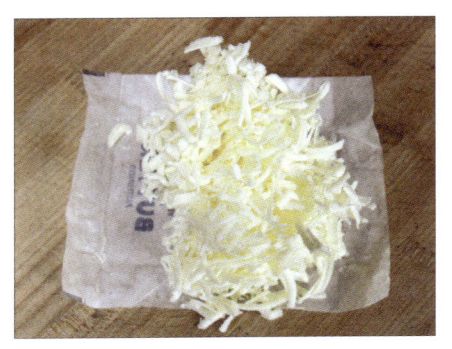

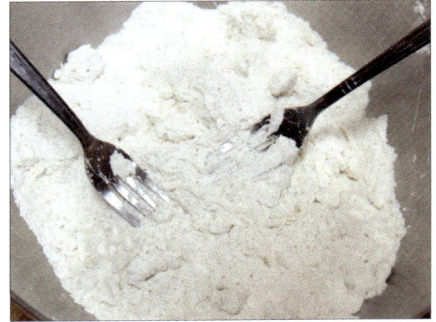

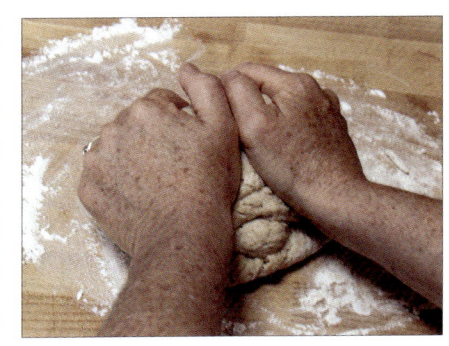

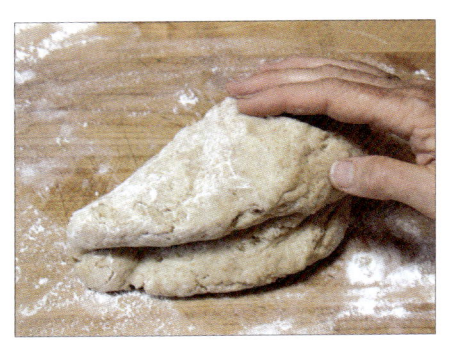

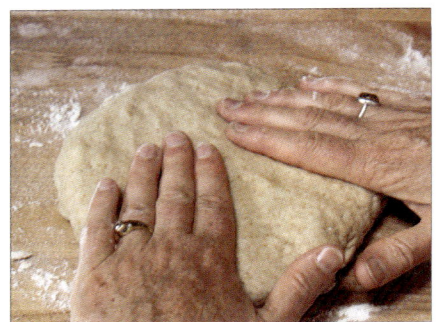

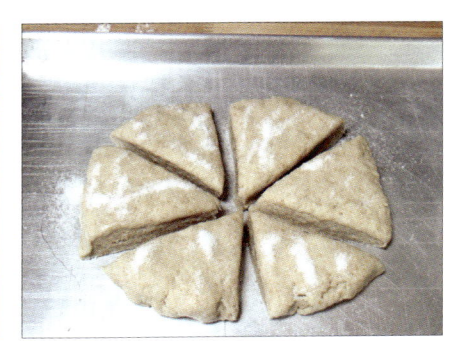

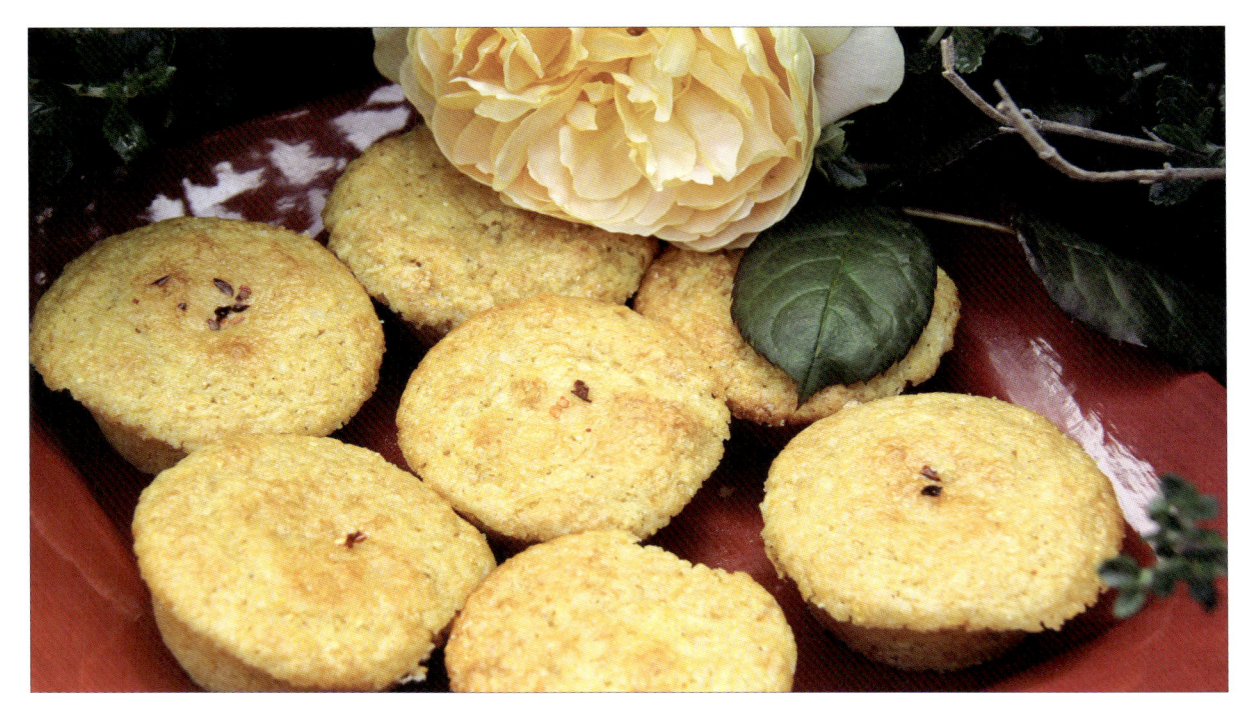

Corn Muffins

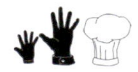

Yield: 12 Muffins

This simple and tasty alternative to cupcakes or cornbread takes 30 minutes to make. For a more adventuresome flavor, add some cayenne pepper or chile flakes.

- 1 cup plain yogurt
- 1 large egg, room temperature
- 3 tablespoons butter
- 1 cup cornmeal
- ¼ cup brown sugar, packed
- 1 tablespoon white sugar
- 1 cup flour
- 2 teaspoons baking powder
- ½ teaspoon baking soda
- ½ teaspoon salt

Preheat oven to 375°

1. Oil muffin cups or use paper muffin-cup liners.

2. Melt butter, then allow to cool slightly.

3. In a bowl combine yogurt, egg and melted butter. Be sure butter isn't too hot. Whisk until mixture is all one color. Set aside.

4. In a large bowl combine the cornmeal and the brown and white sugars.

5. Add the flour, baking powder, baking soda and salt to the cornmeal/sugar mixture. Mix with a spoon until combined.

6. Make a well in the center of the flour mixture. Scrape the yogurt mixture into the well and mix until everything is blended.

7. Spoon the batter into the muffin cups.

8. Bake 20 minutes or until tops are golden brown.

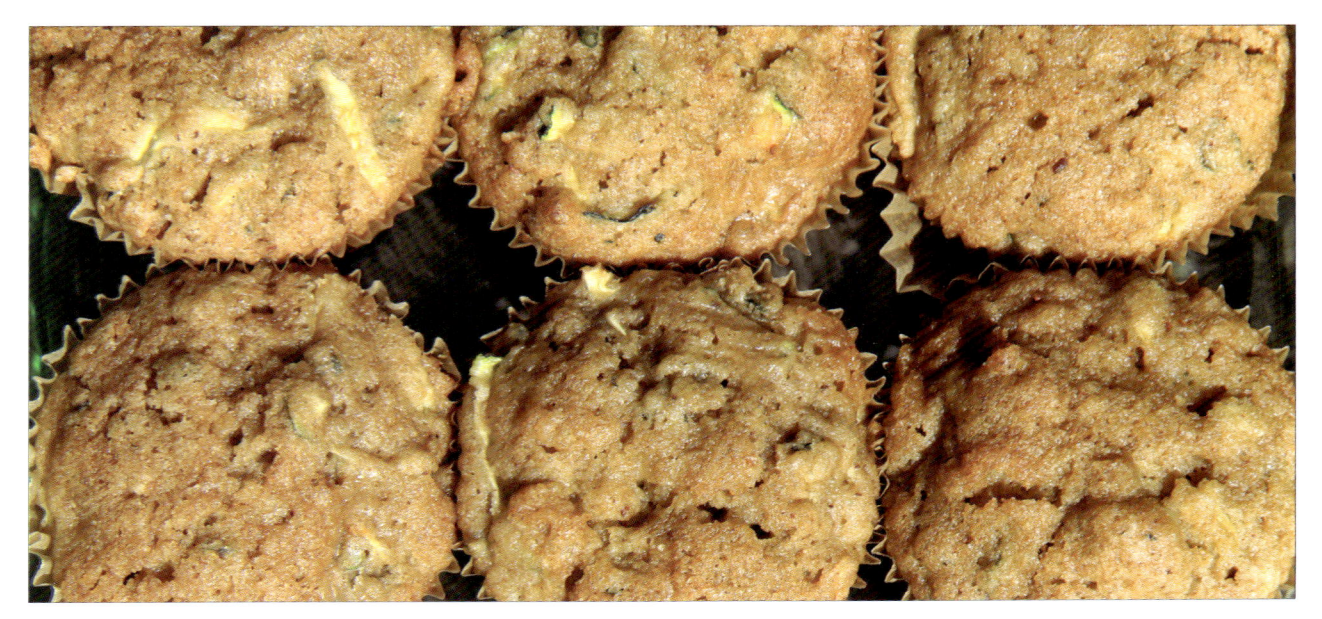

Zucchini or Carrot Muffins

Yield: 12-15 Muffins

Grated vegetables add a punch of nutrition and color to make these muffins a favorite with kids of all ages.

- 2 large eggs
- ¾ cup brown sugar, packed
- ½ cup vegetable oil
- 2 cups grated zucchini or carrots (about 2 small zucchini or 4 medium carrots)
- 2 cups whole wheat flour
- 1 teaspoon baking powder
- 1 teaspoon baking soda
- 1 teaspoon ground cinnamon
- ½ teaspoon salt

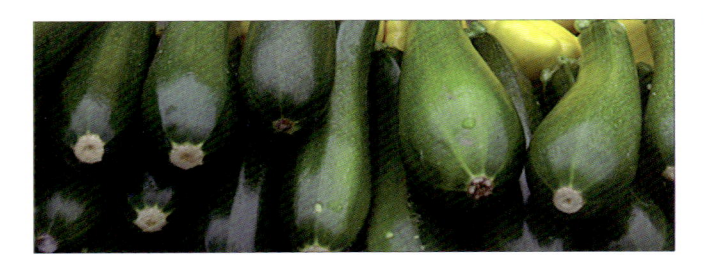

Preheat oven to 350°

1. Oil muffin tins or use paper muffin-cup liners.
2. Whisk eggs, sugar and oil in a medium bowl. Stir in zucchini.
3. Mix flour, baking powder, baking soda, cinnamon and salt in a large bowl. Add wet ingredients to dry ingredients and stir until just combined.
4. Spoon the batter evenly into the muffin tins.
5. Bake until muffins are a rich golden brown and a wooden toothpick inserted in the center comes out clean, about 20-30 minutes.
6. Cool in pan 5 minutes. Remove muffins from tin and cool.

Options:

- At Step 3, add ½ cup chopped walnuts or ½ cup raisins.
- At Step 3, add additional spices such as 1 teaspoon of ground ginger, nutmeg or cloves.

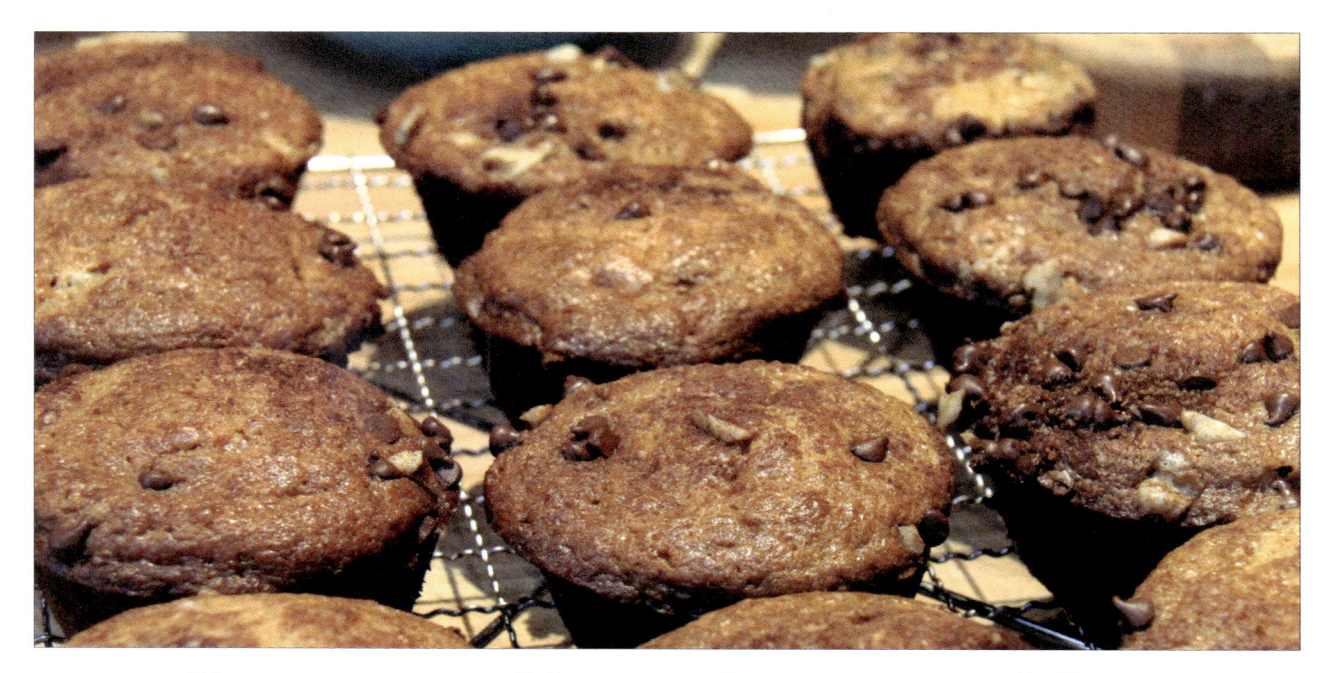

Banana-Chocolate Muffins

Yield: 24 Muffins or 2 Loaves

There is always one banana in the bunch that's been around too long. No one will eat it with brown spots. Here's a perfect solution.

Batter
- ½ pound butter (2 sticks), softened
- 2 cups sugar
- 3 eggs
- 2 very ripe bananas, peeled and mashed
- 1 teaspoon vanilla extract
- 2 teaspoons baking powder
- 2 teaspoons baking soda
- ⅛ teaspoon salt
- 3 cups all-purpose flour
- 1 pint sour cream

Filling
- ⅓ cup brown sugar, packed
- 1 tablespoon ground cinnamon
- 1 cup chopped walnuts
- 2 cups chocolate chips

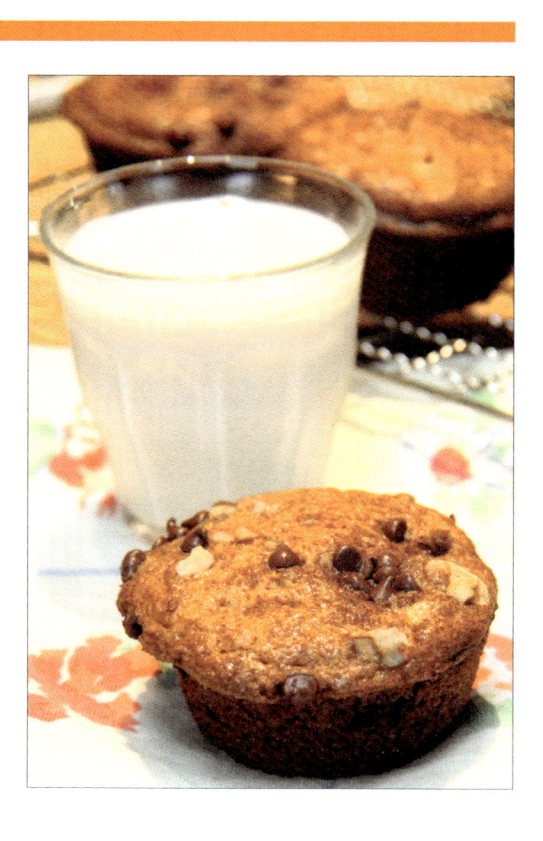

Preheat oven to 350°

1. Oil muffin tins or use paper muffin-cup liners. If using loaf pans, oil them well.

2. Combine softened butter, sugar, eggs, bananas and vanilla until light and fluffy.

3. Combine baking powder, baking soda, salt and flour in a separate bowl.

4. Add half of the sour cream to the dry ingredients, then add half of the banana mixture. Repeat until everything has been added and mixed completely.

5. Mix brown sugar, cinnamon, walnuts, chocolate chips and set aside.

6. Fill each cup ¼ full with the banana mixture. If using loaf pans, fill pans ¼ full.

7. Sprinkle half the chocolate chip mixture evenly over the banana batter in the muffin tins or loaf pans.

8. Cover with remaining banana mixture, then cover with remaining chocolate chip mixture.

9. Bake 30 minutes for cupcakes and 45 minutes for loaves, or until a toothpick inserted in the center comes out clean.

10. Remove from the oven and cool.

Overripe Fruit

Bananas are picked while they are still green because they only grow in tropical places and have to take a very long journey to get to the continental United States.

Sometimes they don't get eaten before they become covered with brown spots. Don't worry, the brown spots are the banana's starches turning completely into sugars. This is why ripe bananas are much sweeter than green ones. Therefore, overripe bananas and other fruits are a great source of sugar for recipes.

Of course, there is a difference between overripe and rotting, but your nose and taste buds will be able to tell that.

Uses for overripe fruit:

- bananas in banana bread, muffins or smoothies
- apples in applesauce (see page 136) or baked apples
- watermelon in ice cube popsicles

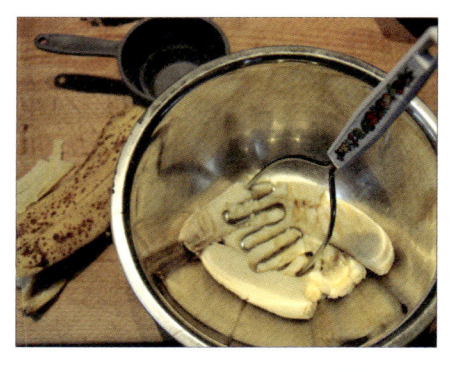

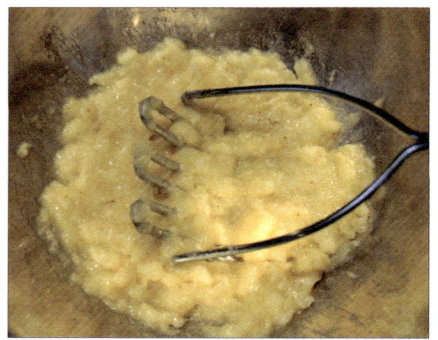

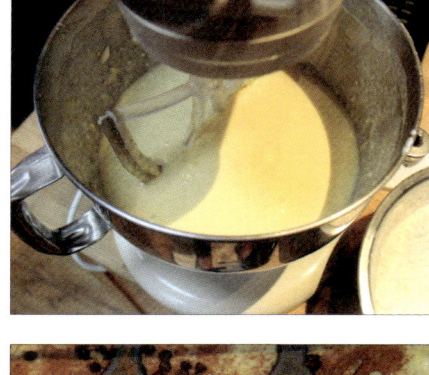

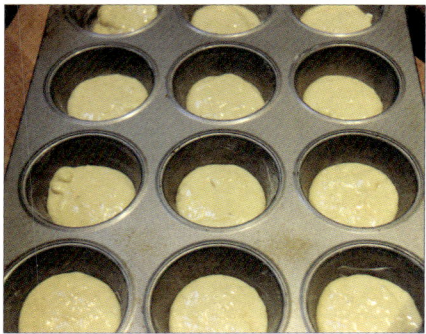

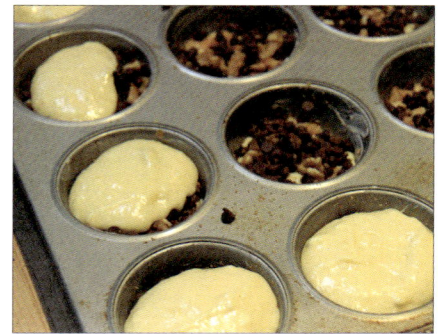

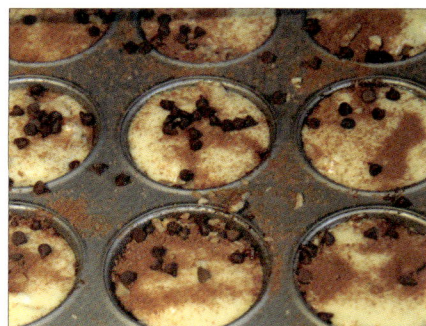

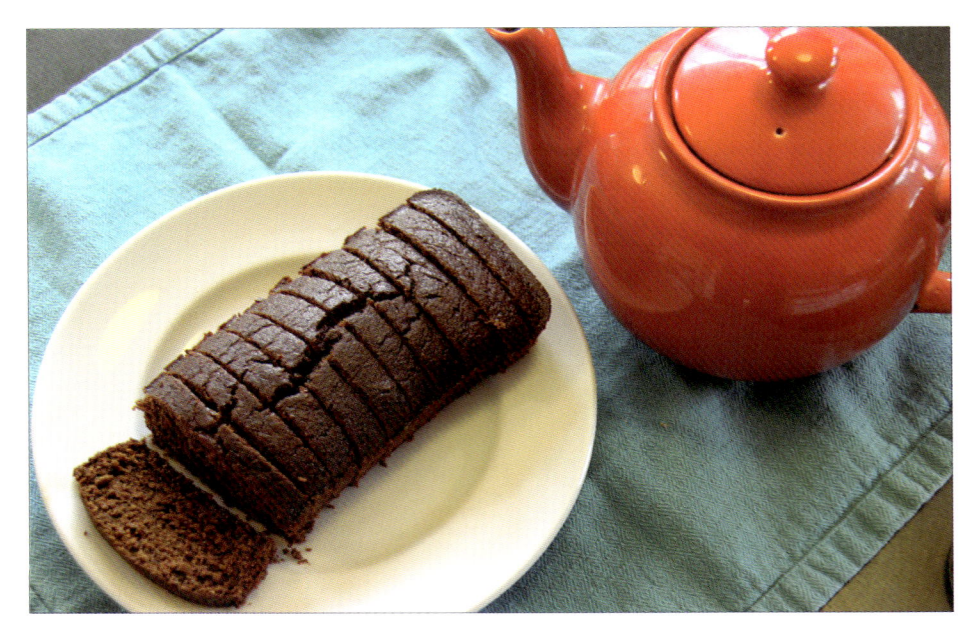

Gingerbread

9-12 servings

Delicious during the holiday season or any time of the year, this hearty, not-too-sweet bread tastes great smeared with cream cheese.

- 1½ cups unbleached all-purpose flour
- 1½ cups whole wheat flour
- 1½ teaspoons ground ginger
- 1½ teaspoons ground cinnamon
- ½ teaspoon baking powder
- ½ teaspoon baking soda
- ½ teaspoon salt
- ½ cup butter
- ¼ cup brown sugar, packed
- 1 egg
- ½ cup light molasses
- ½ cup boiling water

Preheat oven to 350°

1. Oil and flour a 9-inch loaf pan.

2. Mix the flours, ginger, cinnamon, baking powder, baking soda and salt. Set aside.

3. In a large bowl, cream butter and brown sugar until light and fluffy.

4. Beat in the egg and molasses.

5. Add flour mixture and water to egg mixture. Mix until smooth.

6. Pour batter into pan and bake 30-35 minutes, or until a toothpick inserted into cake comes out clean.

7. Cool in the pan 10-15 minutes.

8. Run a knife between loaf and edge of pan all the way around. Turn pan over onto a rack and tap firmly on the bottom to loosen loaf from pan. Slice and serve warm or cooled.

Options:

- Use all whole wheat flour. Increase other quantities to: 1 cup boiling water, 1 cup molasses, 2 eggs. Everything else stays the same.
- Use an oiled 9-inch square baking pan instead of the loaf pan. Bake 25-30 minutes.

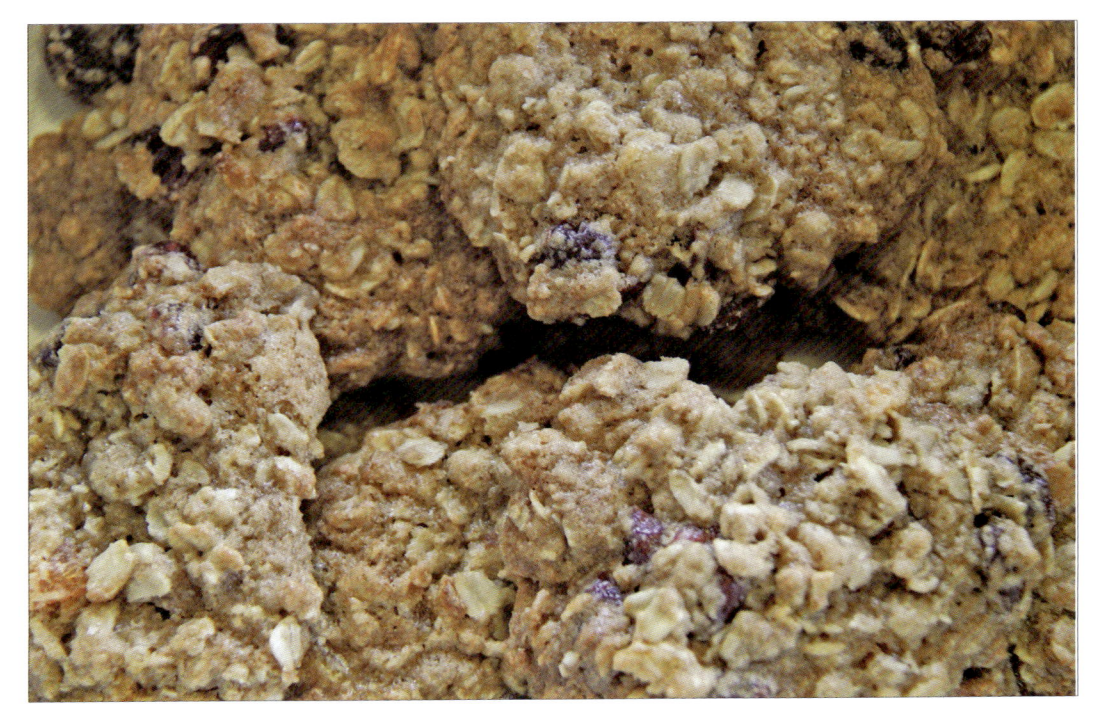

Chewy Fruity Cookies

Yield: 24 Cookies

These cookies are a burst of energy—dense, sweet, and chewy. They hit the spot when you've got a cookie craving. Look for a variety of dried fruit in bulk bins, where it is often cheaper, or dry your own (see page 137).

⅓	cup all-purpose flour
⅓	cup whole wheat flour
1½	cups old-fashioned rolled oats
1	teaspoon baking soda
½	teaspoon salt
6	tablespoons butter
¾	cup brown sugar, packed
1	cup dried fruit of your choice, chopped into small pieces
1	teaspoon vanilla extract
1	large egg, lightly beaten
1	teaspoon vegetable oil

Preheat oven to 350°

1. Oil 2 baking sheets. Chop fruit. In a small bowl, beat egg.

2. Combine flours and oats, baking soda and salt in large bowl.

3. Melt butter in a small pan over low heat or in a dish in the microwave (start with 20 seconds).

4. Add the brown sugar to the butter. Stir until smooth.

5. Add the sugar mixture to the flour mixture and mix until well blended.

6. Add fruit, vanilla and beaten egg; mix just until combined.

7. Drop dough, 1 tablespoon at a time, 2 inches apart onto baking sheets.

8. Bake 12 minutes. Cool on pans 3 minutes or until almost firm. Remove cookies from pans with a spatula and cool.

Dips and Spreads

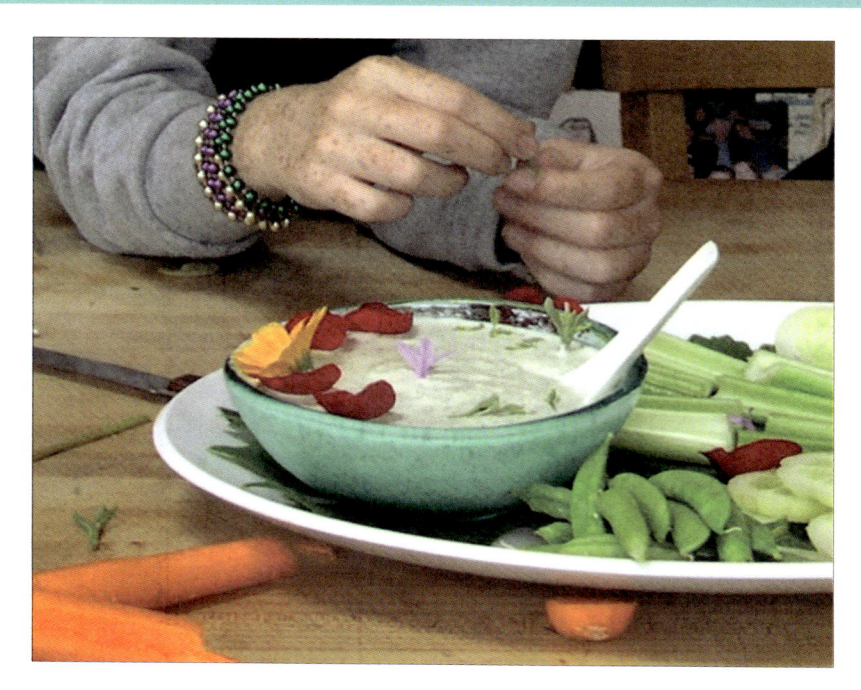

Dips and spreads go great with lunches. Some dips can serve all by themselves as one of the MyPlate components. Hummus (see page 167) or Black or White Bean Spread (see page 163) can be the main protein for lunch, in a sandwich or wrap. Yogurt Dip (see page 164) can provide calcium as a creamy addition to pita sandwiches and salads.

Other dips and spreads don't provide enough nutrition to have any MyPlate icons, but some kids who are resistant to vegetables will eat them with their favorite dip.

Be careful of the extra fat, salt and sugar added to purchased products. One tablespoon of bottled ranch salad dressing contains approximately 70 calories, most of which is fat. Compare this with homemade oil-and-vinegar salad dressing, at about 20 calories per tablespoon.

No-Prep

- Peanut butter
- Sunflower butter
- Cashew butter
- Almond butter
- Jam and jelly
- Hummus—purchased
- Bean spread—purchased
- Salsa—purchased
- Baba ganoush—purchased

Blenders and Food Processors

Smoother dips and spreads are made possible by the use of a blender or food processor. Without one of them, many spreads can be made by finely chopping, such as Pesto (page 165) and Salsa (page 159). But to get things creamy and smooth, you really need one of these tools.

Look for them at second-hand or thrift stores, garage sales, estate sales, or on craigslist.org. Make sure to test the appliance before buying, or come to an agreement with the seller that you can return it if it doesn't work.

A word of warning: The blades of a food processor are extremely sharp! To handle them, hold them carefully. Never put the blade into dirty dishwater so that it's invisible. Always put the blade in the same place to dry, so you know where it is.

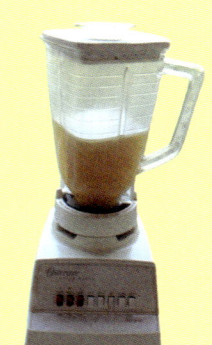

Low-Prep

- Mashed avocado
- Mashed banana
- Mashed beans

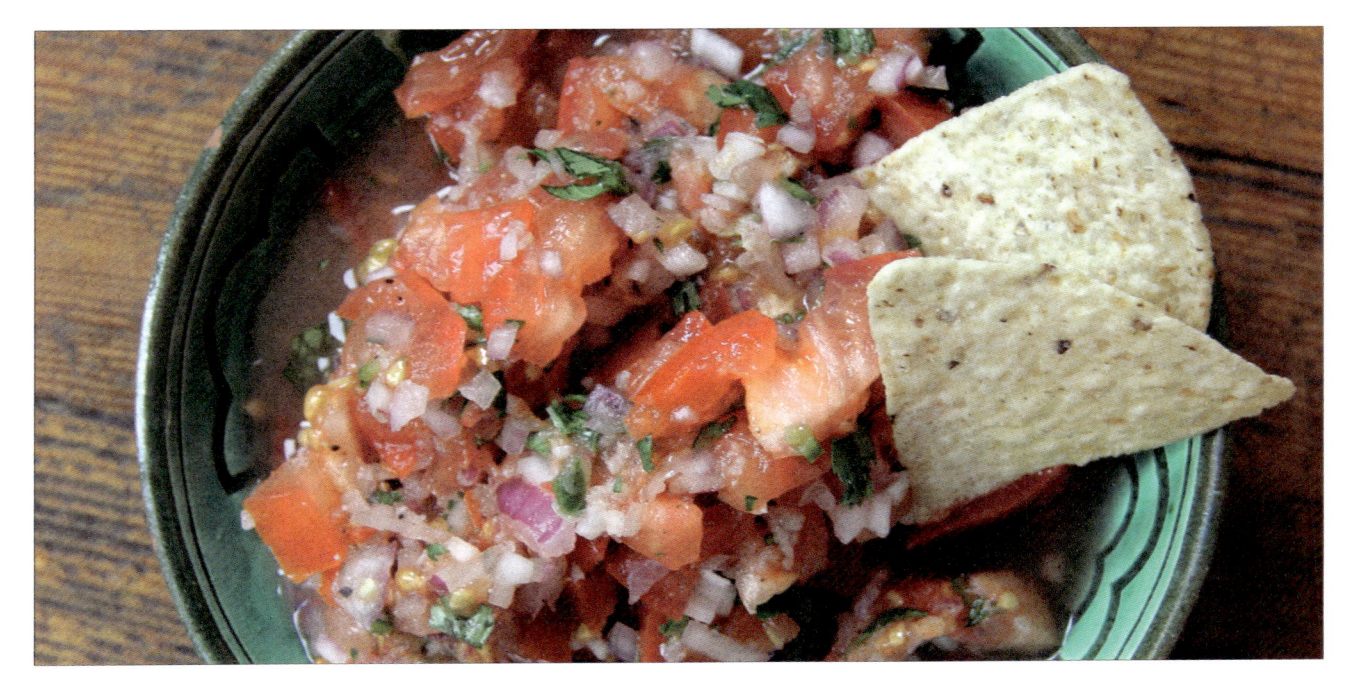

Fresh Tomato Salsa

Yield: 2-3 cups

Ripe, in-season tomatoes, bursting with flavor, are perfect candidates for this salsa. You can grow some of the ingredients yourself in a "Yarden" (see page 183).

- 1 fresh chile of your choice, chopped
- 2 large tomatoes
- 1 small red onion, cut into ¼-inch-thick slices
- 3 garlic cloves, peeled and mashed
- 1½ teaspoons chopped fresh cilantro
- Juice of 1-2 limes
- Salt and pepper to taste

1. Chop tomatoes, onion, garlic and cilantro. Remove stem from chile. Cut the chile in half and remove the seeds. Wear gloves if you have sensitive skin, and don't touch your eyes or face.

2. Mix all ingredients together in a bowl. Adjust taste by adding more lime juice, salt or pepper

Option:

- If you want a hotter kick, leave the seeds in the fresh chile, or add ¼ teaspoon cayenne or chile pepper flakes.

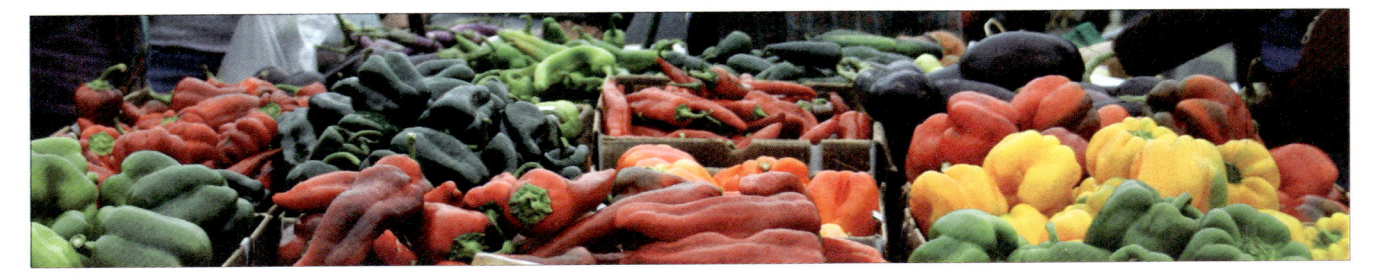

Sassy Summer Watermelon Salsa

Yield: 3 cups

This salsa was created by Arcata Elementary School students under the guidance of Rosa Dixon, owner of Natural Decadence Catering. It was created for the Harvest of the Month North Coast Youth Culinary AllSTARS Salsa Competition, coordinated by the Humboldt County Office of Education.

2	cups seedless watermelon, chopped into ½-inch cubes
1	cup cucumber, peeled and diced
½	cup seedless red grapes, quartered
¼	cup red bell pepper, finely chopped
⅓	cup minced cilantro
3	tablespoons minced basil
2	tablespoons minced mint leaves
1½	tablespoons fresh lime juice
1	tablespoon jalapeño chile pepper, seeded and minced
1	teaspoon champagne vinegar or rice vinegar
⅛	teaspoon salt

1. Wash, peel and chop watermelon, cucumber, grapes, bell pepper, cilantro, basil, and mint. Juice the lime.
2. Remove stem, cut chile in half, remove seeds and chop. Wear gloves if you have sensitive skin, and keep your hands away from your face.
3. Combine all ingredients, except watermelon, in a large bowl. Then gently mix in watermelon. Chill for 24 hours.

Option:
- Garnish with lime zest and fresh mint.

Salsa Competition

"On a sunny September morning at the Arcata Farmers' Market, a joyous community event takes place: The Annual North Coast Youth Culinary AllSTARS Salsa Competition, held during peak season for local produce.

Kids in grades 4 through 6, dressed in chef jackets and big smiles, serve the hordes of food enthusiasts and a panel of judges samples of salsas they created with the help of local chefs. The kids are extremely proud of their recipes. Ingredients range from traditional tomatoes, onion, and cilantro to eclectic combinations such as fennel and oranges, pineapple and ginger.

Prior to the competition, the kids practiced their culinary skills in cooking classes and farm field trips. One young girl, who wants to open her own restaurant, made a comment that has really stuck with us: 'I think it was great that we [kids] got to express ourselves through the food we chose.'"

**Linda Prescott,
Nutrition Program Director,
and Megan Russin,
Nutrition Educator,
Humboldt County Office of Education**

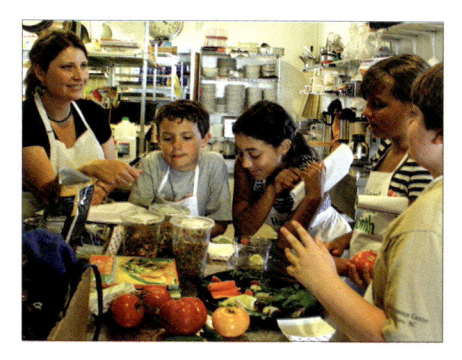

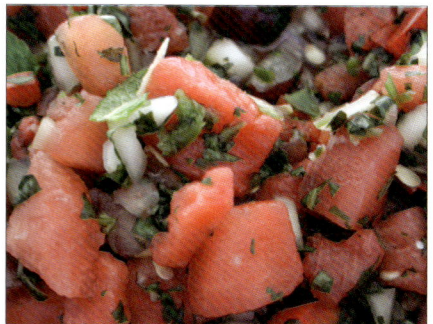

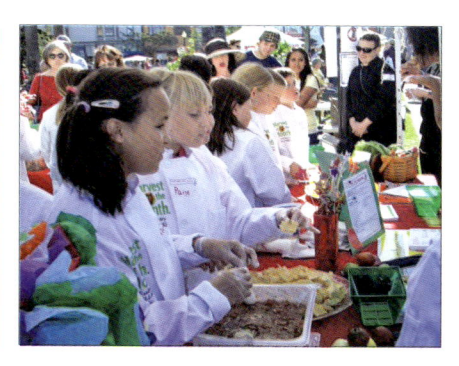

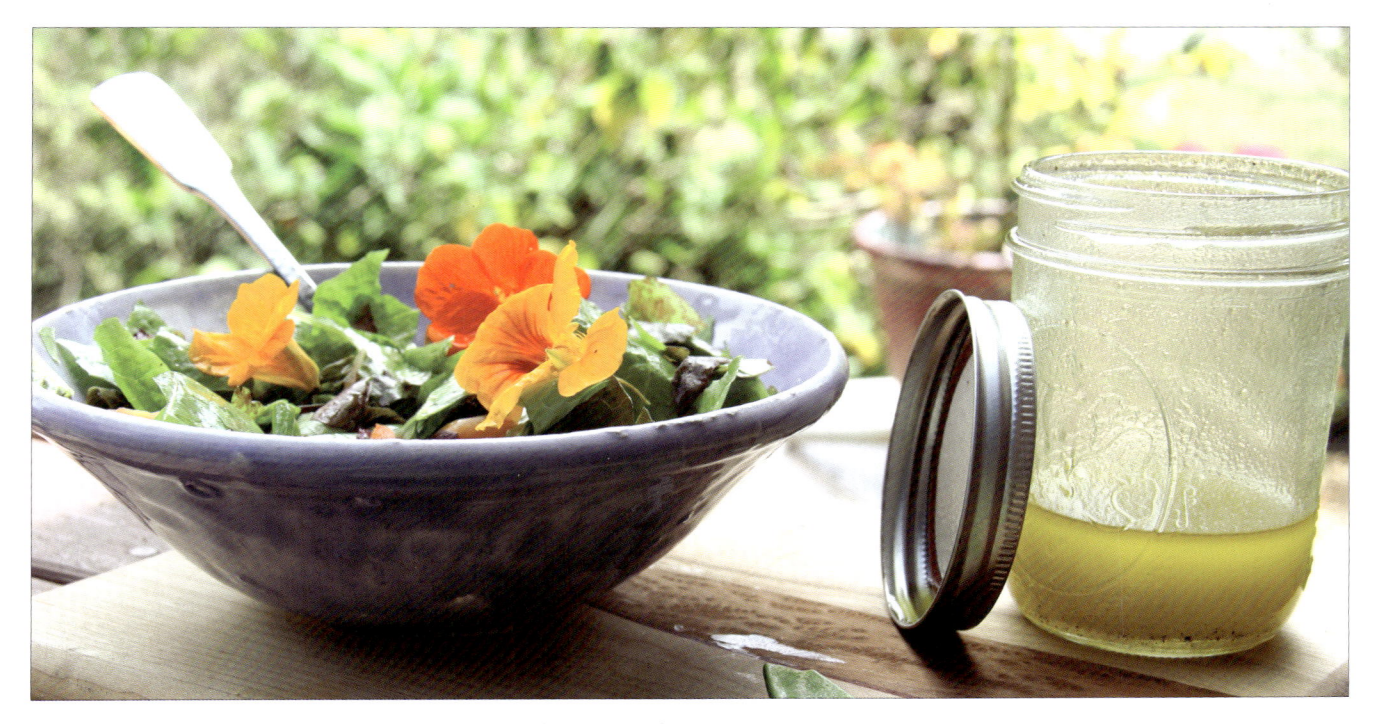

Vinaigrette

Yield: 1 cup

Use this basic dressing (oil and vinegar) for almost any salad, including green, potato, pasta, or grain salads, and almost any vegetable dish.

- ¼ cup vinegar or lemon juice
- ¾ cup olive oil
- ½ teaspoon salt
- ⅛ teaspoon black pepper
- ¼ teaspoon sugar or honey

Options:
- Add 1 clove crushed garlic or garlic powder.
- Add ¼ teaspoon prepared mustard.
- Add chopped parsley, chives, or other herbs.
- Add 1 teaspoon celery seed.

1. Put all ingredients in a jar. Tighten lid and shake.

2. If using honey, first heat it to a thin liquid consistency. **On stove top:** place a small glass container in small pot in 2 inches of water. Warm until honey thins. **In microwave:** heat honey in glass container until thin. Microwaves vary in time and power; start with 5 seconds.

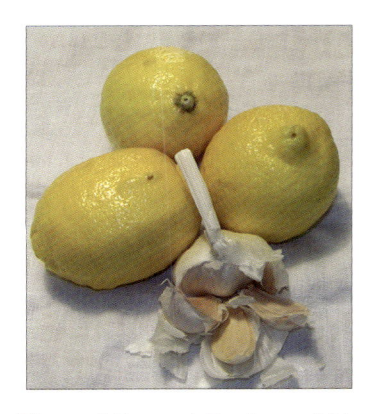

Dip and Spread Recipes

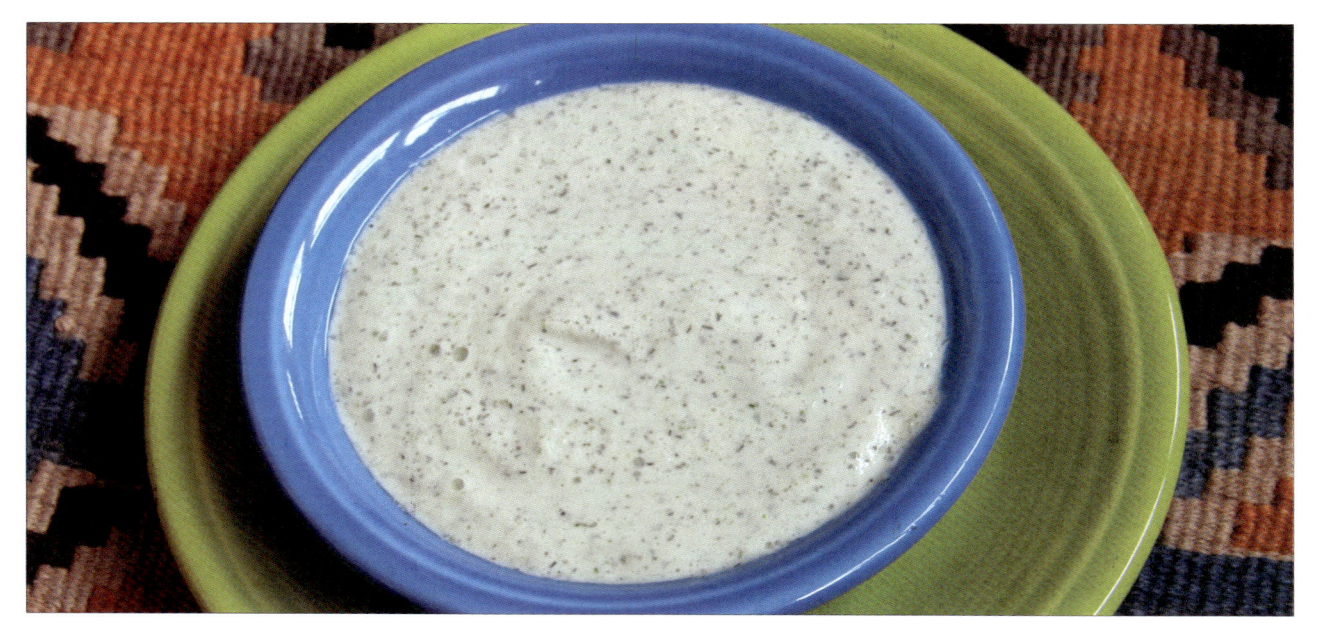

Ranch Dressing

Yield: 1 cup

Ranch dressing is a popular creamy dip for sliced raw vegetables or dressing for a salad. Try this healthier version. Making your own at home means more flavor, fewer additives, less salt and fat, and less waste. However, lots of vegetables, especially when fresh and in season, are sweet and delicious on their own, so make sure to try them plain.

- ½ pound extra-firm silken tofu
- ½ cup mayonnaise
- ¼ cup lemon juice
- ¼ cup sour cream
- 1 teaspoon soy sauce or tamari sauce
- 4 tablespoons chopped green onion
- 2 stalks of celery, chopped
- ½ teaspoon minced garlic
- 1 tablespoon chopped fresh parsley (or 1 teaspoon dried)
- 1 tablespoon chopped fresh dill (or 1 teaspoon dried)
- Salt and pepper to taste

1. Chill tofu in the freezer at least 3 hours.
2. Stir mayonnaise, lemon juice, sour cream and soy sauce together in a small bowl.
3. Chop vegetables and herbs.
4. Combine all ingredients in the food processor or blender and process until well blended, about 2 minutes.
5. Unused portion can be stored in the refrigerator, covered, for about a week.

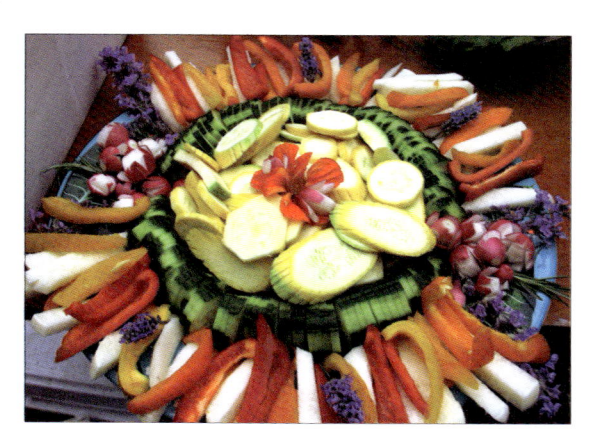

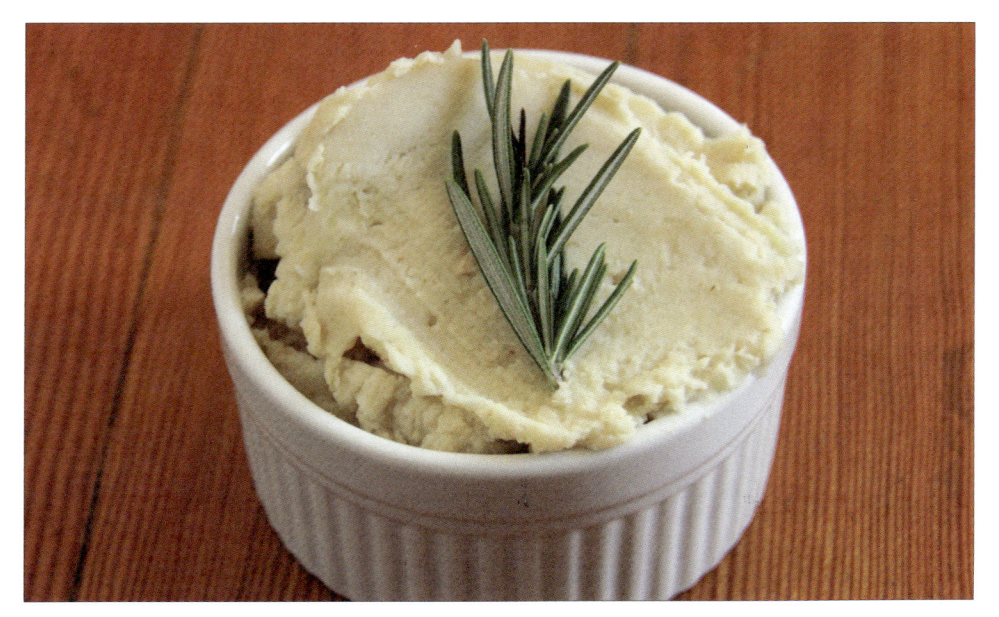

Black or White Bean Dip

Yield: 2 cups

This simple bean dip is about as adaptable as you can get. Use it as the protein in sandwiches or wraps, paired with cheese or avocado; inside burritos, served with chips; or as a dip for vegetables.

- 2 cups cooked white (navy, cannellini) or black beans (1 cup dried or one 14.5- to 16-ounce can)
- 1½ tablespoons water
- 2 tablespoons olive or vegetable oil
- 2 teaspoons lemon or lime juice
- ¼ teaspoon salt

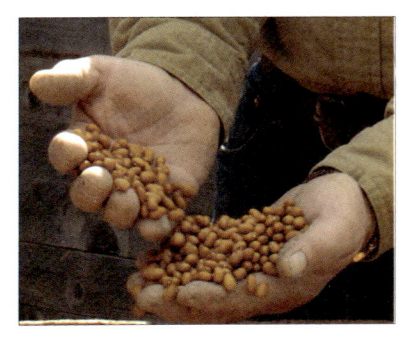

1. Rinse and drain beans.
2. Add all ingredients to a food processor or blender.
3. Process until smooth. If using a blender, blend for a few seconds. Turn off blender; scrape sides and push dip down with a rubber spatula. Repeat until dip is as smooth as you want it. Taste and add more seasonings and/or juice, if desired.

Options:

- If you don't have a food processor or blender, use a potato masher to make a chunky bean dip.
- For a fuller flavor, add ¼ teaspoon each garlic powder and onion powder.
- For a spicy Southwest-style black bean dip, use lime juice, add ½ teaspoon cumin, ¼ teaspoon chile powder, and 1 tablespoon chopped cilantro.
- Add more water and oil for creamier dip.

Dip and Spread Recipes

Yogurt Dip

Yield: 1 cup

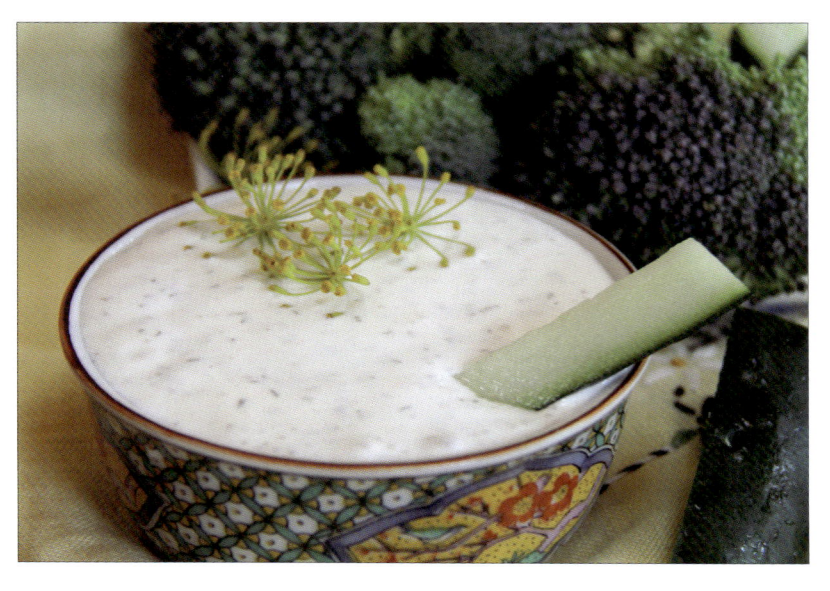

Here is a savory yogurt dip that will go well with vegetables, crackers, or as a dressing for salads.

- ¾ cup plain yogurt
- ¼ cup sour cream
- 3 teaspoons chopped fresh dill (or 1 teaspoon dried)
- ⅛ teaspoon garlic salt or 1 clove garlic, minced
- 1 tablespoon mayonnaise
- pepper to taste

1. Mix yogurt, sour cream, dill and garlic salt in a bowl. Stir vigorously, or blend in a blender or food processor. Stir in the mayonnaise. Chill one hour.

Options:

- Peel, seed and grate one cucumber and add to yogurt mixture.
- For **Greek tzatiki dip**: Add 1 diced cucumber, substitute sour cream for the mayonnaise, and add ½ teaspoon white vinegar.
- For **Indian raita**: Add 1 diced cucumber, ¼ teaspoon cumin, ¼ teaspoon curry powder and 1 teaspoon minced mint leaves.
- To lower the fat content, use non-fat or low-fat yogurt and leave out the mayonnaise.

Yogurt Recipes of the World

Yogurt originally came from Central Asia and the Middle East. The name comes from the Turkish word for "long life."

Yogurt is high in protein and vitamins. It has "active cultures" (called probiotics) or good bacteria your stomach uses to help digest food. Mildly lactose-intolerant people who get an upset stomach from milk can eat yogurt.

Yogurt around the world:

- Raita - Indian and Pakistani sauce to cool down spicy foods
- Tzatzki - Greek and Middle Eastern sauce with cucumber used in salads and wraps
- Kefir - originally a fermented, carbonated sheep milk from the Caucasus Mountains. Now made with sheep, cow, or goat milk and widely available.
- Kumis - from Central Asia; a fermented mare's milk drink
- Lassi - Indian yogurt drink blended with fruit.

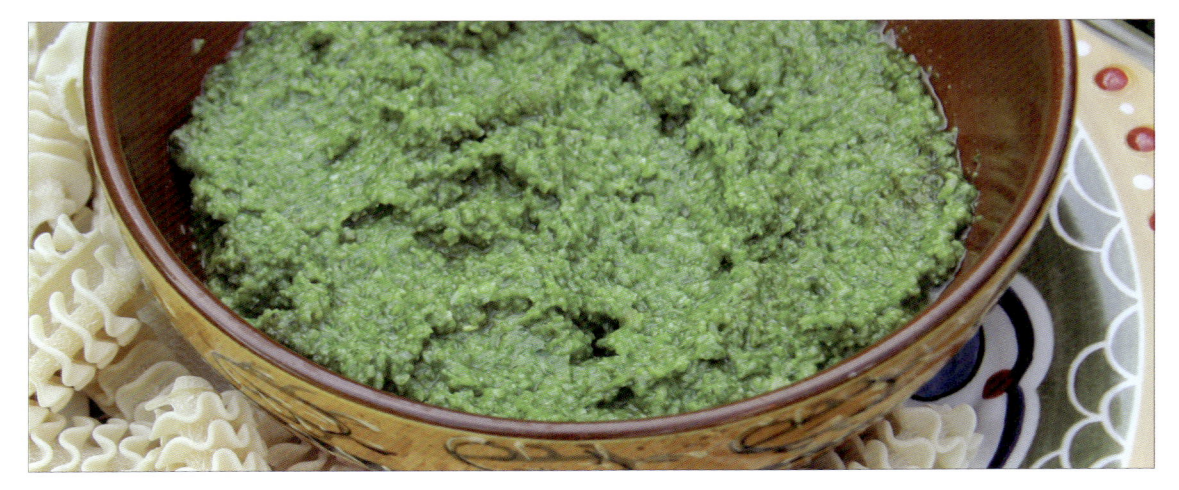

Classic Italian Pesto

Yield: 1 cup

The term "Pesto" comes from an Italian word meaning to pound. You can "pound" or blend together almost any herb or leafy green. This is a classic Italian pesto made with basil leaves. Pesto is super easy to make in a blender or food processor, but if you don't have either one, you can just chop the basil and nuts very small.

- 3 cups of fresh basil, washed and patted dry
- 1 large garlic clove
- ¼ cup olive oil
- ½ cup walnuts or pine nuts
- 1 teaspoon salt
- ¼ cup Parmesan cheese

Process everything in a blender or food processor. The finished pesto should be smooth.

Adjust ingredients to your taste.

Options:

- Substitute spinach, parsley or cilantro for half or all of the basil.

Caution: Nutritional yeast is **not** the same as the yeast used for baking. Do **not** use baker's yeast in this recipe.

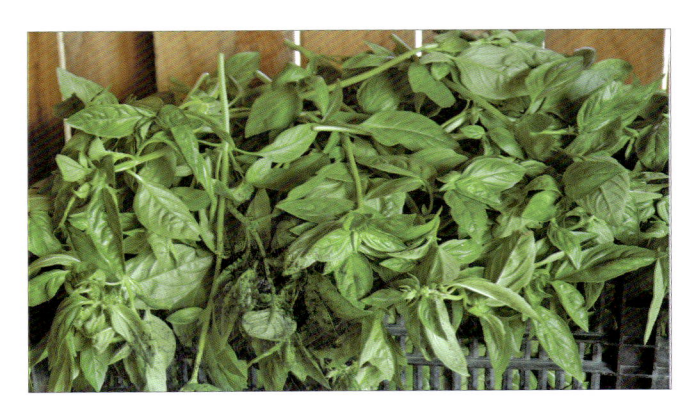

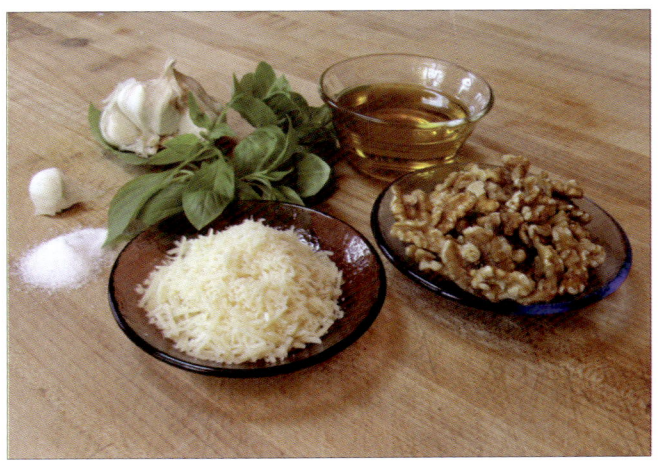

Pea Pesto

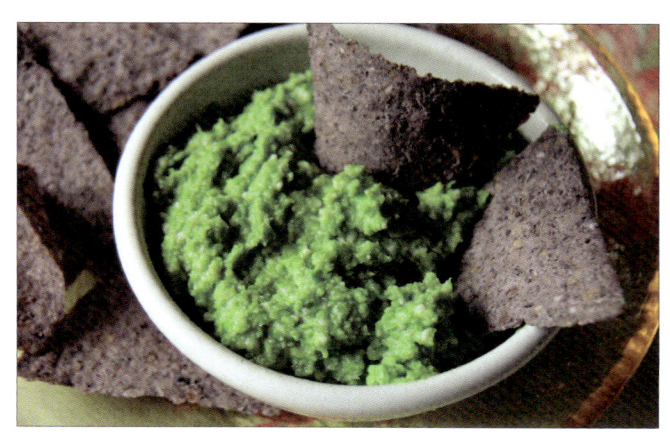

Yield: 2 cups

1. Defrost peas overnight in the refrigerator.
2. Combine all ingredients in a medium bowl and stir.
3. Put mixture into a blender or food processor and process until smooth.
4. Test and add more garlic, salt or pepper as needed.

Options:

- If you don't have a blender or food processor, chop the garlic very finely and put all ingredients in a big zippered plastic bag. Push extra air out of bag and check the seal, then roll with rolling pin or bottle on flat surface. It will take a few minutes, but kids love to hear the peas pop!
- For a vegan version, replace cheese with 2 tablespoons of nutritional yeast.

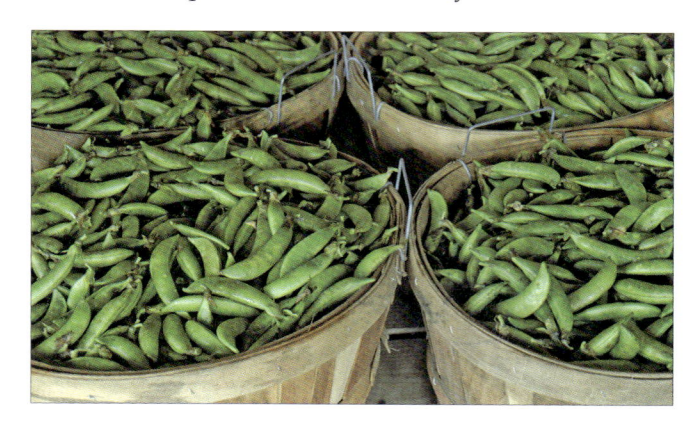

The option for creating this pesto without a food processor or blender is a fun task for kids. Squishing the peas in the bag by hand has some amusing sound effects.

1	(10-ounce) bag of frozen peas (about 1½ cups), defrosted
½	cup Parmesan or Romano cheese, grated
1-2	cloves of garlic, peeled and finely chopped (or 1 teaspoon powdered garlic)
¼	teaspoon salt
¼	cup olive or vegetable oil
	Pepper to taste

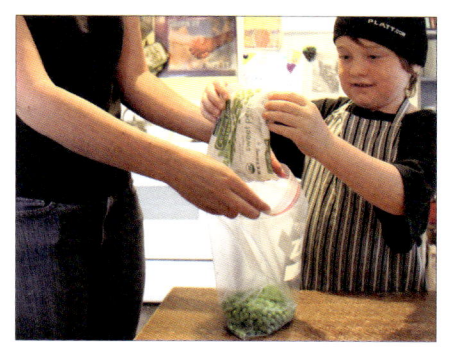

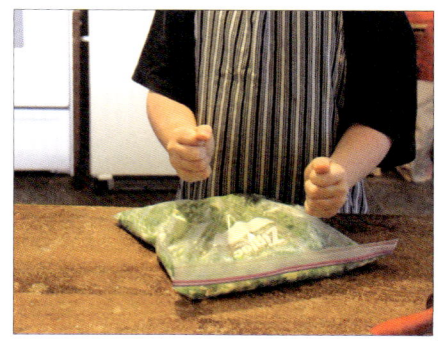

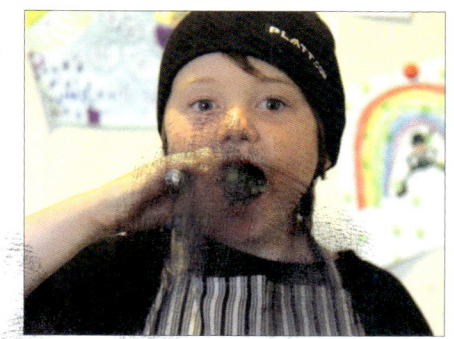

166 Dip and Spread Recipes

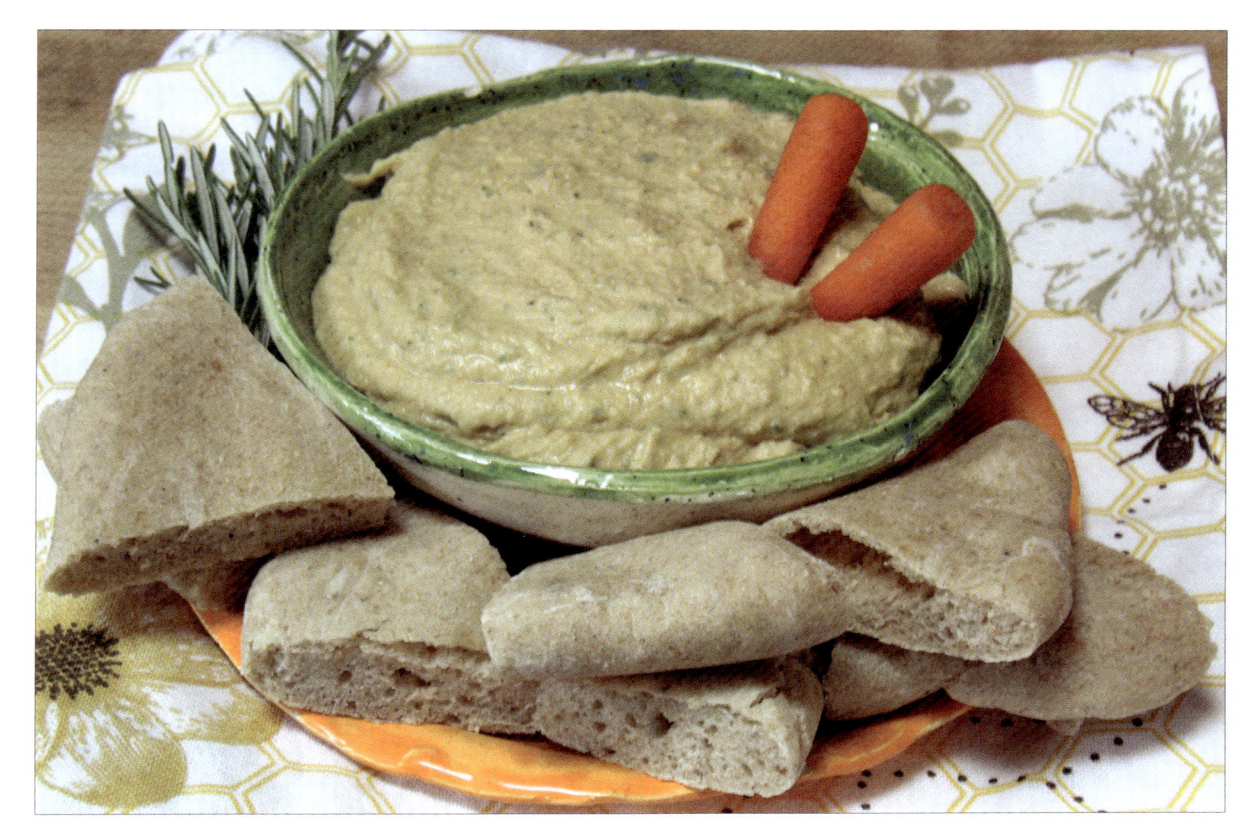

Hummus

Yield: 2 cups

A classic Middle-Eastern favorite that makes an excellent dip for vegetables or crackers, spread on sandwiches and wraps or as a filling for pita pockets. A food processor or blender is necessary.

- 2 cups cooked garbanzo beans (1 cup dried or one 14.5- to 16-ounce can)
- 3 medium garlic cloves, peeled and chopped
- ¼ cup olive oil
- ¼ cup chopped parsley
- ¼ cup roasted tahini (sesame paste)
- 1 teaspoon salt
- 2 tablespoons lemon juice
- 1 teaspoon soy sauce
- 1 tablespoon paprika

1. Cook beans (see page 54) if necessary. Rinse and drain canned beans. Peel garlic and chop.

2. Place all ingredients in food processor or blender. Blend until the hummus is a smooth paste, about 2 minutes.

3. Adjust the thickness with more olive oil, to suit your taste. The consistency should be like smooth peanut butter. Adjust the flavor with more lemon juice or salt.

Cream Cheese Spreads

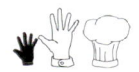

Yield: About ½ cup for each recipe

The following recipes work best with the use of a food processor, but it is possible to hand stir the ingredients together. If you are hand stirring, it's easier if the cream cheese is softened. You can do so by placing the cream cheese in a small glass bowl in the microwave at a low setting (10 percent power) for 10 to 20 seconds, or leave at room temperature for half an hour.

Cream Cheese Spread Directions

Place everything in the bowl of the food processor and puree until all ingredients are well incorporated into the cream cheese. There might be some bigger chunks—you can continue to puree if you want it smoother. If mixing by hand, stir everything until very well blended.

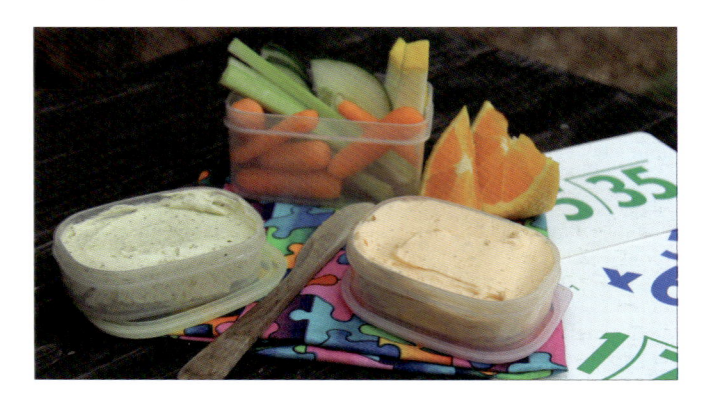

Fruit Spread

- 3 ounces plain cream cheese
- 1 small piece of fresh fruit, finely chopped or 5 pieces dried fruit, finely chopped
- ¼ cup chopped walnuts
- 1 tablespoon honey

Ginger and Preserves

- 4 ounces plain cream cheese
- 2 tablespoons peach, apricot or strawberry jam
- ⅛ teaspoon ground ginger

Pesto

- 3 ounces plain cream cheese
- 1 teaspoon pesto (see page 165)

Sun-dried Tomato

- 3 ounces plain cream cheese
- 1 teaspoon sun-dried tomatoes in oil

Drain the tomatoes well, then measure and chop them.

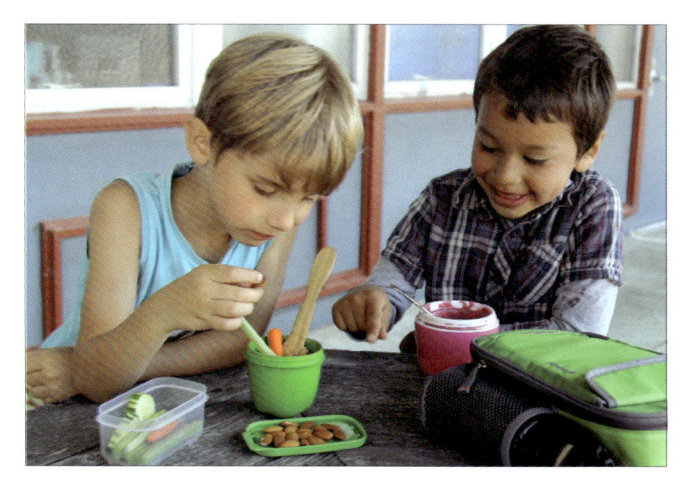

Chapter 6
Do It Yourself Projects

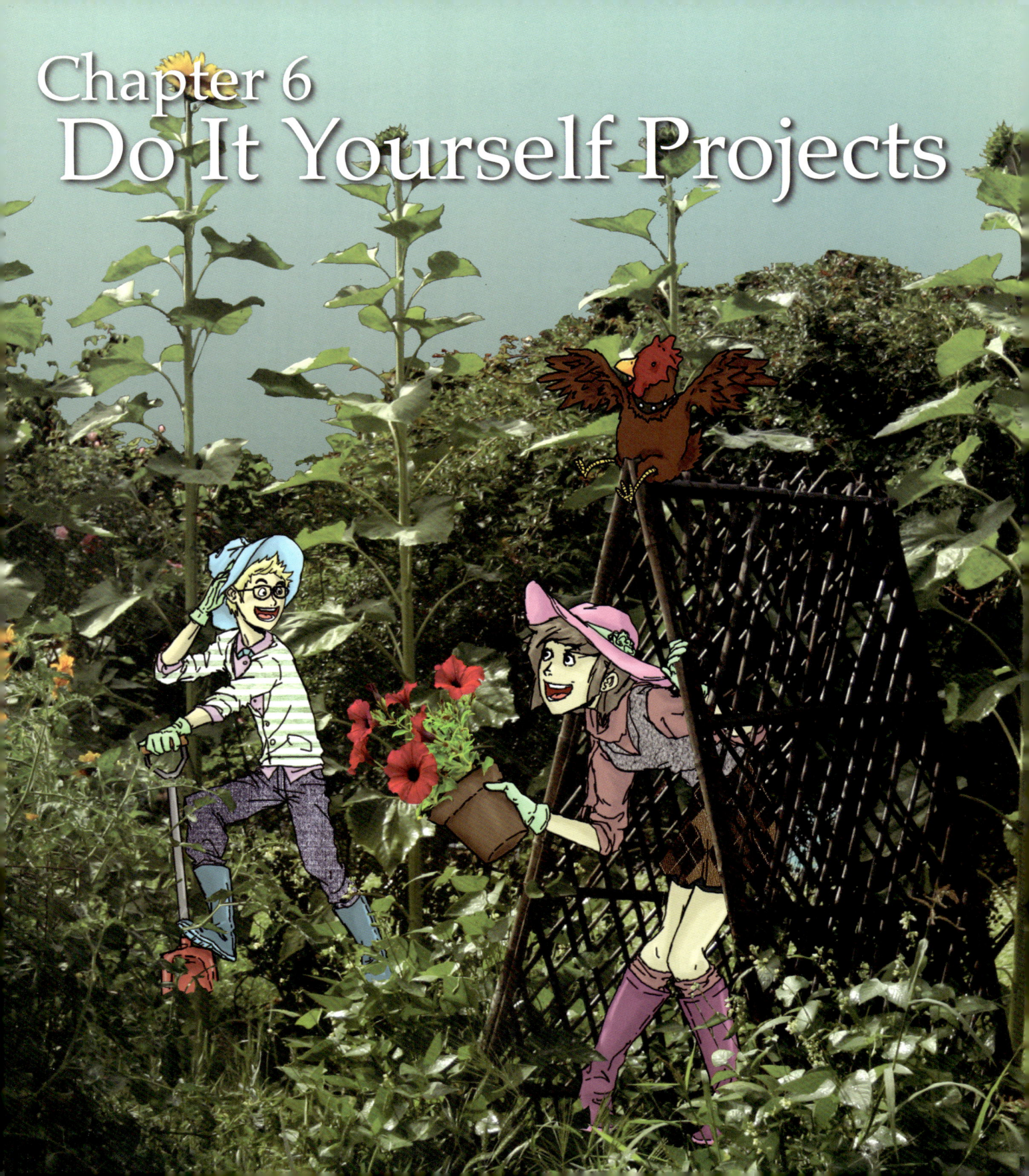

Worm Bin Composter

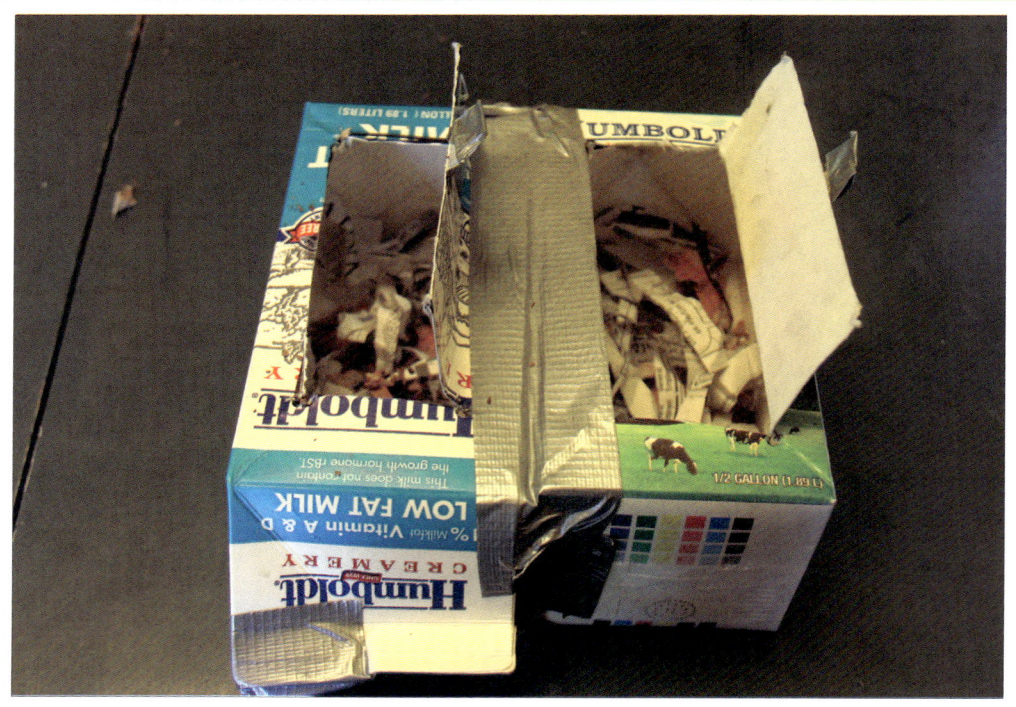

Compost is an excellent natural fertilizer that's easy to make from garden debris and kitchen scraps. Composting recycles valuable organic material. A compost area can be in the garden if it's protected from digging animals, contained in bins or fencing, and turned occasionally with a hay fork or shovel.

If outdoor composting is not practical, a worm bin will convert food waste to worm castings, which makes an excellent fertilizer.

This worm bin composter is designed to turn food waste into compost for your small garden. It shows how composting works on a small scale. Once you see this and grow your garden, you may wish to create a larger composting system.

Age: 8+   Some adult supervision required   Time to complete: Less than an hour

Here's what you'll need:

Materials:

- Two half-gallon waxed cardboard juice or milk cartons
- Duct tape
- Newspaper
- Garden debris (leaves and grass)
- Red worms (buy at local nursery or bait shop)

Tools:

- Scissors
- Several sharp pencils

Worm Bin Composter

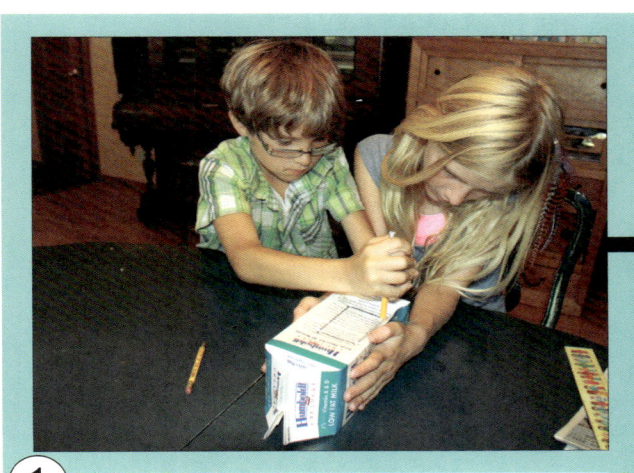

1 Rinse and dry the cartons. **Make a 2" x 3" worm migration hole between the cartons.** At the same place on one side of each carton, use a sharp pencil to poke four holes marking the corners for the migration hole. Make the hole 1" from the edge.

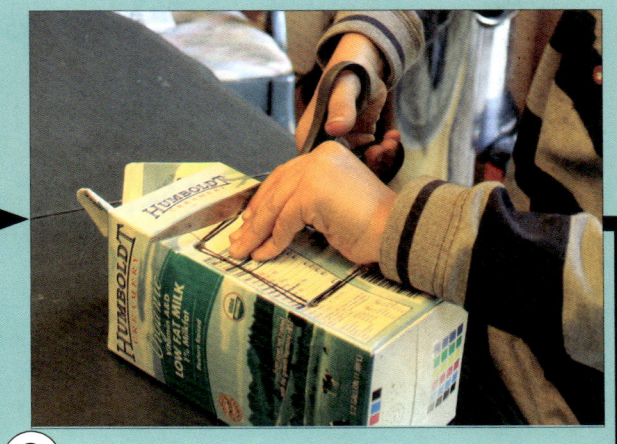

2 **Use scissors to cut the rectangular opening.** Check to make sure you are cutting the holes in the same place on each carton. They need to match up so the worms can migrate from carton to carton.

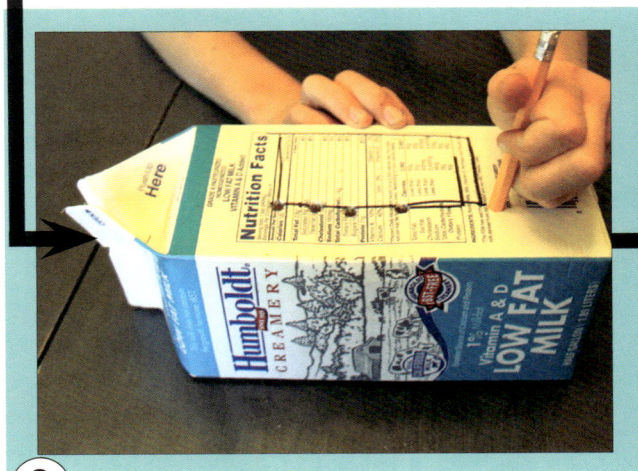

3 **Poke holes for ventilation and drainage.** Poke holes along the opposite side of the migration hole and on the bottom of each carton. Three holes along the middle of the sides and five along the bottom are sufficient.

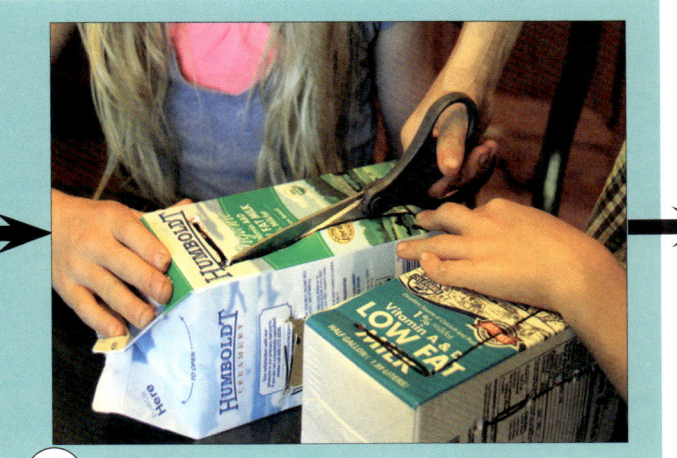

4 **Cut flaps into the top side of each carton.** The flaps should be almost as big as the side of the carton. Poke four holes in the shape of a rectangle near the corners of the cartons. Cut along only three of the four corner holes to make each flap.

Do It Yourself Projects 171

Worm Bin Composter

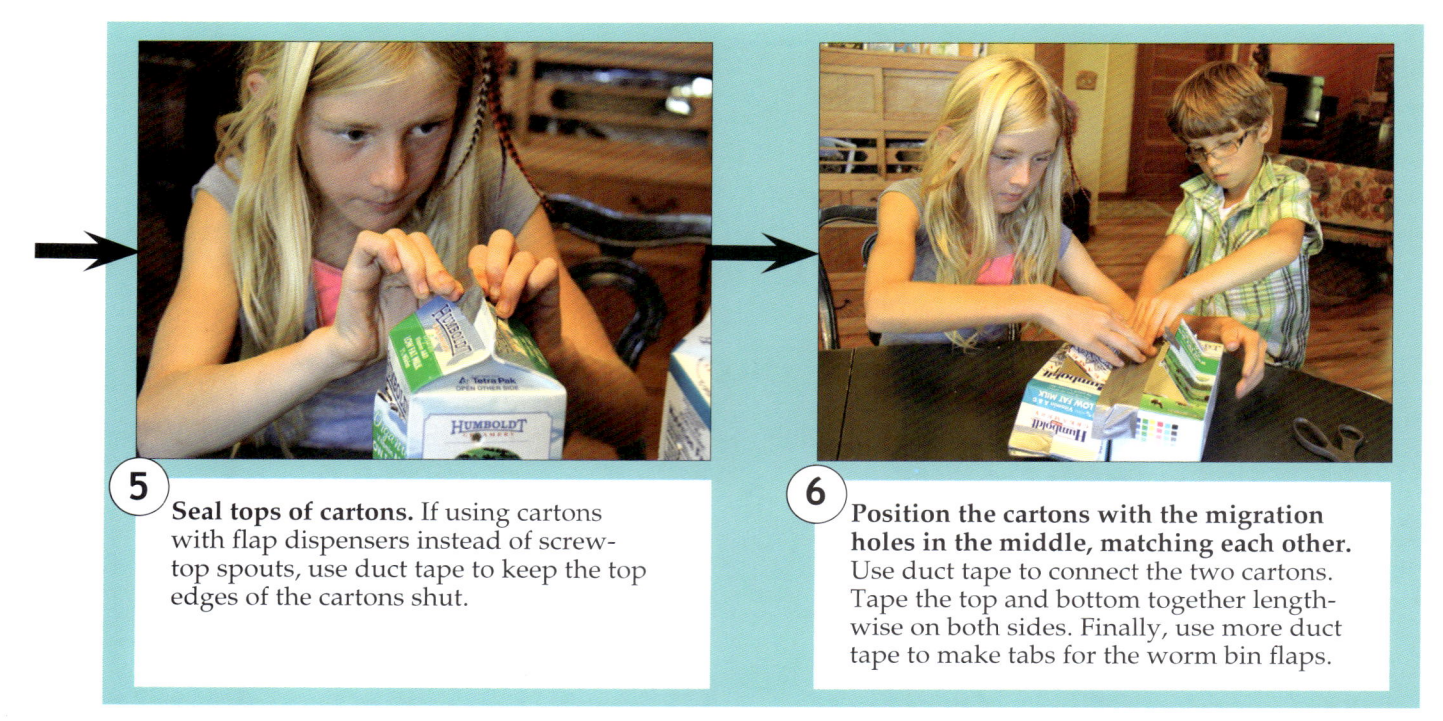

5. Seal tops of cartons. If using cartons with flap dispensers instead of screw-top spouts, use duct tape to keep the top edges of the cartons shut.

6. Position the cartons with the migration holes in the middle, matching each other. Use duct tape to connect the two cartons. Tape the top and bottom together lengthwise on both sides. Finally, use more duct tape to make tabs for the worm bin flaps.

How to Use the Worm Bin

1. Start by putting a small amount of damp shredded newspaper and a handful of dirt or dead leaves to make bedding in both sides of your bin. Add a rough handful of food scraps into one side (See: What to feed your worms, on the next page.)

2. Leave your worm bin for about a week or so without worms in it so that the contents of the bin can begin the decomposition process.

3. Gently add 100 to 250 worms (a rough handful) to the side of your bin that contains the food scrap mixture.

4. Once a week, use a spoon to gently mix up ("aerate") the side of the bin that contains the worms to keep harmful gases from building up. Also once a week, add a small amount, about a half a handful, of food to the bin.

5. Check the worm bin every few days. If it is dry, spray in some water to keep it moist.

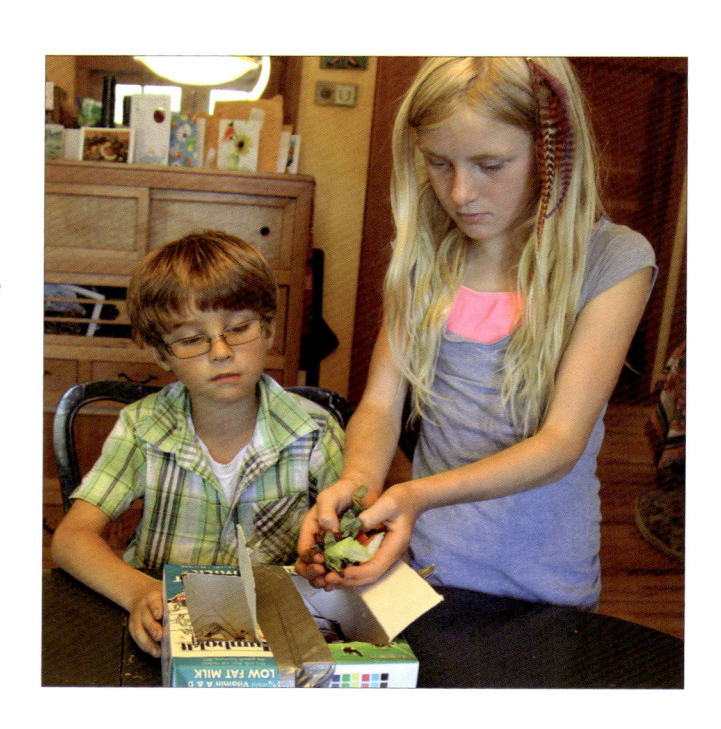

Worm Bin Composter

6. After 2-3 months, the bin will start to accumulate castings (worm poop). When this starts to happen, add food scraps to the side of the bin containing bedding but no food. The worms will then migrate (via the migration hole) to where more food is provided.

   The picture to the right shows what busy worms look like. They have turned the food, garden waste and paper into castings. It's now time to put food into the second bin so they will migrate. We removed the worms and castings from the bin so you could see them better.

7. After the worms have migrated to the fresh side of the bin, remove the castings from the first side and use them in your garden to produce bigger, healthier plants. Put fresh bedding into the first side.

The projected lifetime of the bin is six months to a year. Due to the simple design, however, it is easy to make another worm bin to replace the old one!

Modular Design

A modular design means that you can expand your worm bin to the size you want.

1. Get another juice or milk carton and place it next to your 2-carton bin.
2. Follow steps 1-5 on pages 171-172 to add the new carton.
3. Cut an extra migration hole into your existing worm bin.
4. Make sure the migration holes line up, then tape the new bin in place next to the old one.
5. Repeat as necessary until you reach your desired worm bin size.

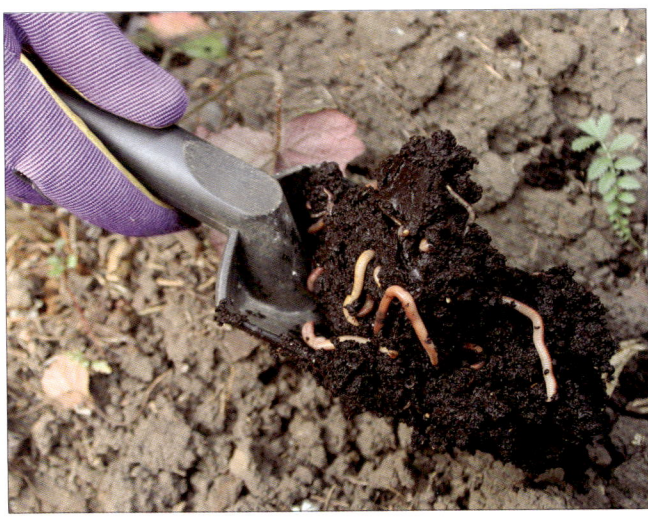

What to feed your worms	What not to feed your worms
Vegetable scraps	Meat
Coffee grounds and filters	Fish
Tea bags	Dairy products
Old bread	Greasy or oily foods
Fruit peels or pulp	Pet waste

The Wormland Worm Bin was designed by students Delo Freitas, Dylan Child, Brett Manus and Kusondra King in Humboldt State University's Engineering 215 Class in the Spring of 2011 under the direction of their instructor, Lonny Grafman.

Instructions from the students and a "how to" video are available at www.appropedia.org/Locally_Delicious_Kids_Worm_Bin_inst

The full student report is available at: www.appropedia.org/Locally_Delicious_Kids_Worm_Bin

Solar Dehydrator

Dehydrator with Solar Collector

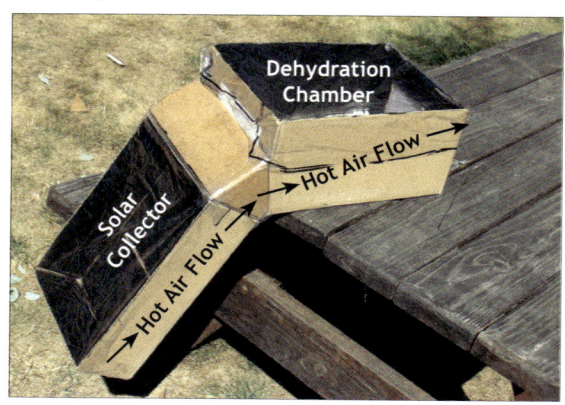

Dehydrator without Solar Collector

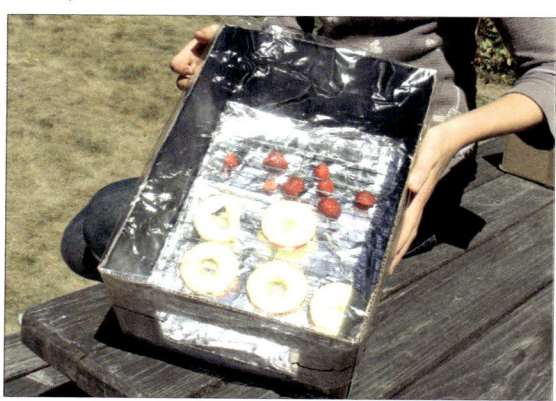

Build a solar dehydrator, face it toward the sun and you have a functional food preservation machine for a little work and a little money.

The Solar Dehydrator can have two chambers connected by a cardboard triangle. Air flows into the Solar Collector (SC) through holes at its bottom edge. The air heats as it flows through this hot chamber, and then into the Dehydration Chamber (DC). A mesh-covered hole in the DC allows moist air to escape. The food inside the DC dries. If you live in a hot climate, the Solar Collector may not be needed. Instructions start with a Dehydrator without the Solar Collector and then show how to build and add the Solar Collector for use in cooler climates.

Age: 8+   Adult help required for cutting with box cutter

Time to complete: About 1½ hours

Here's what you'll need for the Dehydrator Chamber (May be all that is needed in hot climates.)

Materials:
- Oven cooling rack (See photo, page 50) Racks are usually between 10" x 10" and 11" x 14"
- A box that is at least 1" larger than the oven cooling rack and between 6" and 9" deep. Deeper boxes can be cut down.
- Plastic kitchen food wrap
- Clear packing tape and cellophane tape
- 2-ounce bottle of black water-based tempera paint
- Aluminum foil
- An 8" x 10" piece of netting or mesh

Tools:
- Ruler
- Box cutter
- Scissors
- Pen or pencil
- Small paint brush or foam paint applicator

Here's what you'll need in addition for the Solar Collector:

- A second box the same size as the first box. The box needs to be cut down to 4" deep.
- A piece of cardboard at least 4" x (the width of the box + 6") Example: If your box is 12" across on the narrow end, the cardboard needs to be 4" x (12" + 6") which is 4" x 18"
- More plastic kitchen food wrap

Caution: Cutting with a box cutter should be done by an adult or older child with supervision

Solar Dehydrator

Making the Dehydration Chamber (DC)

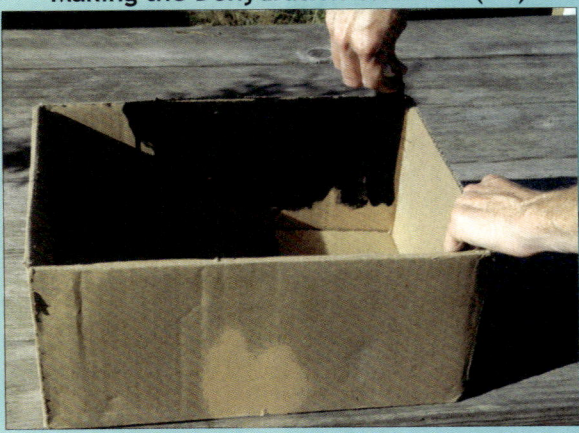

1. If the box has flaps, cut them off. Cut the box to between 6" and 9" deep. Use black tempera paint to paint the inside walls of the DC.

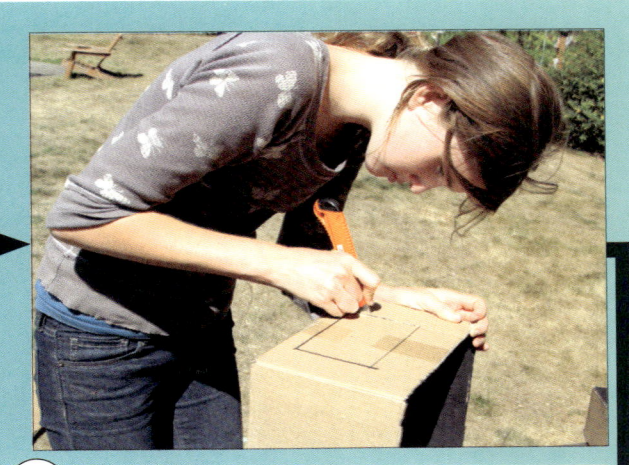

2. Mark a rectangular hole 6" wide x 3.5" high at about the middle of one narrow side of the DC. The hole will let the hot, moist air escape.

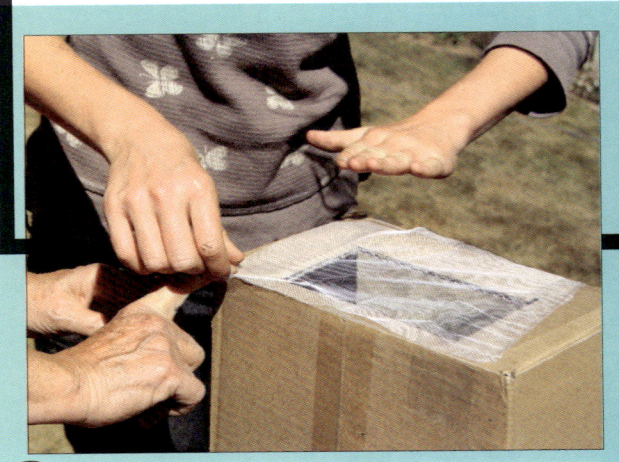

3. Use scissors to cut a piece of netting about 6" x 8", big enough to cover the hole. Tape the netting to the outside of the box to cover the hole. The netting prevents bugs from getting in, but lets the hot air escape.

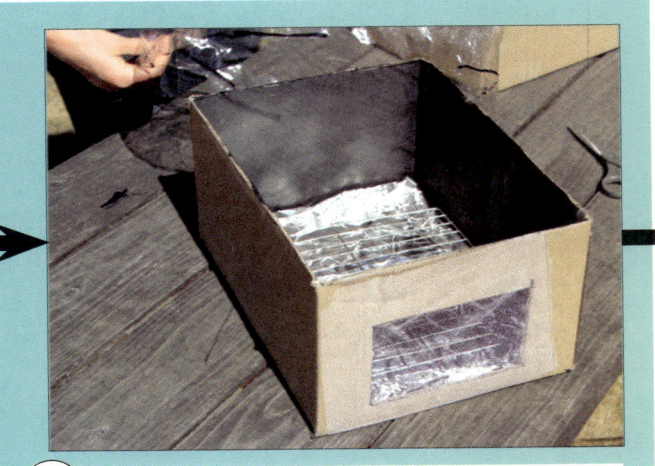

4. Line the bottom of the DC with aluminum foil. Place the cooling rack on top of the foil. If you live in a hot climate, the dehydrator is ready to use. Go to Step 5. If you live in a cool climate go to Step 6.

Solar Dehydrator

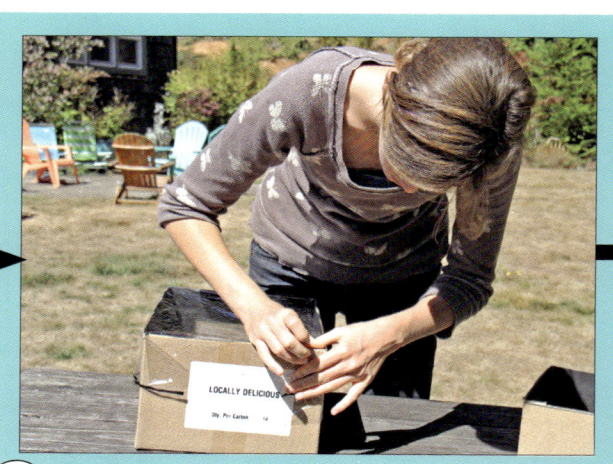

Making Solar Collector (SC)

5) When you use the dehydrator you will cut pieces of plastic kitchen food wrap and cover the box. Tape the pieces together if necessary. Use cellophane tape to tape edges of plastic to the box as you will remove the plastic wrap to remove the food.

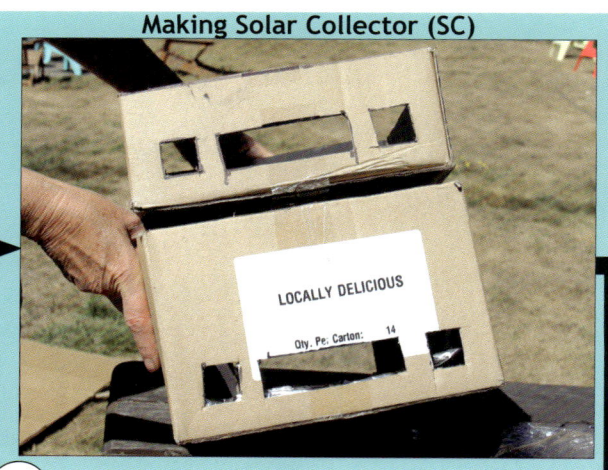

6) Mark and cut 3 holes **at the same place** on one narrow end of both the SC and DC boxes. Make the middle hole 1.5" high x 3.5" wide. Make the two side holes 1.5" square. Cut the holes about 1" from the bottom edge of each box.

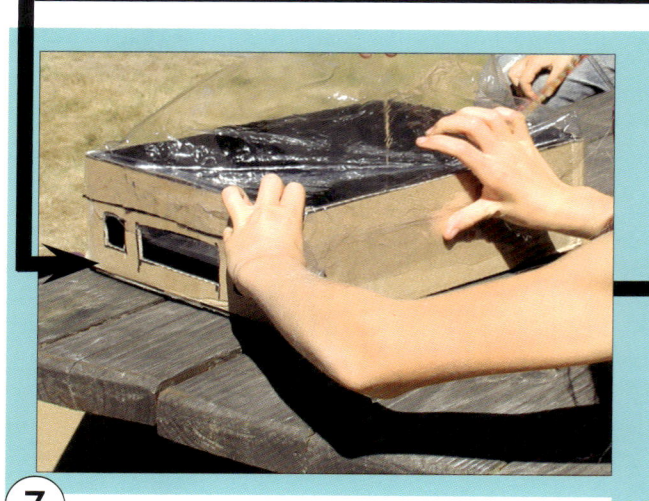

7) Paint the entire inside of the 4" deep box with black tempera paint. Cut pieces of plastic wrap and tape them permanently to the SC box using packing tape.

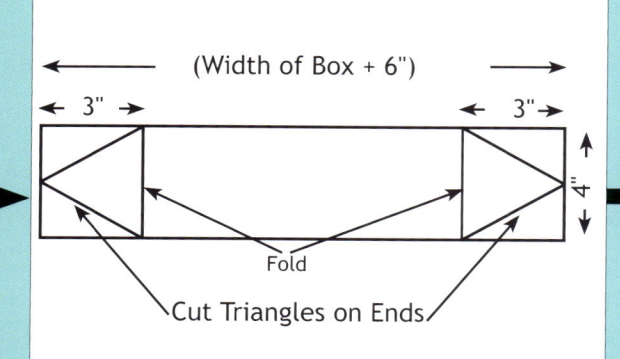

8) Cut a piece of cardboard the width of your box (on the side with the holes) plus 6" wide by 4" high. Mark a line 3" from each end. Fold on line. Mark and cut a triangle shape on each end. The triangles start at the folded line and are centered on each end.

176 Do It Yourself Projects

Solar Dehydrator

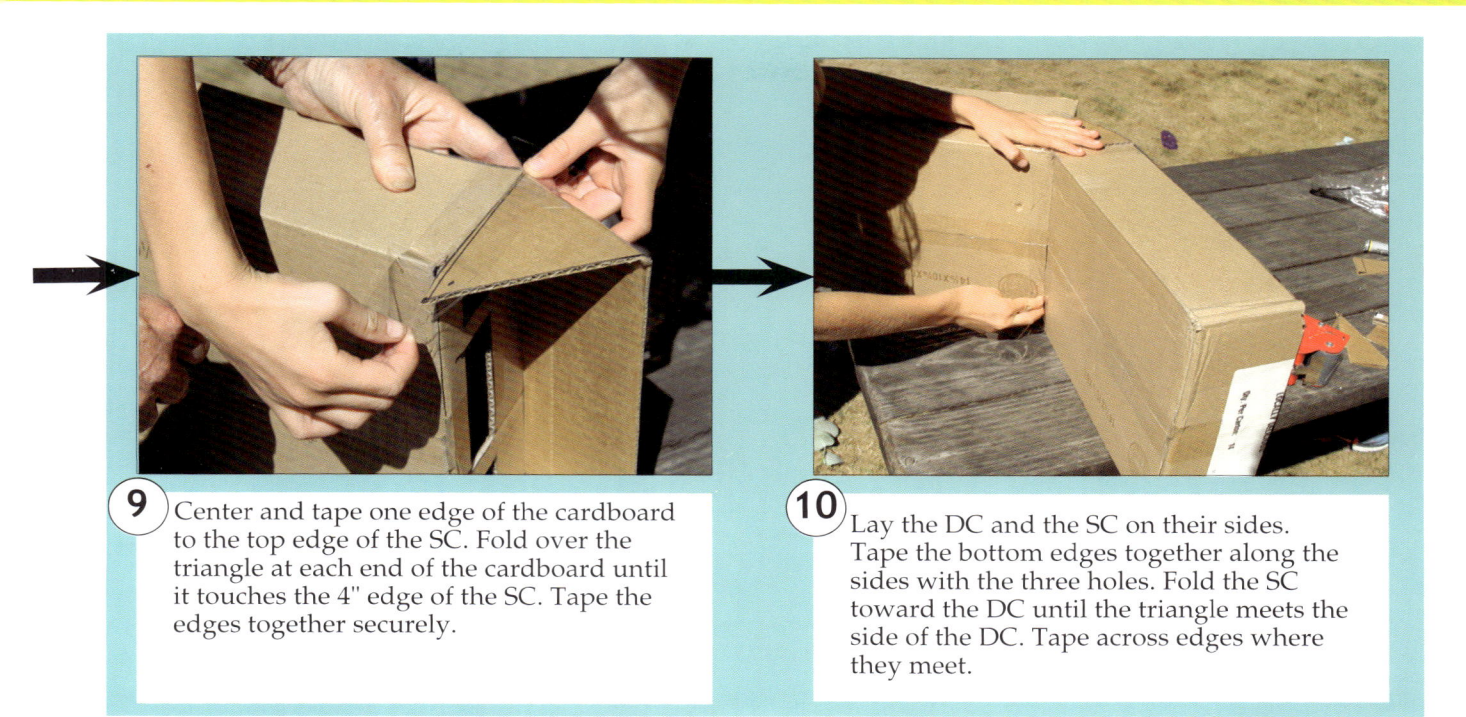

9 Center and tape one edge of the cardboard to the top edge of the SC. Fold over the triangle at each end of the cardboard until it touches the 4" edge of the SC. Tape the edges together securely.

10 Lay the DC and the SC on their sides. Tape the bottom edges together along the sides with the three holes. Fold the SC toward the DC until the triangle meets the side of the DC. Tape across edges where they meet.

How to Use the Solar Dehydrator

If the solar dehydrator does not have an SC, just put it on a table and put in cut fruit or vegetables. If it has an SC, put the DC portion of the dehydrator on a table or chair so the SC can hang down. Position the dehydrator so the SC is facing the sun.

Cut fruit into thin (about ¼") slices for large fruit such as apples, pears, bananas or peaches, or into halves for small fruit such as plums or apricots. Dip apples and pears into lemon juice mixed with water to prevent the fruit from turning brown. Berries with thicker skins such as cranberries, blueberries and grapes will dry faster if cut in half. Vegetables can also be dehydrated. See further instructions for dehydrating fruit on page 137.

Place fruit or vegetables onto the cooling rack. Place the rack into the DC. Cover the DC with two layers of plastic kitchen food wrap and use cellophane tape to keep the plastic wrap in place.

Drying time will vary with the thickness of the fruit and the temperature in the DC and will likely take 8 hours or more. The DC will get to over 100° with outside temperatures of at least 55° and hotter as the outside temperature increases.

To decide if the food is done, first cool a test piece of fruit or vegetable a few minutes. Consider fruit dry when no wetness can be squeezed from a piece which has been cut—it should be rather tough and pliable. Consider vegetables dry if they're brittle.

Fruit leather puree should be placed on a solid surface to dry, such as a lightly oiled pan with edges. (See recipe for Fruit Leather on page 134.)

Solar Food Warmer

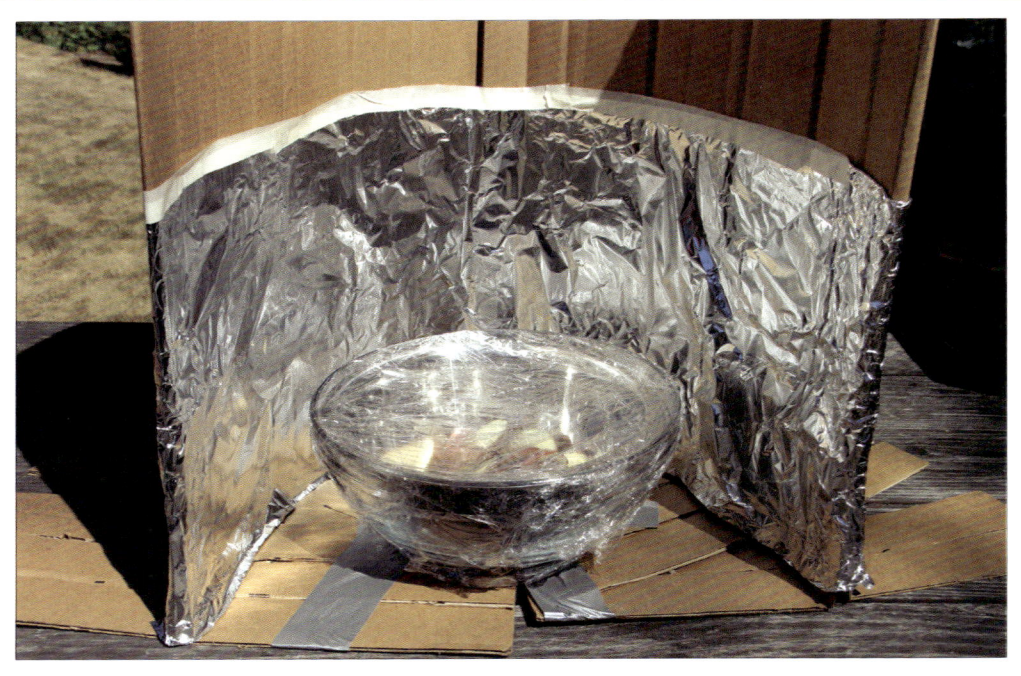

The Solar Food Warmer is designed to heat food using air trapped between two bowls and heated by reflected sunlight.

Age: 8+ Some adult help required for spray painting and cutting   **Time to complete: 1 hour**

Here's what you'll need:

Materials: (You'll probably find many of these items at home. If not, try shopping at a thrift store or a garage or yard sale. Reusing materials will save money and is better for the environment.)

- Large (about 15" in diameter) glass bowl, preferably with handles
- Metal bowl—about ½" to 1½" smaller in diameter than the glass bowl
- Glass lid or plastic kitchen wrap cover for outer bowl; any kind of cover for inner bowl
- Black barbecue paint (essential, because it is not toxic when heated)
- Black electrical or duct tape
- Aluminum foil
- Masking tape
- Cardboard box—18" x 18" x 18" is ideal but any size between 12" x 12" x 12" and 24" x 24" x 24" will work fine. It doesn't have to be square.
- Oven mitts

Tools

- Scissors or box cutter

Caution: Cutting with a box cutter should be done by an adult or older child with supervision

Solar Food Warmer

Making the Solar Reflector

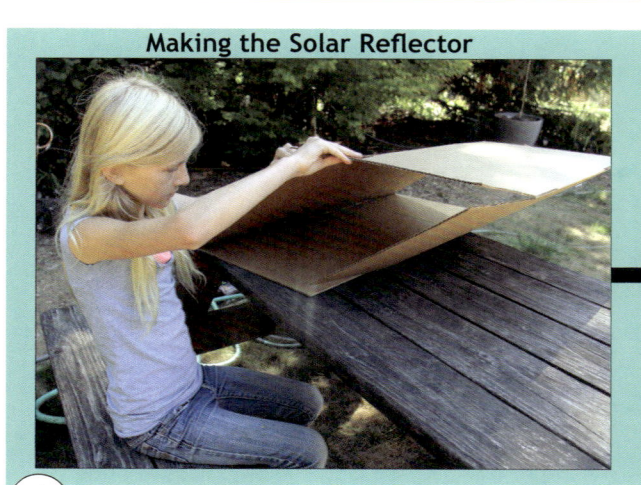

1 Unfold the top and bottom flaps of the cardboard box. Do not cut box yet. Place the cardboard box on its side so that it lies flat.

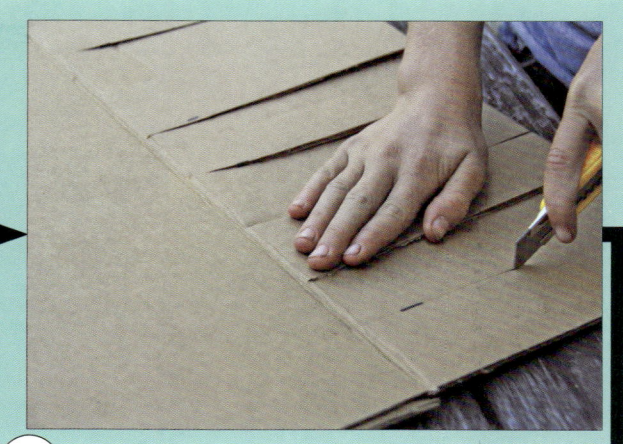

2 Use scissors or a box cutter to cut slits 2 inches apart on the top two flaps at the bottom of the box. The cuts should go up to the top edges of the flaps. Turn the box over or hold the top flaps up and cut 2-inch slits on the bottom flaps.

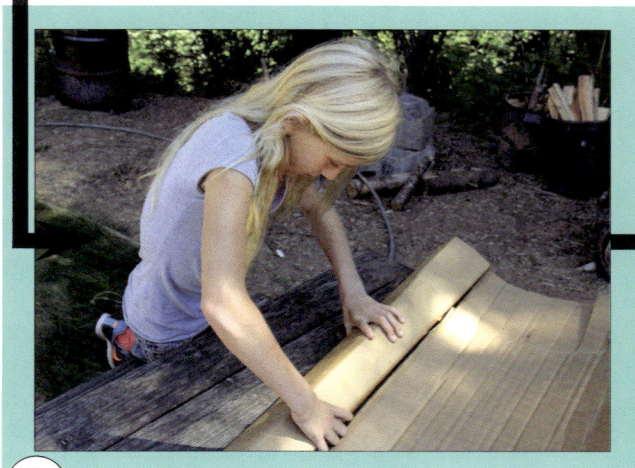

3 Bend the box close to the slits so that you have creases in the cardboard all the way up the box. Continue bending until it forms a roll. Unroll so that the whole box curves inward into a semi-circle.

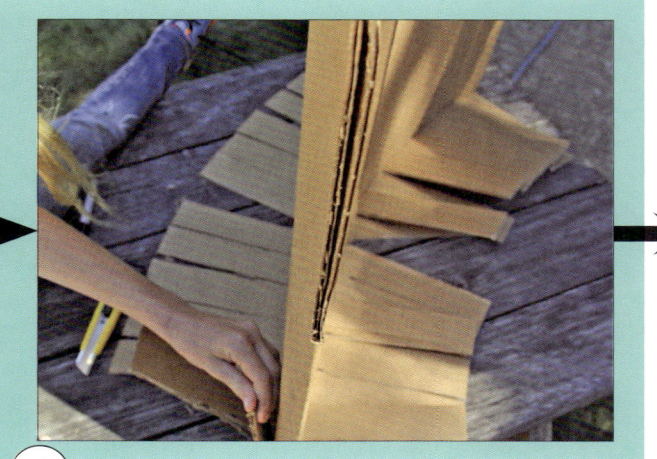

4 Stand the reflector panel up so that there are flaps on each side with the box formed into a curved shape.

Do It Yourself Projects 179

Solar Food Warmer

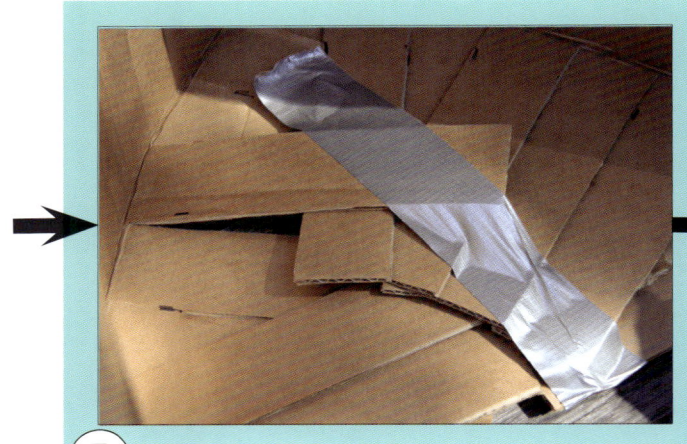

5 Hold the box in its curved shape by pulling together the tabs created by the 2-inch slits on the top side and taping them in place with duct or electrical tape. The final shape will be a semi-circle.

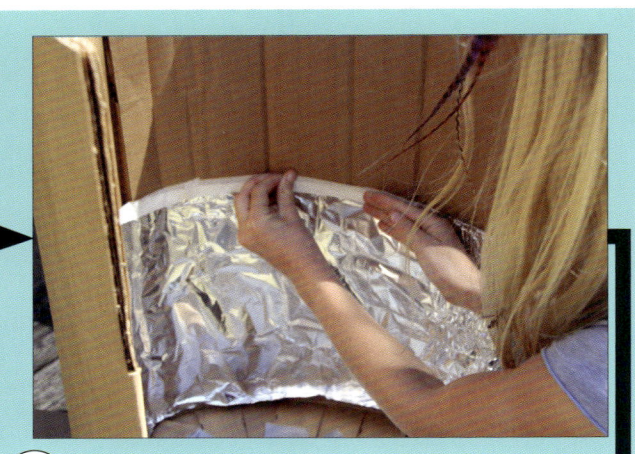

6 Roll out and cut a long piece of aluminum foil. Use masking tape to secure the aluminum foil (with the shinier side up) to the inside of the curved cardboard. The solar reflector is now finished.

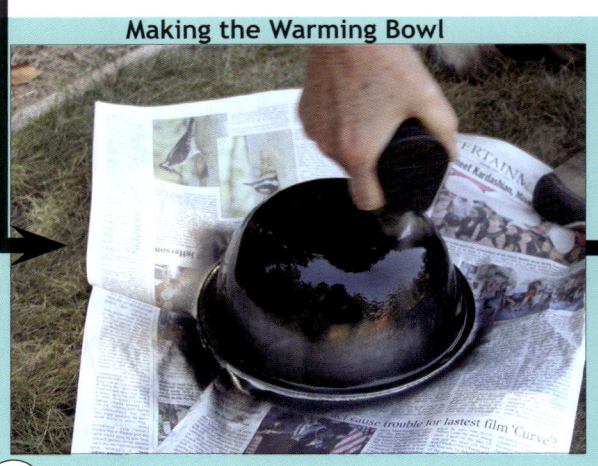

Making the Warming Bowl

7 Have an adult spray-paint the outside of the smaller (metal) cooking bowl with the black paint. Read the paint label instructions for the drying time. If the inner bowl has a lid, spray-paint it on the outside.

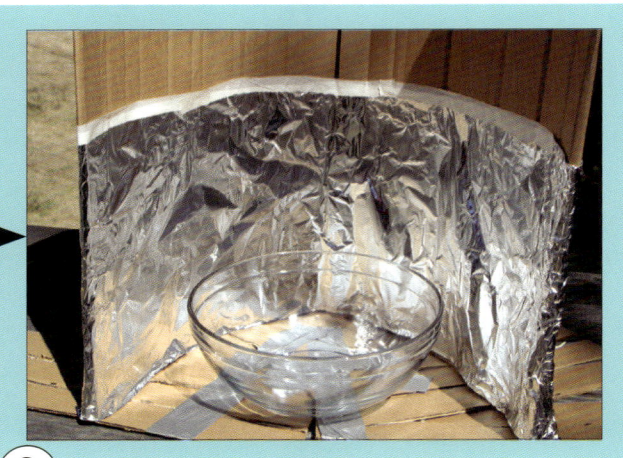

8 Place the larger glass bowl inside the curve of the solar warmer.

Solar Food Warmer

Using the Solar Warmer

1. Place the food in the smaller bowl.
2. Put a lid onto the smaller bowl, or cover the bowl with plastic wrap.
3. Put the smaller bowl inside the larger glass bowl and cover the larger bowl with a lid or plastic wrap. If the lids or plastic wrap don't provide a tight enough seal, use masking tape to create a seal.
4. Place the reflector panel in a sunny area and angle the reflector toward the sun.
5. Place the bowls in the middle of the reflector panel.
6. Leave the reflector panel and warming bowls in the sun. Our warming chamber reached 150° in 30 minutes on a overcast day with an outside temperature of 57°. If you live in a sunny area, your food warmer may become hotter.

What to Cook?

The solar food warmer described here can be used by children.

Use it to heat prepared foods such as soup, chili or stew. Grate cheese and use the food warmer to melt it on corn chips or toast. Warm up some leftover pizza. Melt some chocolate to dip fresh strawberries or bananas into.

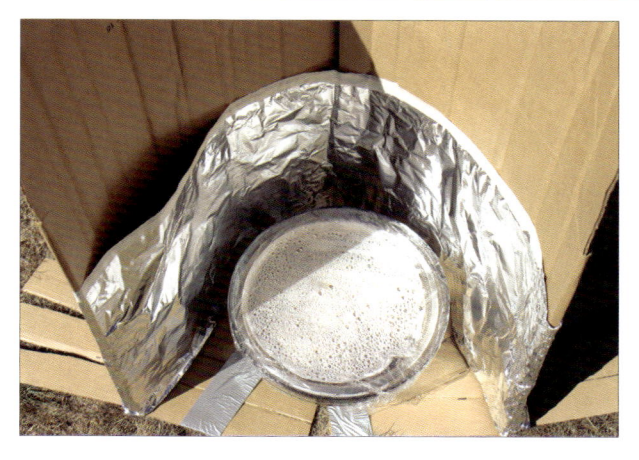

Always use a pot holder to handle the bowls after they have been in the sun.

If you like this project, you can check out other solar ovens described on the web. Many can be used to boil and bake food. They can get really hot!

The Solar Food Warmer was designed by students Shelly Dean, Matt McCammon, Josue Candelario, and Jill Hauck in Humboldt State University's Engineering 215 Class in the Spring of 2011 under the direction of their instructor, Lonny Grafman.

You can see the full student report and "how to" video at www.appropedia.org/Locally_ Delicious_solar_ oven_for_kids

Additional Do It Yourself Projects

The students at Humboldt State University created additional projects for home and school. Instructions for making the projects are available at www.appropedia.org/Locally_Delicious

Tear the Roof Off
Sliced apples dry in 18 hours of sunlight with this legless solar dehydrator

The GnomeTainer
Modular, raised garden with integrated rain catchment that can be installed on a porch

Catch and Cook
A solar oven capable of reaching 160° in 20 minutes

Row Blender
Row yourself a smoothie with an exercise-powered blender

Sodhoppers' Solar Dehydrator
Durable food dehydrator, using a discarded kitchen cabinet

Interactive School Garden
Modular garden design incorporating several different garden styles

The Solar Swing
Solar oven reaching 200° in 30 minutes

Worm Bin
Large worm bin built from a 55-gallon drum

Grow Your Own Food

Food always tastes better when you grow it yourself. Kids who grow their own food have more connection to it and most kids love to eat what they grow.

Gardening provides a multitude of opportunities. Before the first carrot has been pulled out of the soil, children can have hours of fun getting their hands dirty, playing with water, examining insects and learning how to use garden tools. They learn how to make their own choices, empowering them to take control of their food. Gardening gives children the opportunity to take care of their own little piece of the Earth, awakening them to the beautiful world we share, and creating Earth stewards from an early age.

Grow food in the ground, in a "Yarden" (a 3 x 3-foot garden), or in pots or other containers. If you don't have your own garden space, think about joining a Community Garden in your neighborhood. They are sprouting up in small towns and large cities. This is a good way to get to know your neighbors, to share gardening experience and to teach kids how to garden.

To grow food, all you need is healthy soil, water and plenty of sunlight. To get started, seek out gardening classes in your community and ask advice at your local nursery about what vegetables and fruit to grow in your area. Seed catalogs are also a great source of information about gardening, as are websites and books.

What to grow. Plant seeds, seedlings ("starts") or both. By far the easiest seeds to sprout are radishes and beans. Time spent looking over seed catalogs is a wonderful way for kids to get acquainted with all the possibilities. Think about the foods you like to eat and grow those. If you have a yard, you can grow anything that works with your climate. Examples of what to grow in the ground, in a Yarden or in containers are described in the next couple of pages.

What the plants need

Soil. Soil needs to be loose. If it's hard and clay-like, replace it with loamy soil mixed with compost. If the soil is crumbly, just mix in some compost. Don't skimp on good soil. Healthy soil, full of minerals and organic matter, makes strong, healthy plants and good-tasting food.

For growing in containers, mix some dirt with a good-quality mix of peat moss and perlite, and blend in a complete fertilizer. If you plan to water by hand, add a soil polymer that will help keep the roots moist.

Feeding. Feeding is an important part of growing healthy plants. Organic fertilizer is best. Be sure to follow the directions on the fertilizer package. The soil can be kept healthy by adding compost on a regular basis. Compost can easily be made by composting fruit and vegetable scraps and garden debris, or from worm castings. Check out the simple Worm Bin Composter described on page 170.

Watering. Make sure your plants get enough water. A simple method for container gardening is to water until the water comes out of the bottom of the pot. For plants in the ground, stick your finger into the soil about one inch to see if it's moist. Don't over-water. Generally most plants are watered at their base. Some vegetables do not like being watered on their tops, including tomatoes, eggplant, basil and peppers. Water by hand or use a drip irrigation system.

Sunlight. Most vegetables need at least 6 hours of sun a day. It is worth your time to observe the path of the sun when deciding where to put your garden. Take into consideration the time of the year. In some areas, gardens can flourish year round, but in colder climates, gardening can be limited by season.

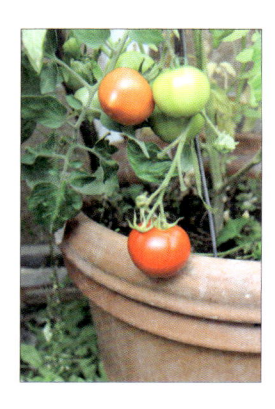

Grow Your Own Food

Making a Yarden

It doesn't take an acre or an entire backyard to create a garden. A Yarden is a 3 x 3-foot-square garden in which a lot of food can be grown. Yardens can be planted with various themes and can contain vegetables, fruits or flowers. Kids can design their own Yardens based on their general interest or the types of foods they like to eat.

Start by measuring out the space with a yardstick. Create a border of rocks, wood, bricks, or anything you might have on hand. Be creative.

Dig out the dirt about a foot deep and place the soil on a tarp. Amend the soil as described on the previous page. Put the amended soil back into the Yarden and add more if needed. Plant seeds, seedlings or both.

Growing Herbs

Growing an herb garden provides you with delicious additions to your recipes. Herbs can be grown in the ground, in a Yarden or in containers. More information on herb gardens is available at www.designing-edible-gardens.com/BasicHerbGarden.html.

Basil (Hot weather)

Oregano (Perennial* - hot or cool weather)

Chives (Hot or cool weather)

Cilantro (Cool weather)

Dill (Hot or cool weather)

Mint (Perennial - hot or cool weather)

Parsley (Hot or cool weather)

Rosemary (Perennial - hot or cool weather)

Thyme (Perennial - hot or cool weather)

*Perennial plants live for several years.

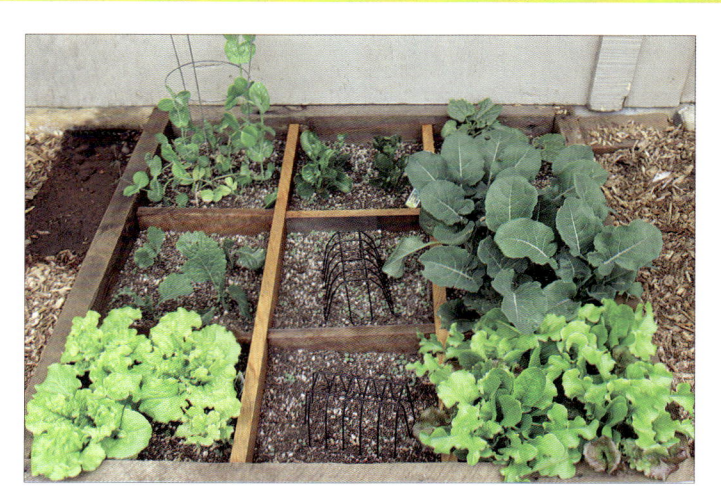

Growing Plants in the Ground

If you have space in your yard, the following are some examples of plants that are best grown directly in the ground, as they are too large for pots:

- Berries and grapes
- Rhubarb
- Artichokes
- Asparagus
- Corn
- Pumpkins and other winter squash
- Trees (apple, pear, plum, peach, and citrus)

Growing Plants in Containers

Many plants that grow in the ground can also grow in a container. All you need are good-sized containers such as recycled garden pots, wooden tubs, recycled plastic bins or trash cans with a few holes drilled in the bottom of them. Don't use old tires, because they release toxic gas.

The table on the next page has information on plants you can grow in containers. It shows how deep the container needs to be and how close the plants can be grown together, along with helpful notes. As with all gardening projects, consult with your local nursery to find out which plants grow best in your area and to learn about specific needs for the plants you want to grow.

What to Plant in Containers

Plant	Pot Depth	Spacing	Notes
"Green" Beans	12"-18"	Direct sow seeds 3" apart, or plant starts 4" apart	Pole beans and bush beans are easy to grow. Pole beans will need to be trellised up to 6-8 feet. Beans can be yellow, green, purple and bicolored.
Carrots	14"	Sow seeds ½" to 1" apart. Thin to 2" apart.	Plant seeds only. Kids love to pull carrots right out of the ground and eat them immediately.
Chard	18"	18" per plant	Chard can overwinter in many places. Chard stalks can be white, red, yellow, magenta or dark orange.
Cucumbers	18"	One plant per pot (In a big tub, plant 2)	Try growing Armenian cucumbers. They're delicious and don't need peeling. Lemon cucumbers look like lemons.
Garlic	10"-12"	4" apart	Separate garlic bulb into cloves and plant only the largest. Plant 2-3" below the surface. Plant in fall and harvest in summer. When the top produces a small bud, clip off and don't water.
Kale	14"	12" apart	Kale is a great fall/overwintering vegetable. It can grow year round in many cool coastal areas
Lettuce	12"	8" apart	Easy to grow from seed or from starts. Experiment with different varieties.
Onions	18"	Plant 1" apart. Thin to 4-6"	Use thinned plants as green onions. Onions are ready when the tops look dried out and an onion bulb is sticking out of the ground.
Peppers	16"	One plant per pot (In a big tub, plant 3)	There is a wide variety of peppers, from very sweet and mild to very hot, and very small to very large. Many peppers start out green, then turn color as they ripen.
Potatoes	18"	6" apart	Potatoes can be prolific, grown in a pot or tub. Plant the tubers in about 8" of soil in the bottom of the pot. As the plant grows, add more soil to the top set of leaves until your pot is full. After the blossoms have died and the plant starts to yellow, tip the pot over and be ready for a big harvest.
Radishes	12"	Sow seeds	Radishes grow quickly and easily.
Snap Peas	18"	Sow seeds or plant starts	Pea plants need to be trellised 6-8 feet high. Plant seeds or starts 6" apart. Kids love to eat the peas right off the vines.
Strawberries	18"	12" apart	Plant in spring. They like acidic soil. Mix peat moss with your potting mixture. Kids will love to help pick the berries.
Summer Squash	18"	One plant per pot	Try zucchini, yellow crookneck and scallopini (patty pan). Winter squash and pumpkins do not do well in pots.
Tomatoes	18"	One plant per pot	Plant heirlooms—they're sweet and delicious. Some need trellising and some are bushy. Tomatoes can be red, white, yellow, orange, purply-black, green-striped. Indeterminate tomatoes produce all season, and determinate tomatoes produce all at once.

Resources

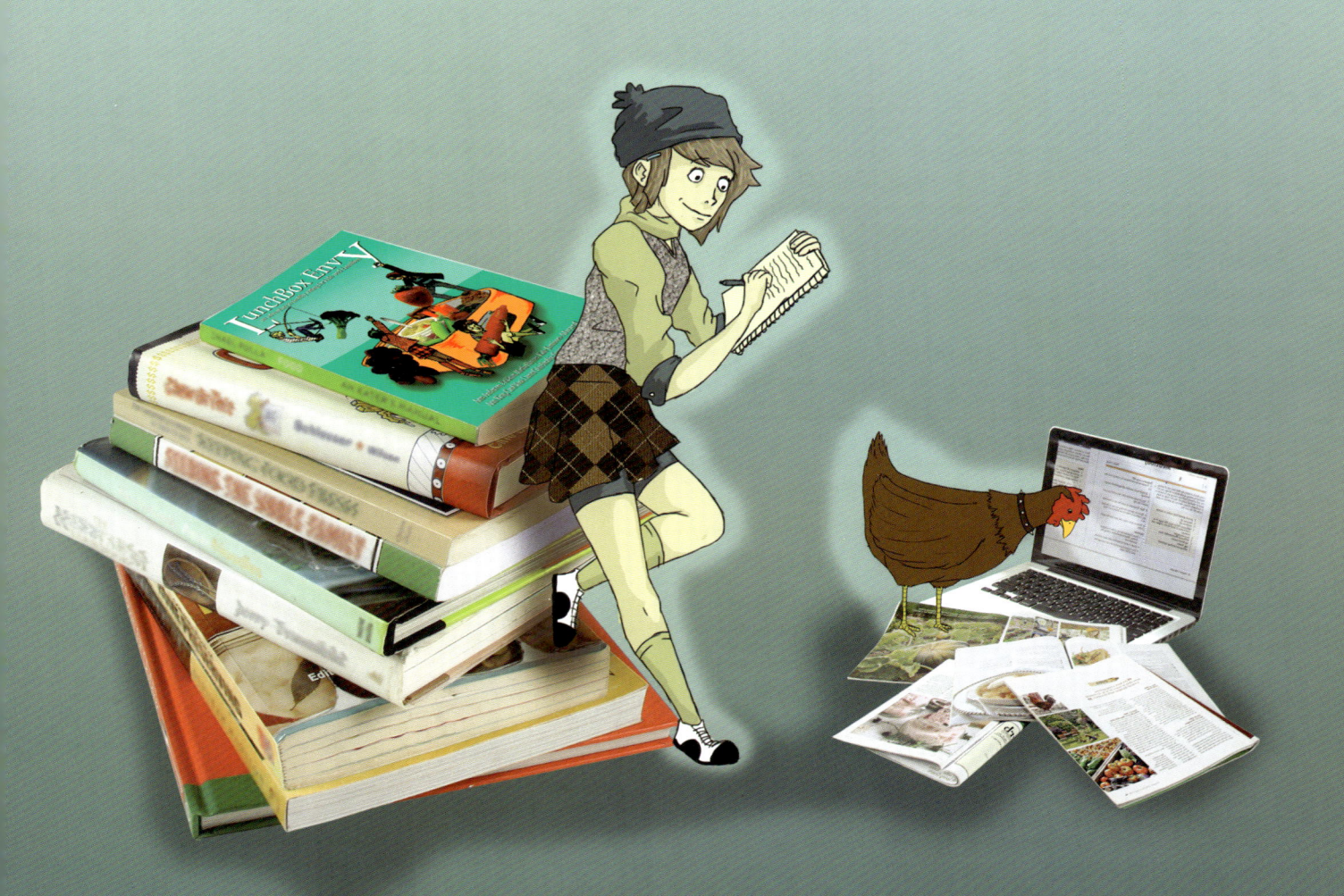

Glossary

General

Agribusiness (see also CAFO, Factory farm): A combination of the words "agriculture" and "business" to describe food production that's treated like any other manufacturing business.

Antibiotic: A medication that kills or slows the growth of bacteria. See "Factory farms."

Bisphenol A: A substance used in the making of plastics. Declared toxic by Canada in 2010. Banned for use in baby bottles in the U.S.

CAFO (Concentrated Animal Feeding Operation, Factory farm): A farm that operates as a factory. Animals are raised in confinement at high density.

Certified organic: A designation applied to food from a farm that has gone through a government-regulated organic certification process.

Diabetes: A disease in which a person has high blood sugar. Serious long-term complications include heart and circulatory disease, chronic kidney failure and damage to vision.

Factory Farm: See CAFO

Farmers' markets: Individual vendors—mostly farmers—who set up booths, tables or stands, outdoors or indoors, to sell produce, meat products, fruits and sometimes prepared foods and beverages.

Fish farms: Where fish are commercially raised in enclosures, usually for human food.

Food bank: An organization that distributes food to those who have difficulty purchasing enough for their needs.

Gleaning: The act of collecting leftover crops from farmers' fields after they have been commercially harvested.

Heart disease (cardiovascular disease): A class of diseases that involves the heart or blood vessels (arteries and veins).

High blood pressure: A condition requiring the heart to work harder than normal to circulate blood through the body.

High-fructose corn syrup (HFCS): Any of a group of corn syrups that have undergone processing to convert some of their glucose into fructose to produce a desired sweetness.

Hormones: Chemical messengers that transport signals from one cell to another. Used in industrial agriculture to stimulate growth in animals.

Industrial agriculture: Food production treated as an industry. Similar to factory farming.

Milling: The process of grinding a solid material, such as oat grains, into smaller pieces or powder, such as oatmeal or oat flour.

Natural flavoring: Flavoring occurring naturally rather than chemically constructed. Can be from unusual sources.

Obesity: A condition in which excess body fat has accumulated, potentially leading to increased health problems and reduced life expectancy.

Organic: Foods produced without the use of synthetic pesticides or chemical fertilizers.

Pasture-raised (grass-fed): Refers to animals raised for food that are allowed to graze naturally in fields.

PCBs (polychlorinated biphenyls): Persistent organic pollutants that cause cancer in laboratory animals. Evidence suggests they can also cause cancer in humans.

Pesticides: Chemicals for destroying plant, fungal or insect pests. Commonly used in industrial agriculture.

Processed food: Commercially prepared food products that require minimal preparation before eating.

Subsidized crops: Crops such as corn and soybeans that the government pays farmers to grow (and sometimes, to not grow).

Wild-caught: Fish caught in the wild rather than taken from a farmed source.

Cooking Terms

Al dente: Pasta or vegetables cooked until tender but still firm to the bite.

Bake: To cook using dry heat, usually in an oven. When applied to meats, poultry or vegetables, the process is called "roasting."

Batter: An uncooked mixture of flour, liquid and other ingredients that is thin enough to be poured or spooned.

Glossary

Beat: To stir or mix ingredients in a continuous circular motion. See also "Blend," "Mix" and "Stir."

Blanch: To drop vegetables or fruit briefly into boiling water, and immediately into ice water.

Blend: To thoroughly combine two or more ingredients. See also "Beat," "Mix" and "Stir."

Broil: Cook by direct heat in an oven, broiler, or on a grill.

Broth: Made by cooking meat, fish, poultry or vegetables in water with seasonings and straining off the liquid for use in recipes.

Brown: To cook food briefly on the stovetop or in the oven until it's brown on the outside.

Brush: To apply a coating with a small brush.

Chevre [pronounced "SHEH-vruh"]: Goat cheese.

Chiffonade [pronounced "shiff-oh-NAHD"]: A French term referring to vegetables cut into thin strips.

Cream: To combine butter and sugar to a fluffy, creamy consistency, using a food processor, a fork or the back of a spoon.

Crimp: To seal two edges of pastry together to keep the filling from leaking out, as with empanadas.

Custard: A mixture of milk, eggs, and flavorings. Used to fill sweet or savory pies.

Cut in: To distribute cold, solid fat into dry ingredients.

Dehydrate: To preserve foods by drying them.

Drizzle: To pour a liquid in a fine stream over food.

Fluff: To separate grains of food such as rice, usually using a fork.

Fritatta [pronounced "free-TAH-tuh"]: A thick omelette-like dish made up of combinations of vegetables, meat and cheese. Includes eggs and milk.

Fry: To cook in hot fat. Also called "sauté," which uses less fat.

Marinade: A liquid mixture, usually with a vinegar or wine base, used to tenderize and to add flavor to food.

Marinate: To soak foods in marinade in a non-reactive container. Follow food safety procedures when marinating raw meats, poultry or seafood.

Mix: To combine two or more ingredients so they are evenly distributed. See also "Beat," "Blend" and "Stir."

Non-reactive: Cookware that does not make a nasty-tasting chemical reaction in the presence of acidic foods such as vinegar or wine. Glass, stainless steel and glazed ceramic or glazed ceramic cast-iron containers are non-reactive.

Peel: To remove the skin or rind from a vegetable or fruit with a peeler or paring knife.

Pinch: An amount that can be pinched between thumb and first finger, usually about ⅛ teaspoon.

Potatoes (baking type): Have a coarse skin and mealy texture but turn light and fluffy when cooked. Ideal for baking, mashing and French fries. Common varieties are Russet and Idaho.

Potatoes (boiling type): Have a thin, smooth skin. Ideal for soups, casseroles, potato salad, roasting and barbecuing because they hold their shape. Common names are White or Red potato.

Preheat: To bring an oven or broiler to the desired temperature before beginning to cook in it.

Puree [pronounced "pure-AY"]: To reduce an ingredient to a smooth, thick mixture, usually with a blender or food processor.

Quiche [pronounced "keesh"]: A savory pie usually made with eggs, milk, vegetables and meat. Has only a bottom crust.

Roast: When applied to meats or vegetables, to cook using dry heat, usually in an oven. See also "Bake."

Roux [pronounced "roo"]: A flour and melted fat mixture used to thicken sauces, soups and gravy.

Sauté [pronounced "saw-TAY"]: To cook in hot fat. Sautéing uses less fat than frying. See also "Fry."

Savory: The opposite of sweet; uses herbs, peppers, onions, etc. to create flavor.

Shred: To cut into thin pieces, using a grater or shredder.

Stew: To cook food slowly in a simmering liquid for a long time. Also refers to foods cooked in this manner.

Stir: To mix ingredients by means of a circular or figure eight movement. See also "Beat," "Blend" and "Mix."

Glossary

Strain: To separate liquids from solids by pouring food through a sieve or colander.
Strata: A layered baked casserole that includes bread, eggs and often cheese, as well as vegetables and meat.
Toast: To brown by direct heat in a toaster or hot oven.
Toss: To mix ingredients lightly with a lifting motion. Usually used with salad and pasta.
Vinaigrette: [pronounced "vin-ay-GRETT"]: A French term for oil-and-vinegar salad dressing.
Wilt: To cook leafy vegetables lightly so they become limp but retain their color.

Nutrition

Calcium: A mineral used by the body to build and strengthen bones and teeth.
Calorie: Nutritionally, a unit of measure used to express the energy-producing qualities of food.
Carbohydrate: Often means any food that is particularly rich in the complex carbohydrate starch (such as cereals, bread and pasta) or simple carbohydrates (such as sugar).
Dietary fibers: Provides dietary bulk in the large intestine. They absorb water as they move through the digestive system, making bowel movements possible.
Fats: Play a vital role in maintaining healthy skin and hair, insulating body organs against shock, maintaining body temperature and promoting healthy cell function. Fats also serve as energy stores for the body.
Gluten: A protein composite found in foods processed from wheat and related grain species, including barley and rye. Oats may contain gluten due to contamination in the field or during processing.
Iron: A mineral that helps red blood cells carry oxygen to all parts of the body.
Magnesium: A mineral that helps the body maintain a steady heartbeat and keeps the muscles and nerves working properly.
Micronutrients: Nutrients required by humans and other living things in small quantities to orchestrate a whole range of physiological functions, but which the organism itself cannot produce. Vitamins are an example.
Minerals: In the nutritional sense, micronutrients such as calcium and iron that help bodies stay healthy.
Phytochemicals: Naturally found in plants. May help prevent disease and promote good health. Different kinds of phytochemicals give fruits and vegetables their bright colors.
Potassium: A mineral that helps the body maintain a healthy blood pressure and keeps muscles and nerves working properly.
Protein: An essential building block for proper nutrition. One of the major nutrients that make cells, protect the body's organs and help absorb certain vitamins. Muscles, organs and the immune system are made up mostly of protein.
Refined grains: Grains or seeds that have been processed so that the nutritious outer coating is lost.
Starches: The most common carbohydrate in the human diet. Contained in large amounts in foods such as potatoes, wheat, corn and rice.
Sugar: A plant-based sweetener usually derived from sugar cane, sugar beets, maple trees, palm trees and other sap-producing plants.
Vitamins: Micronutrients needed to help the human body grow, function and fix itself.
  Vitamin A: Helps the body maintain healthy eyes and skin.
  B vitamins: Folate helps lower a woman's risk of having a child with certain birth defects. **Riboflavin** and **thiamin** help the body turn food into energy. Riboflavin also helps the body maintain healthy red blood cells. Thiamin helps maintain healthy heart, muscles and nerves.
  Vitamin C: Helps the body heal cuts and wounds and maintain healthy gums.
  Vitamin E: Helps maintain healthy cells throughout the body.
  Vitamin K: Helps certain cells in the blood act like glue and stick together at the surface of a cut.
Whole grains: Seeds that retain their original state, including the nutritional outer coatings.
Zinc: A mineral needed for healthy growth and development. Also helps the body maintain a healthy immune system and helps the body heal from cuts and wounds.

Read More

Cookbooks
Katzen, Mollie, *Pretend Soup and Other Real Recipes*. Random House, New York, 1994
Lair, Cynthia, *Feeding the Whole Family: Recipes for Babies, Young Children, and Their Parents*. Sasquatch Books, Seattle, 2008
Madison, Deborah, *Local Flavors*. Broadway Books, New York, 2002
Rombauer, Irma S. and Rombauer-Becker, Marion, *Joy of Cooking*. Bobbs-Merrill, New York, 2006
Rosso, Julie and Lukins, Sheila, *The New Basics Cookbook*. Workman Publishing, New York, 1989
University of Georgia Cooperative Extension and the United States Department of Agriculture, *Complete Guide to Home Canning; So Easy To Preserve, 5th Edition*. 2006

General Food Books
Lappé, Frances Moore, *Diet for a Small Planet*. Ballantine Books, New York, 1991
Pollan, Michael, *The Omnivore's Dilemma: A Natural History of Four Meals*. The Penguin Group, New York, 2006
——*In Defense of Food: An Eater's Manifesto*. The Penguin Group, New York, 2008
——*Food Rules, An Eater's Manual*. The Penguin Group, New York, 2009
Roberts, Paul, *The End of Food*. Houghton Mifflin Harcourt, New York, 2008
Schlosser, Eric and Wilson, Charles. *Chew On This: Everything You Don't Want to Know About Fast Food*. Houghton Mifflin, Boston, 2006 (Written for young teens.)

Online Sources
Buying Clubs and Co-op Groceries: www.coopdirectory.org
Canning and Food Preservation:
  USDA, Canning and Preserving. http://nchfp.uga.edu/publications/publications_usda.html
Environmental Technologies:
  Appropedia: www.appropedia.org
Food:
  Environmental Working Group: www.ewg.org;
    The Dirty Dozen Non-organic Foods: www.organic.org/articles/showarticle/article-214
    Sugar in Cereals: www.ewg.org/report/sugar_in_childrens_cereals
  Mother Earth News: www.MotherEarthNews.com
  Organic food: www.organicconsumers.org
  Protecting organic food: www.cornucopia.org
  Seafood Watch: www.montereybayaquarium.org/cr/seafoodwatch.aspx
  Vegetarian food: www.vegetariantimes.com
Help in Food Deserts. See references on page 22
Gardens:
  Community Gardens: www.acga.localharvest.org
  Organic Gardening: www.organicgardening.com
  The Edible Schoolyard Project: www.edibleschoolyard.org
Nutrition Information and Recipes:
  Champions for Change, Network for a Healthy California: www.cachampionsforchange.cdph.ca.gov
  My Plate: www.choosemyplate.gov
  FDA Food Facts Label: www.fda.gov/Food/ResourcesForYou/Consumers/ucm079449.htm
  USDA Food and Nutrition Information Center: http://fnic.nal.usda.gov
School Lunches:
  Chef Ann Cooper–Lunch Lessons: Changing the Way We Feed Our Children: www.chefann.com

Food Labels

Food labels tell you what is in the package. There are three parts that are important: the Nutrition Facts label, the ingredient list and the product origin. Find more information online, see listings under Nutrition on page 189.

"Nutrition Facts" Label

Serving size shows how much is in a serving and is usually in common units such as cups, number of pieces, etc. There is no legal standard for serving size. Food manufacturers often choose the serving size that makes the amounts of the sugar, fat and salt fall into a range that looks good to the consumer. As an example, a package of cookies may indicate that a serving is **one** cookie so they don't have to report trans fat. Trans fat is generally considered a harmful fat but does not need to be shown on the label if the serving contains less than 0.5 grams. A serving size of two cookies might contain enough trans fat that it would have to be listed. People might not buy that cookie if they knew that it contained trans fat.

Servings per Container shows how many servings are in the package. Some packages will look like one serving, but always check the label. The number of serving listed may be unrealistically high. This allows the food to appear to be lower in calories, sugar, fat and salt. So before you look at the other numbers, consider the serving size and number of servings and multiply the other numbers as appropriate.

Calories shows you how much energy is provided in **each serving**—not the whole package. The number of calories required for children varies from a little more than 1,000 calories a day to almost 3,000 depending the age, gender and activity level of the child. www.MyPlate.gov provides detailed information.

% Daily Values show percentages of daily requirements for fats, carbohydrates, fiber, protein, vitamins and minerals. Are based on what a healthy person needs each day. The percentages are based on a 2,000 calorie a day diet.

Total Fat shows total fat and types of fat. Trans fat, hydrogenated and partially hydrogenated fats should to be avoided or kept to a minimum. Cholesterol is another type of fat that may be of concern for people with heart disease.

Sodium shows the amount of sodium (salt). High levels can be a problem for people with high blood pressure.

Total Carbohydrates includes sugar, starch and fiber. High fiber has many benefits. High sugar can contribute to obesity.

Protein shows the amount and percentage of daily requirements for a healthy adult.

Vitamins and Minerals shows the percentage of each for a healthy person.

Food Labels

Ingredient list

The ingredient list shows ingredients in order of content by weight.

The information below was taken from three cereal containers and demonstrates what to look for on ingredient lists.

Cereal 1: INGREDIENTS: SUGAR, WHOLE GRAIN CORN FLOUR, WHEAT FLOUR, WHOLE GRAIN OAT FLOUR, OAT FIBER, SOLUBLE CORN FIBER, PARTIALLY HYDROGENATED VEGETABLE OIL, (ONE OR MORE OF: COCONUT, SOYBEAN, AND/OR COTTONSEED OILS), SALT, SODIUM ASCORBATE, AND ASCORBIC ACID (VITAMIN C), NIACINAMIDE, REDUCED IRON, NATURAL ORANGE, LEMON, CHERRY, RASPBERRY, BLUEBERRY, LIME, AND OTHER NATURAL FLAVORS, RED #40, BLUE #2, TURMERIC COLOR, YELLOW #6, ZINC OXIDE, ANNATTO COLOR, BLUE #1, PYRIDOXINE HYDROCHLORIDE (VITAMIN B6), RIBOFLAVIN (VITAMIN B2), THIAMIN HYDROCHLORIDE (VITAMIN B1), VITAMIN A PALMITATE, BHT, [PRESERVATIVE], FOLIC ACID, VITAMIN D, VITAMIN B12

The first ingredient is sugar, meaning there is more sugar in the package than anything else. Next are four kinds of grains (two are whole grains), then hydrogenated fat (See "fat" on previous page.) This cereal also has many kinds of flavoring including "natural flavoring" (see page 36), and several kinds of food dyes and added vitamins. The Nutrition Facts label (not shown here) shows 14 grams of sugar for a 29 gram (1 cup) serving, **which means this cereal is 48% sugar.**

Cereal 2: INGREDIENTS: WHOLE WHEAT OATS, WHOLE WHEAT FLOUR, UNSULPHURED MOLASSES, BARLEY MALT EXTRACT, BAKING SODA, SALT, VITAMIN C (ASCORBIC ACID), NATURAL VITAMIN E (MIXED TOCOPHENOLS TO MAINTAIN FRESHNESS)

The first two ingredients, by weight, are whole grains, the third and forth are sugars, followed by baking soda, salt, vitamins and a preservative. The Nutrition Facts label (not shown here) shows 12 grams of sugar in a 58 gram (1¼ cup) serving, **which means this cereal is 20.7% sugar.**

Cereal 3. INGREDIENTS: 100% WHOLE WHEAT

Contains only whole wheat. The Nutrition Facts label (not shown here) shows **0 grams sugar in a 40-gram serving or 0% sugar**. For some sweetness, add some cut up fruit or even a teaspoon of sugar. There are 4 grams of sugar in a teaspoon.

Product Origin

Where was the food grown or processed? This is probably different from the location of the distributor. Look for words like: "product of," or "made in." This is important if you want to support local agriculture, to buy in season or to buy food that is produced in the U.S. under regulation by the FDA or USDA.

Other Label Cautions

If the words "All Natural" are printed on a box of crackers, we are led to believe that the ingredients are all natural. The label might tell us that the crackers also contain high-fructose corn syrup, which is not a natural product. Immediately we see that it is not an "All Natural" product. Any ingredient that does not roll off of your tongue, like flour, or peas or honey, is probably not a natural ingredient. It is a chemical. The word "natural" has no legal meaning.

Look at the Nutrition Facts label to find the total amount of sugar. To find the percentage of sugar, look for grams of sugar and divide the number of grams of sugar by the total number of grams in a serving. For the label on page 190, that math is 5 grams sugar/228 grams per serving, or 2% sugar. Remember to look at all the names for sugar. See some names on page 33, and here are more: galactose, glucose solids, glycerine, maltose, mannitol, rapadura, sorbitol, turbinado, can-juice crystals, caramel, cane juice, dextran, diastatic malt, ethyl maltol, fruit juice concentrate.

Don't assume the picture on the package is what is really in the package. We found a package of guacamole that contained hydrogenated soy beans and food coloring. There were NO avocados!

Be a smart consumer and read the labels.

Portions

How Much is Enough?

It's a tricky thing to decide how much is enough. Restaurant servings can have enough food in one portion to feed two or three people. The lasting impression is that that is what a serving size should be. There is no legal definition for "serving size." Below are some general guidelines for serving size and the number of servings appropriate for a school-age child.

A range of servings is given. Older children need more than younger children, boys need more than girls and very active children need more than less active. Use the table below as a starting point. More information can be found at www.MyPlate.gov. Search for portion sizes for each type of food.

Food Group		Number of Servings per Day	Serving Size
	Fruit	3-4	¾ cup fruit juice, 1 medium size piece of fruit (apple, orange, pear, banana), ½ cup chopped raw or canned fruit, ¼ cup dried fruit
	Grain	8-11	½ cup cooked grain, rice or pasta, ½ cup cereal, 1 slice whole wheat bread
	Dairy or Calcium Source	3	1 cup milk, 1½ ounces cheese, ½ cup tofu, ½ cup cooked dark green vegetable
	Vegetable	4-5	½ cup raw or cooked vegetables, 1 cup leafy vegetables
	Protein	2-3	2-3 ounces of meat, poultry, fish or tofu ½ cup cooked beans or peas, 1 egg, 2 tablespoons nut butter, ⅓ cup nuts

You don't need to carry a measuring cup with you—just use your hands for easy estimates.

One handful is about ½ cup. Two hands cupped together is about 1 cup. The size of your palm is about a serving of protein.

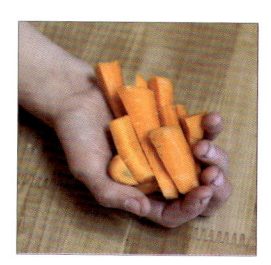

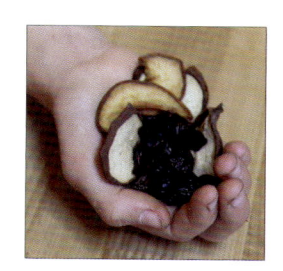

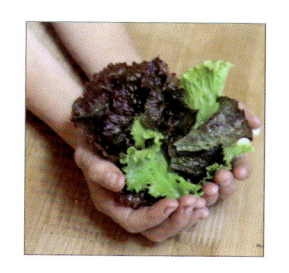

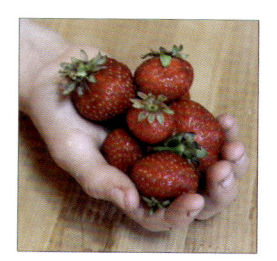

Spice Mixes

The spice combinations below can add variety to your cooking. Pre-made mixes are handy, but spices bought in bulk are fresher. All spice mixes should be kept in a cool, dry place in a container with a tight-fitting lid. Ingredients can be ground in a coffee grinder, a spice grinder, or with a mortar and pestle. Cook whole seeds in a dry frying pan until they start to pop; remove, grind them to powder, then mix with the rest of the ingredients. Experiment with different flavors, but begin cautiously; it is easy to add more, but impossible to remove. The recipes below are suggestions. You may wish to start with just some of the spices on each list.

Cajun
Yield: ¼ cup
Use for beans and rice, fish stews or soups, casseroles
2½ teaspoons paprika
1¾ teaspoons onion powder
1¾ teaspoons garlic powder
1½ teaspoons salt
1½ teaspoons dry mustard
1½ teaspoons dried basil
1 teaspoon thyme
½ teaspoon black pepper
¼ teaspoon white pepper
¼ teaspoon cayenne

Thai
Yield: almost 1 cup
Use in sauce for Asian noodle dishes, meat, seafood, vegetables, or rice dishes
½ tablespoon cumin
1 tablespoon salt
1 tablespoon white pepper
1 tablespoon black pepper
1 tablespoon ground dried hot Thai chilies, or to taste
2 tablespoons dried lemongrass
2 tablespoons dried lime peel
2 tablespoons garlic powder
2 tablespoons ginger
2 tablespoons dried mint
2 tablespoons toasted unsweetened ground coconut

Chinese
Yield: ¼ cup
Use as a rub or in a marinade for meat; add to stir-fry or roasted vegetables; try a pinch in fruit pies, cakes or cookies
2 tablespoons ground ginger
1 tablespoon ground cinnamon
1½ teaspoons ground allspice
1 teaspoon ground anise seed
¾ teaspoon cloves

Mexican
Yield: ¼ cup
Use for tacos, burritos, empanada filling, chicken or bean dishes, seafood, ground meat
¼ teaspoon salt
¼ teaspoon pepper
1 teaspoon cumin
1 teaspoon oregano
1 teaspoon coriander
1 teaspoon thyme
1 teaspoon powdered allspice
1 teaspoon onion powder
1 teaspoon garlic powder
1 teaspoon paprika
1 teaspoon chili powder

Italian
Yield: less than ½ cup
Use for pasta dishes and rice dishes like risotto, roasted vegetables, meat and chicken
1 tablespoon oregano
1 tablespoon basil
1 tablespoon marjoram
1 tablespoon coriander
1 tablespoon thyme
1 tablespoon rosemary
1 tablespoon savory
¼ teaspoon red pepper flakes

Indian - Garam Masala
Yield: ¼ cup
Use for soup or stews, with roasted vegetables and meat
1¼ tablespoons cumin
1¼ tablespoons coriander
1 teaspoon cardamom
1 teaspoon cinnamon
½ teaspoon powdered cloves
1 tablespoon black pepper
⅛ teaspoon ground mace

Index

Ants On A Log 147
Apples
   2-in-1 Chicken & Fruit "Saladwich" 76
   Applesauce 136
   Dehydrating Fruit 137
   Fruit Leather 134
   Fruit Salad with Honey & Yogurt 132
Asian Noodles
   Asian Noodles Formula 92
   Sesame-Peanut Noodle Salad 94
Bacon
   Broccoli & Bacon Salad 129
Bananas
   Banana-Chocolate Muffins 154
   Fruit Smoothie 133
   Overripe Fruit 155
   PBJ Pinwheels 72
Basil
   Classic Italian Pesto 165
Beans
   Beans and Rice 96
   Bean Soup 123
   Black or White Bean Dip 163
   Cooking dry beans 54
   Corn and Black Bean Salad 111
   Cost Comparison: Beans 75
   Hummus 167
   Ideas for beans 79
   Minestrone Soup 122
   Reducing Bean Farts 54
Beef
   Empanadas 86
   Meatloaf 73
Bell peppers. *See* **Peppers**
Berries
   Fruit Leather 134
   Fruit Salad with Honey & Yogurt 132
   Fruit Smoothie 133
Black-Eyed Pea Cakes 74
Bread
   No-Knead Bread 58
   Strata with Meat 104
Broccoli
   Broccoli & Bacon Salad 129
Broth
   Making broth 62
Bulgar
   Tabouli 115
Bulk buying 74
   Why Buy in Bulk? 16
Burritos 78

Buying Clubs 15
Cabbage
   Chicken or Tofu Cabbage Salad 112
   Japanese Griddle Cakes 105
   Three-Color Coleslaw 127
Calzones 84
Canning 136
Carrots
   Carrot and Raisin Salad 130
   Japanese Griddle Cakes 105
   Three-Color Coleslaw 127
   Zucchini or Carrot Muffins 153
Celery
   Ants On A Log 147
Chard
   Strata with Meat 104
Cheese. *See also* **Cream cheese**
   Corn and Pepper Quiche 103
   Mac & Cheese 90
   Pea Pesto 166
   Simply Scrumptious Scones 150
   Strata with Meat 104
Chicken
   2-in-1 Chicken & Fruit "Saladwich" 76
   Chicken Noodle Soup 124
   Chicken or Tofu Cabbage Salad 112
   Empanadas 86
   Meatloaf 73
   Sesame-Peanut Noodle Salad 94
Chocolate
   Banana-Chocolate Muffins 154
   Chocolate Peanut Butter Spread 72
Collard greens
   Fake Grass Salad 128
Compost
   What the plants need 182
   Worm Bin Composter 170
Cookies
   Chewy Fruity Cookies 157
   Granola Bars 148
Cooking Techniques
   Roasting Meat 70
   Stove Top Cooking Techniques 46
   Techniques for Preparing the Ingredients 44
Co-op Grocery Store 15
Corn
   Corn and Black Bean Salad 111
   Corn and Pepper Quiche 103
   Corn Muffins 152
   Popcorn 144
Cornmeal. *See* **Polenta**

Index

Couscous with Peas 98
Cranberries
   Broccoli & Bacon Salad 129
   Chewy Fruity Cookies 157
   Fake Grass Salad 128
Cream cheese
   Ants On A Log 147
   Crunchy Creamy Wrap 77
   Fruit Spread 168
   Ginger and Preserves 168
   Pesto Spread 168
   Sun-dried Tomato Spread 168
CSA (Community Supported Agriculture) 20
Cucumbers
   Greek Tzatiki Sauce 164
   Indian Raita Sauce 164
Dairy Products 35
Dehydrating Fruit 137
   Solar Dehydrator 174
Dips and Spreads 158–168
   Greek Tzatiki Sauce 164
   Indian Raita Sauce 164
Dried fruit
   Chewy Fruity Cookies 157
   Dehydrating Fruit 137
   Fruit Leather 134
   Granola Bars 148
   Granola Cereal 149
Drinks 140
   Delicious snack and drink options 32
   Flavored Water 140
   Fruit Smoothie 133
EBT (Electronic Benefits Transfer Card). *See* **SNAP**
Eggs 100–107
   Egg safety 55
   Hard-cooked Eggs 55
   Scrambled Eggs 55
Empanadas 86
Fairtrade 24
Farmers' Markets 19
Farm Stands 20
Fish 31
   Tuna and pasta salad 110
Food Carving
   Food Carving Fruits & Vegetables 138
   Quick Food Carving 125
Food Desert 22
Food Labels 190
Food Stamps. *See* **SNAP**

Formula Recipes
   Asian Noodles 92
   Italian Pasta 88
   Main Dish Salad 108
   Pizza 82
   Quiche/Frittata/Strata 100
   Sandwich and Wrap 68
   Soup 116
Fresh and In-Season Food 29
Fruit 131–137
   Low- and No-prep fruits 131
   Overripe Fruit 155
Fruit Leather 134
Fruit Salad with Honey & Yogurt 132
Games and Activities
   Find the Hidden Sugar 33
   Food Carving Fruits & Vegetables 138
   Grocery Store Scavenger Hunt 17
   Kid Challenge 2
   Kitchen Test 33
   Rethink Your Drink 34
Garbanzo beans
   Couscous with Peas 98
   Hummus 167
   Tabouli 115
Gardening
   Growing Plants in Containers 183
   Grow Your Own Food 23, 182
   Making a "Yarden" 183
   What the plants need 182
   What to Plant in Containers 184
Genetically Modified (GM) Food 38
Gingerbread 156
Glossary 186
GMO. *See* **Genetically Modified Food**
Grains of the World 96
Granola
   Granola Bars 148
   Granola Cereal 149
Green beans
   Sesame Green Beans 126
Green peppers. *See* **Peppers**
Hummus 167
Hygiene, Kitchen. *See* **Kitchen Hygiene**
Kale
   Fake Grass Salad 128
   Kale Chips 146
   Kale Crust 103
   Strata with Meat 104
Kitchen Hygiene 42
Kitchen Safety 43

Index

Kitchen Tools. *See* **Utensils**
Kiwi
   Fruit Salad with Honey & Yogurt 132
Local Food 24
Low-prep Foods. *See* **No- and Low-prep Foods**
Lunchbox Ideas 11
Lunch Planning
   Weekly Lunch Plan 10
Mac & Cheese 90
Mandarin oranges
   Fake Grass Salad 128
Measurements 53
Meatloaf 73
Minestrone Soup 122
Muffins
   Banana-Chocolate Muffins 154
   Corn Muffins 152
   Zucchini or Carrot Muffins 153
MyPlate 4–5. *See also* **Nutrition**
   Check MyPlate 6
   Examples of MyPlate Foods 5
   What's on MyPlate? 4
Natural
   Weird Source of Natural Fruit Flavors 35
   What About Buying Products labeled "Natural"? 36
No- and Low-prep Foods
   Dips and Spreads 158
   Drinks 140
   Fruits 131
   The Main Dish 67
   Treats and Snacks 141
   Vegetables 125
Noodles. *See also* **Pasta**
   Asian Noodle Formula 92
   Chicken Noodle Soup 124
   Chicken or Tofu Cabbage Salad 112
   Cooking Noodles 57
   Sesame-Peanut Noodle Salad 94
Nori
   Nori Snacks 81
   Sushi 80
Nutrition. *See* **MyPlate**
   Food Labels 190
   Nutritional Glossary 188
Nuts
   BBQ Peanuts or Pecans 143
   Broccoli & Bacon Salad 129
   Classic Italian Pesto 165
   Crunchy Walnuts or Pecans 142
   Fast Roasted Nuts 142
   Go Nuts! 142
   Granola Bars 148
   Granola Cereal 149
   Sesame-Peanut Noodle Salad 94
   Tamari Almonds 143
Oats
   Granola Bars 148
   Granola Cereal 149
Online Recipes 67
Online Sources 189
Oranges
   Fruit Salad with Honey & Yogurt 132
Organic 36–37
   Ways to Reduce Pesticide Exposure 37
   Where to Put Your Money If You Can't Buy All Organic 37
   Why Buy Organic? 36
Pasta
   Cooking Pasta 57
   Italian Pasta Formula 88
   Mac & Cheese 90
   Sugar Snap Peas & Grain Salad 99
   Tuna and Pasta Salad 110
Peaches
   Dehydrating Fruit 137
   Fruit Leather 134
Peanut butter
   Ants On A Log 147
   PBJ Pinwheels 72
Pears
   Dehydrating Fruit 137
Peas
   Couscous with Peas 98
   Pea Pesto 166
Peppers
   Bean Soup 123
   Corn and Black Bean Salad 111
   Corn and Pepper Quiche 103
   Stackable Sandwiches 70
   Three-Color Coleslaw 127
Pesticides
   Ways to Reduce Pesticide Exposure 37
Pesto
   Classic Italian Pesto 165
   Pea Pesto 166
Pie dough
   Empanadas 86
   Making Pie Dough 63
Pita bread
   2-in-1 Chicken & Fruit "Saladwich" 76
   Making Pita Bread 66

Index

Pizza
    Making Pizza Dough 64
    Pita Bread from Pizza Dough 66
    Pizza Formula 82
Planning
    The Planning Process 3
    Weekly Lunch Plan Example 8–10
    What to Put into the Lunchbox 6
Plums
    Dehydrating Fruit 137
Polenta 60
    Quiche Crust 61
Popcorn 144
Pork
    Empanadas 86
    Meatloaf 73
    Strata with Meat 104
Portions 192
    How Much to Put into the Lunchbox 7
Potatoes
    Empanadas 86
    Potato Salad 114
Processed Food 27–28
    What's bad about processed food? 27
    Extra Ingredients in Packaged Food 28
Protein 30
    Benefits of Pasture-raised Meat 30
    Problems with Factory-farmed Meats 30
    Protein from Meat and Poultry 30
    Protein from Plants, Eggs, Dairy and Fish 31
Pumpkin
    Sweet Squash Soup 118
Quiche
    Corn and Pepper Quiche 103
    Polenta Quiche Crust 61
    Quiche Formula 100
Quinoa
    Cooking Quinoa 56
    Sugar Snap Peas & Grain Salad 99
    Tabouli 115
Raisins
    Ants On A Log 147
    Carrot and Raisin Salad 130
    Empanadas 86
Ramen noodles
    Chicken or Tofu Cabbage Salad 112
Rice
    Beans and Rice 96
    Brown Rice 56
    Cooking Rice 56
    Fried Rice 95
    Mexican Rice 97
    Sugar Snap Peas & Grain Salad 99
Roasting Meat 70
Safety, Kitchen. *See* **Kitchen Safety**
Salads
    Salad Dressing
        Ranch Dressing 162
        Simple Vinaigrette 161
    Salad, Main Dish 108–115
    Salads, Fruit 132
    Salads, Grain 98–100
    Salads, Vegetable 127–130
Salsa
    Fresh Tomato Salsa 159
    Sassy Summer Watermelon Salsa 160
Salt 32–33
Sandwiches 68–76
Sauces
    Simple Tomato Sauce 65
Saving Money
    At a grocery store 15
    Bulk Snack Bins 141
    Buying at a Farmers' Market 19
    Cooking with Friends 18
    Cost Comparison: Beans 75
    Cost Comparison: Granola 16
    Cost Comparison: Plain Yogurt 133
    General Tips for Saving Money 14
    How Can Whole, Unprocessed Food be
        Less Expensive? 27
    Pasture-Raised Meat Can Be Affordable 30
    Save Money on Bread 58
    Saving Money on Organic Food 36
    Tips for Shopping at Big-box Stores 18
    Where to Put Your Money If You Can't Buy
        All Organic 37
Scones
    Simply Scrumptious Scones 150
Seasonality 132
    Fresh and In-season Food 29
Serving Sizes. *See* **Portions**
Shopping Tips. *See* **Saving Money**
Skill levels
    Cooking skill levels 53
Smoothies 133
SNAP (Supplemental Nutrition Assistance Program) 21
Soup 116–124
    Keeping Soup Warm for School 119
    Making Soups Thick and Creamy 121
Spice Mixes 193

Index

Spinach
  Strata with Meat 104
Squash. *See* **Summer squash, Winter squash**
Staples 47
Strata
  Strata Formula 100
  Strata with Meat 104
Strawberries. *See* **Berries**
Sugar 32–34
Sugar Snap Peas & Grain Salad 99
Summer squash
  Japanese Griddle Cakes 105
Sushi 80
Sweet potatoes
  Japanese Griddle Cakes 105
Tabouli 115
Tofu
  Chicken or Tofu Cabbage Salad 112
  Ranch Dressing 162
  Sesame-Peanut Noodle Salad 94
  Tofu Sticks 145
Tomatoes
  Fresh Tomato Salsa 159
  Simple Tomato Sauce 65
  Sun-dried Tomato Spread 168
  Tomato Soup 120
Tools. *See* **Utensils**
Tortillas
  Burritos 78
  Crunchy Creamy Wrap 77
  How to Make Flour Tortillas 59
Treats and Snacks 141–157
  Bulk Snack Bins 141
  Delicious snack and drink options 32
  Nori Snacks 81
Tuna
  Tuna and Pasta Salad 110
  Tuna Sandwich 71
Turkey
  Empanadas 86
  Meatloaf 73
Turnips
  Japanese Griddle Cakes 105
Unprocessed Food 27
Utensils
  Basic Cooking Tools 48
  Blenders and Food Processors 158
  Nice-to-Have Tools 50
Vegetables 125–130
  Leafy greens 128
  No-prep Vegetables 125

Vegetarian Diet 31
Waste 12
Watermelon
  Sassy Summer Watermelon Salsa 160
Whole Grains 35
Whole, Unprocessed Food 27. *See* **Unprocessed Food**
WIC (Special Supplemental Nutrition Program for Women, Infants and Children) 21
Winter squash
  Japanese Griddle Cakes 105
  Sweet Squash Soup 118
Wraps 77–87
Yeast 66
Yogurt
  Fruit Salad with Honey & Yogurt 132
  Fruit Smoothie 133
  Yogurt Dip 164
  Yogurt Recipes of the World 164
Zucchini
  Japanese Griddle Cakes 105
  Zucchini or Carrot Muffins 153

About the Artists

Arcata Arts Institute (AAI)
Arcata High School, Arcata, California

Directed by Anne Bown-Crawford, the Arcata Arts Institute offers a unique balance of tradition and innovation, liberal arts and visual arts, technology and touch, performing arts and design. The Institute community is committed to expanding boundaries and vision through rigorous study.

It provides an interdisciplinary, pre-professional arts program—visual, performing and theater arts—within an exemplary comprehensive public high school.

AAI gathers strength and nourishment through partnerships with the community such as the collaboration with Locally Delicious Inc. in the graphic design of *LunchBox Envy*.

Illustration Team

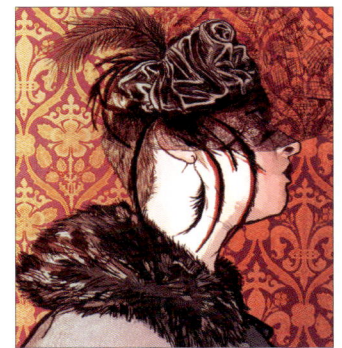

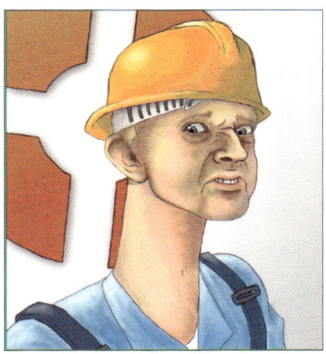

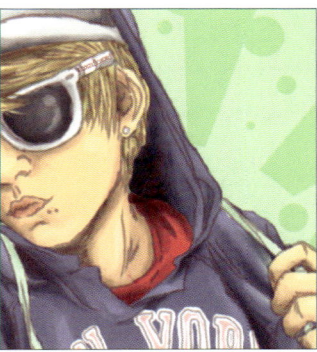

Morgan Tomfohr   John Nordberg   Kelsey Tomfohr

Graphic Design Team

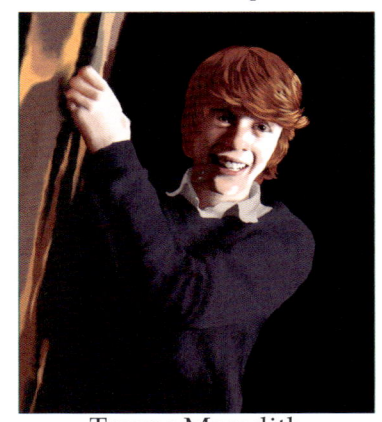

Treyce Meredith   Mahayla Camp

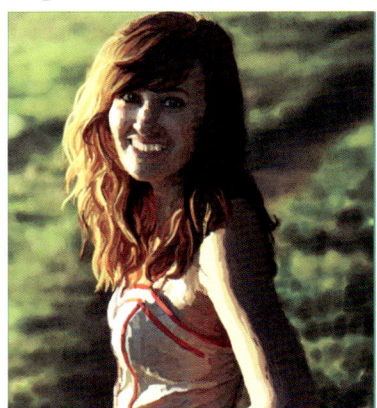

Portrait credits: Morgan and Mahayla by Morgan Tomfohr, Kelsey by Kelsey Tomfohr, John and Treyce by John Nordberg

About the Authors and Locally Delicious, Inc.

The main goal of Locally Delicious, Inc. is to educate children and adults about how to improve personal health, the health of the community and the Earth, through the food choices we make.

LunchBox Envy is our second book and all profits fund community food, farming and nutrition development projects throughout Northern California. We serve as networking agents for sustainable food system development efforts and are involved in policy-making councils and networks. We hope that *LunchBox Envy* will inspire people elsewhere to do the same within their own communities.

The authors are collectively known as the "Heirloom Tomatoes." Pictured clockwise from left:

Carol Moné is a school teacher and is a long-term community activist and serious locavore.

Suzanne Simpson is an artist and a passionate gardener, cook and canner. She is part of the change in what our children eat.

Ann Anderson is a retired publisher of books and patterns on quilting. She spent most of her career in computer sales and marketing after earning a Master's Degree in Cellular and Molecular Biology.

Pat Bitton is British by birth and has been living, growing food, and cooking on the North Coast since 2005. She is a freelance technical writer and also works part-time at Humboldt State University.

Ann King "Retired" from the publishing industry, she's looking hungrily toward the leisure of actual retirement and the pursuit of art, which is her real love.

Kate Jamison-Alward has a B.A. in Cultural Anthropology, and a love for nature, family, community, hiking, cooking, playing music, and "social justice."

Martha Haynes grew up in the Garden State and is a retired educator. Work on this book has made her a more discerning shopper as she has learned how to use labels to determine what goes in her shopping basket.

Lauren Cohn-Sarabia is a professional caterer in Humboldt County. She enjoys teaching cooking to children and adults, taking photographs and growing vegetables for her family in her home garden.

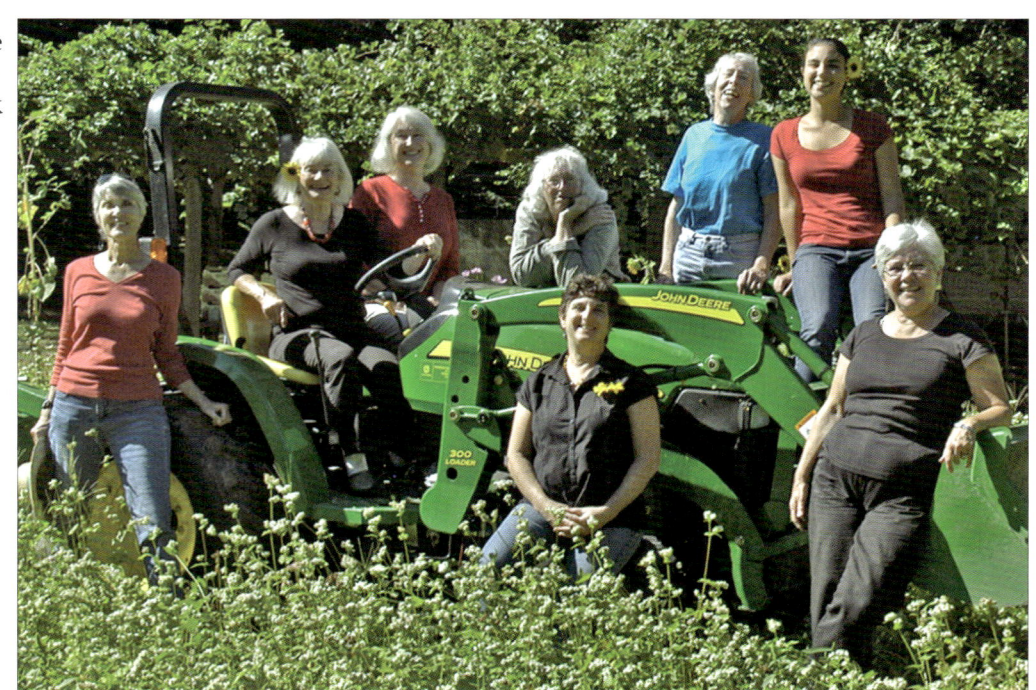